Methods in Pharmacology and Toxicology

Series Editor
Y. James Kang

For further volumes:
http://www.springer.com/series/7653

Cancer Prevention

Dietary Factors and Pharmacology

Edited by

Ann M. Bode and Zigang Dong

The Hormel Institute, Austin, MN, USA

Humana Press

Editors
Ann M. Bode
The Hormel Institute
Austin, MN, USA

Zigang Dong
The Hormel Institute
Austin, MN, USA

ISSN 1557-2153 ISSN 1940-6053 (electronic)
ISBN 978-1-4614-9226-9 ISBN 978-1-4614-9227-6 (eBook)
DOI 10.1007/978-1-4614-9227-6
Springer New York Heidelberg Dordrecht London

Library of Congress Control Number: 2013954409

Printed on acid-free paper

Humana Press is a brand of Springer
Springer is part of Springer Science+Business Media (www.springer.com)

Dedication

We dedicate this volume to The Hormel Foundation and especially Mr. Gary Ray, Chair of The Hormel Foundation, and Mr. Richard Knowlton, former CEO Hormel Foods Corporation and former Chair of The Hormel Foundation. Mr. Ray and Mr. Knowlton have provided unwavering support and guidance to The Hormel Institute and its faculty and staff for many years, and we sincerely thank them.

Preface

Despite the intensive efforts and substantial advances that have occurred by focusing on improving treatments, cancer is still one of the primary causes of death in many countries around the world. This disease is the foremost public health threat wielding major physical, social, and economic burdens worldwide. However, cancer is mostly preventable. In fact, the World Health Organization (WHO) indicates that one-third of all cancer deaths are preventable. Based on this idea and numerous epidemiological findings, attention has centered on dietary phytochemicals and other natural compounds as an effective intervention in cancer development. However, the failure of many large-scale clinical trials worldwide has raised doubts as to whether diet-based cancer prevention can be clinically successful. Because these trials were not designed on mechanism-based preclinical studies, identifying cancer-preventive dietary agents or functional foods that have specific molecular or cellular targets is thought to be essential to move forward. Every individual has a different and unique risk of cancer incidence, prognosis, and response to treatment. Indeed, the necessity of personalized therapy for treatment of lung or breast cancer, for example, is well established. Such reports indicate a trend toward personalized cancer treatment as a requirement for effective cancer therapy. Conversely, a personalized diet for cancer prevention has not been well documented, although prescribing a personalized diet for cancer prevention might make sense. Unfortunately, this will not likely happen anytime soon because, beyond unhealthy eating and lack of exercise, a valid link between diet and cancer has been elusive.

Cancer prevention has been categorized into three main types that include primary (e.g., avoiding carcinogens), secondary (e.g., screening for premalignant lesions), and tertiary (e.g., preventing recurrence). Each type of cancer has its own particular characteristic genes and proteins that regulate its growth. Therefore, knowing the specific gene(s) or protein target(s) of a phytochemical chemopreventive agent increases the probability of the agent exerting efficacy in high-risk individuals. Although reports have suggested benefits and targets of phytochemicals, these studies mainly rely on cell and animal models. In order to apply phytochemicals or other natural compounds as personalized cancer-preventive agents, the effects of these compounds in humans will need to be assessed. In the future, personalized prevention methods using natural compounds could play a crucial role in cancer prevention, especially in high-risk populations. Rigorous research in identifying molecular targets and conducting human studies with phytochemicals would provide an enhanced approach to personalized cancer prevention. Similar to the development of cancer therapeutic drugs, the development of the recent cancer-preventive agents is based on the discovery of precise molecular targets.

The prevention of cancer begins with state-of-the-art research to identify the essential factors that protect against cancer and those that cause or increase the risk of cancer. The most advanced scientific methods or protocols are the keys to obtain such knowledge. The aim of this volume is to provide researchers and non-researchers with practical methodologies for developing and validating small molecule- and phytochemical-derived drug discovery and mechanisms by which these compounds can modulate distinct target proteins involved in oncogenic signaling. While this volume is primarily focused toward cancer prevention research, the range of techniques demonstrated in the book also provides an introduction of cancer prevention research methods to researchers outside the field. Chapters deal with a critical discussion of both laboratory and clinical topics, with each chapter containing both a discursive section and a detailed methods section.

The book begins with a chapter detailing the methods for successfully combining computational and experimental methods for identifying molecular targets of phytochemicals. These strategies are based on the idea that targeting specific and multiple cancer genes, signaling proteins, and transcription factors to prevent cancer is now considered to be a very effective means by which to prevent cancer. Nutrients and dietary factors have attracted a great deal of interest because of their perceived ability to act as highly effective chemopreventive agents by targeting protein kinases and/or transcription factors, with very few adverse side effects. However, understanding the precise molecular mechanisms of nutrients in preventing cancer is imperative in the quest to identify key molecular targets for the development of more effective, less toxic anticancer agents ultimately leading to the eradication of cancer as a life-threatening disease. Combining in silico screening methods with laboratory validation methods is a powerful means to accomplish this goal. The second chapter expands on the most common laboratory methods utilized in laboratory validation studies.

Chemoprevention can involve precluding carcinogens from reaching their molecular target sites, from undergoing metabolic activation, or from subsequently interacting with crucial cellular macromolecules, such as genes and proteins, at the initiation stage. Thus, the induction of phase II/detoxifying enzymes can be an effective means for achieving protection against a variety of carcinogens in animals and humans. Thus, the third chapter focuses on basic methods used to study the cancer chemopreventive potential of dietary phytochemicals acting by stimulating the transcription factor, nuclear factor erythroid 2-related factor 2 (Nrf2 or NFE2L2), that regulates the expression of many phase II detoxifying/antioxidant enzymes. The next chapter zooms in on methods used to screen and validate the effect of natural chemopreventive agents, such as silibinin from milk thistle, on the protein expression of various prostate cancer-related biomarkers for proliferation, apoptosis, angiogenesis, and metastasis. Notably, the methods to study cancer biomarker protein expression described in this chapter are very useful in many types of cancer chemopreventive studies. Similarly, Chap. 5 focuses on a food-based approach to cancer prevention using freeze-dried berries and describes methods used to harvest the berries, grind them into a powder, and determine the nutrient, chemical, and microbial content of the powder before use in both preclinical and clinical studies. The authors provide details regarding the ability of black raspberries and strawberries to modulate the development of premalignant lesions, including Barrett's esophagus and esophageal dysplasia, in the esophagus. The hope is that the information and methods in this chapter will greatly facilitate those who are interested in applying food-based approaches to cancer prevention.

The next two chapters provide details on specific animal models useful in chemoprevention studies. First, the use of mouse lung tumor models, which are widely used in lung cancer chemopreventive studies, is described. The authors provide comprehensive instructions for the selection of mice, genotyping, and induction of lung tumors and details of the histological features of specific lung tumors. They also provide material on the application of these features in lung cancer chemoprevention studies and information on how to semiquantitatively phenotype lung tumor development. The next chapter in this group of two describes the azoxymethane (AOM) plus dextran sulfate sodium (DSS)-induced mouse colon carcinogenesis model, which is considered to be a powerful tool for investigating the pathogenesis and chemoprevention of colitis-associated colorectal cancer. Authors provide not only the optimized protocol for effective induction of colon tumors in mice by treatment with AOM plus DSS but also detailed specific protocols, all of which can be used for investigating the inflammation-associated colon carcinogenesis and the chemopreventive effect of dietary phytochemicals.

The next five chapters focus more on specific methodologies and/or new technologies of which all can be applied to studies focusing on the mechanism(s) of action of small molecules and natural compounds in chemoprevention. Cellular metabolic pathways and bioenergetics were studied in great detail many years ago. However, diseases such as cancer are now known to exhibit aberrant metabolism and energy production, and certain natural compounds can cause apoptotic cell death by interfering with their mitochondrial energy production. The first chapter in this group of five details a relatively new approach based on the Seahorse Extracellular Flux Analyzer, which obtains real-time measurements of oxidative phosphorylation and glycolysis in living cells, facilitating mechanistic studies of cancer chemopreventive agents. Next, the use of the specific high-throughput sequencing method, RNA-seq, to study the impact of phytochemicals on growth factors, such as insulin-like growth factor, that have been shown to play a primary role in both cancer development and progression is described. This technology is a method of high-throughput sequencing of cDNA utilized to gain information about a sample's RNA content. RNA-seq is a powerful technique that can provide information regarding an organism's transcriptome, such as abundances of transcripts, mutations, fusion transcripts, noncoding RNA, transcriptional modification, gene regulation, and protein information. Preparations of freshly harvested epidermal cells from adult mice treated or untreated with chemopreventive agents can be extremely useful for downstream applications such as clonal culture, flow cytometry, molecular biology, or other assays involving adult tissue stem cells in the context of carcinogenesis or chemoprevention. The third chapter in this group describes the harvesting methods that have been developed to provide reproducible yields of highly viable cells with the goal of authenticating their functions. The equipment and techniques presented here are also useful for the preparation of enriched stem cells for further study in molecular and cellular biology. DNA adduct measurements can provide valuable information regarding DNA damage associated with exposure to specific carcinogens and effectiveness of chemopreventive agents in alleviating this damage. Chapter 11 provides detailed step-by-step information on analysis of N^2-ethyl-dGuo, the major DNA adduct formed when acetaldehyde reacts with DNA. This adduct has been used to study mechanisms of alcohol carcinogenesis, but the protocol described can be applied to small amounts of DNA isolated from many different tissues and cell types and the effect of chemopreventive agents. Imaging technologies provide invaluable tools for developing and validating phytochemical-derived drug discovery and parsing out the molecular mechanisms by which these natural compounds can modulate distinct target proteins involved in oncogenic signaling. The last chapter in this group of five provides detailed steps in preparing relatively thick tissue samples for microscopy using multiple biomarkers providing unprecedented imaging information on pathophysiology, localization, and co-localization of target structures and signaling components.

Of course, the ultimate goal is to translate the basic findings regarding chemopreventive agents into the human or the clinical condition. The final chapter in this volume discusses each of the "five cardinal elements of trial design" denoted as "ABCDE" or agent, biomarker, cohort, design, and endpoint. In addition, authors provide a detailed evaluation of previous trials in the context of these five elements. The goal is to garner examples that are informative and can facilitate an improved design and conduct of future clinical trials.

Finally, we are grateful to all of the contributors, each of whom is an internationally recognized expert in the field of cancer prevention. We thank them for their enthusiasm, professionalism, and enormous insight and, importantly, their punctuality in submitting their chapters in a timely manner. To work with each of them was a great pleasure and an invaluable experience. We also thank David Casey (Springer US) for his support and assistance in this project.

Austin, MN, USA

Ann M. Bode
Zigang Dong

Contents

Contributors

RAJESH AGARWAL • *Department of Pharmaceutical Sciences, Skaggs School of Pharmacy and Pharmaceutical Sciences, Aurora, CO, USA; University of Colorado Cancer Center, University of Colorado, Aurora, CO, USA*

SILVIA BALBO • *Masonic Cancer Center, University of Minnesota Cancer Center, Minneapolis, MN, USA*

HEATHER BECKWITH • *Hematology, Oncology, and Transplantation, Department of Medicine, University of Minnesota, Minneapolis, MN, USA*

ANN M. BODE • *The Hormel Institute, University of Minnesota, Austin, MN, USA*

YA CAO • *Key Laboratory of Carcinogenesis and Cancer Invasion, Cancer Research Institute and Molecular Imaging Center, Ministry of Education, Central South University, Changsha, Hunan, China*

STEVEN CARMELLA • *Department of Laboratory Medicine and Pathology, University of Minnesota Cancer Center, Minneapolis, MN, USA*

GAGAN DEEP • *Department of Pharmaceutical Sciences, Skaggs School of Pharmacy and Pharmaceutical Sciences, Aurora, CO, USA; University of Colorado Cancer Center, University of Colorado, Aurora, CO, USA*

ZIGANG DONG • *The Hormel Institute, University of Minnesota, Austin, MN, USA*

MARNA ERICSON • *Department of Dermatology, Academic Health Center, University of Minnesota, Minneapolis, MN, USA*

FRANCISCO FUENTES • *Center for Cancer Prevention Research, Department of Pharmaceutics, Ernest Mario School of Pharmacy, Rutgers, The State University of New Jersey, Piscataway, NJ, USA; Department of Desert Agriculture and Biotechnology, Arturo Prat University, Iquique, Chile*

EUN-RYEONG HAHM • *Department of Pharmacology and Chemical Biology and Cancer Institute, University of Pittsburgh School of Medicine, Pittsburgh, PA, USA*

ERNEST HAWK • *Division of Cancer Prevention and Population Sciences, MD Anderson Cancer Center, Houston, TX, USA*

STEPHEN S. HECHT • *Department of Laboratory Medicine and Pathology, Masonic Cancer Center, University of Minnesota Cancer Center, Minneapolis, MN, USA*

YI-WEN HUANG • *Department of Obstetrics and Gynecology, Medical College of Wisconsin, Milwaukee, WI, USA*

SWETHA INTURI • *Department of Pharmaceutical Sciences, Skaggs School of Pharmacy and Pharmaceutical Sciences, Aurora, CO, USA; University of Colorado Cancer Center, University of Colorado, Aurora, CO, USA*

YIQUN JIANG • *Key Laboratory of Carcinogenesis and Cancer Invasion, Cancer Research Institute and Molecular Imaging Center, Ministry of Education, Central South University, Changsha, Hunan, China*

KELLY M. JOHNSON • *The Hormel Institute, University of Minnesota, Austin, MN, USA*

AH-NG TONY KONG • *Department of Pharmaceutics, Center for Cancer Prevention Research, Ernest Mario School of Pharmacy, Rutgers, The State University of New Jersey, Piscataway, NJ, USA*

LAURA A. KRESTY • *Division of Hematology and Oncology, Department of Medicine, Medical College of Wisconsin, Milwaukee, WI, USA*

CHIEH-TI KUO • *Division of Hematology and Oncology, Department of Medicine, Medical College of Wisconsin, Milwaukee, WI, USA*

HA-NA LEE • *Tumor Microenvironment Global Core Research Center, College of Pharmacy, Seoul National University, Seoul, South Korea*

JONG HUN LEE • *Department of Pharmaceutics, Center for Cancer Prevention Research, Ernest Mario School of Pharmacy, Rutgers, The State University of New Jersey, Piscataway, NJ, USA*

KYEONG-RYOON LEE • *Department of Pharmaceutics, Center for Cancer Prevention Research, Ernest Mario School of Pharmacy, Rutgers, The State University of New Jersey, Piscataway, NJ, USA*

WEI LI • *Key Laboratory of Carcinogenesis and Cancer Invasion, Cancer Research Institute and Molecular Imaging Center, Ministry of Education, Central South University, Changsha, Hunan, China; The Hormel Institute, University of Minnesota, Austin, MN, USA*

XIAOLAN LIU • *Key Laboratory of Carcinogenesis and Cancer Invasion, Cancer Research Institute and Molecular Imaging Center, Ministry of Education, Central South University, Changsha, Hunan, China*

KAREN COLBERT MARESSO • *Division of Cancer Prevention and Population Sciences, MD Anderson Cancer Center, Houston, TX, USA*

REBECCA J. MORRIS • *The Hormel Institute, University of Minnesota, Austin, MN, USA*

MICHELLE B. MOURA • *Department of Pharmacology and Chemical Biology and Cancer Institute, University of Pittsburgh School of Medicine, Pittsburgh, PA, USA*

HEUIJOON PARK • *Laboratory of Lymphocyte Signaling, The Rockefeller University, New York, NY, USA*

DAN PEIFFER • *Division of Hematology and Oncology, Department of Medicine, Medical College of Wisconsin, Milwaukee, WI, USA*

BEN RANSOM • *Department of Laboratory Medicine and Pathology, University of Minnesota Cancer Center, Minneapolis, MN, USA*

NYSSA READIO • *The Hormel Institute, University of Minnesota, Austin, MN, USA*

LUCINA C. ROUGGLY • *Department of Surgery and The Alvin J. Siteman Cancer Center, Washington University School of Medicine, St Louis, MO, USA*

TODD F. SCHUSTER • *The Hormel Institute, University of Minnesota, Austin, MN, USA*

YING SHI • *Key Laboratory of Carcinogenesis and Cancer Invasion, Cancer Research Institute and Molecular Imaging Center, Ministry of Education, Central South University, Changsha, Hunan, China*

LIMIN SHU • *Department of Pharmaceutics, Center for Cancer Prevention Research, Ernest Mario School of Pharmacy, Rutgers, The State University of New Jersey, Piscataway, NJ, USA*

ANUPAMA SINGH • *Department of Human Oncology, School of Medicine and Public Health, University of Wisconsin, Madison, WI, USA*

ASHOK SINGH • *Department of Human Oncology, School of Medicine and Public Health, University of Wisconsin, Madison, WI, USA*

SHIVENDRA V. SINGH • *Department of Pharmacology and Chemical Biology and Cancer Institute, University of Pittsburgh School of Medicine, Pittsburgh, PA, USA*
GARY D. STONER • *Division of Hematology and Oncology, Department of Medicine, Medical College of Wisconsin, Milwaukee, WI, USA*
ZHENG-YUAN SU • *Department of Pharmaceutics, Center for Cancer Prevention Research, Ernest Mario School of Pharmacy, Rutgers, The State University of New Jersey, Piscataway, NJ, USA*
YOUNG-JOON SURH • *Tumor Microenvironment Global Core Research Center, College of Pharmacy, Seoul National University, Seoul, South Korea*
MIN TANG • *Key Laboratory of Carcinogenesis and Cancer Invasion, Cancer Research Institute and Molecular Imaging Center, Ministry of Education, Central South University, Changsha, Hunan, China*
BENNETT VAN HOUTEN • *Department of Pharmacology and Chemical Biology and Cancer Institute, University of Pittsburgh School of Medicine, Pittsburgh, PA, USA*
DIAN WANG • *Department of Radiation Oncology, Medical College of Wisconsin, Milwaukee, WI, USA*
LI-SHU WANG • *Division of Hematology and Oncology, Department of Medicine, Medical College of Wisconsin, Milwaukee, WI, USA*
YIAN WANG • *Department of Surgery and The Alvin J. Siteman Cancer Center, Washington University School of Medicine, St Louis, MO, USA*
DOUGLAS YEE • *Masonic Cancer Center, University of Minnesota, Minneapolis, MN, USA*
MICHAEL S. YOU • *Department of Surgery and The Alvin J. Siteman Cancer Center, Washington University School of Medicine, St Louis, MO, USA*
MING YOU • *Department of Pharmacology and Toxicology, Medical College of Wisconsin, Milwaukee, WI, USA*
XINFANG YU • *Key Laboratory of Carcinogenesis and Cancer Invasion, Cancer Research Institute and Molecular Imaging Center, Ministry of Education, Central South University, Changsha, Hunan, China*
HYE-WON YUM • *Tumor Microenvironment Global Core Research Center, College of Pharmacy, Seoul National University, Seoul, South Korea*

Chapter 1

Combining Computational and Experimental Methods for Identifying Molecular Targets of Phytochemicals

Ann M. Bode and Zigang Dong

Abstract

Targeting specific and multiple cancer genes, signaling proteins, and transcription factors to prevent cancer is now considered to be the most effective means to prevent cancer. Proteins that bind to a specific DNA gene sequence and act to initiate transcription of the distinct protein gene product are referred to as transcription factors. Transcription factors such as activator protein-1 (AP-1), nuclear factor-kappaB (NF-κB), p53, nuclear factor of activated T cells (NFAT), and cAMP response element-binding (CREB) protein have been shown to play a critical role in carcinogenesis and all are regulated by the mitogen-activated protein (MAP) kinase cascades. The activation of these or other transcription factors results in transcription of genes that encode proteins that regulate a multitude of cellular responses including apoptosis, differentiation, development, inflammation, and proliferation. Nutrients and dietary factors have attracted a great deal of interest because of their perceived ability to act as highly effective chemopreventive agents by targeting protein kinases and/or transcription factors, with very few adverse side effects. In the last few years, we have successfully combined computational biology and experimental validation to identify specific molecular targets of a variety of nutrients/phytochemicals, including EGCG, [6]-gingerol, resveratrol, and various flavonoids such as kaempherol, quercetin, and myricetin, to prevent cancer. Understanding the precise molecular mechanisms of these and other nutrients in preventing cancer may reveal key molecular targets for the development of more effective, less toxic anticancer agents ultimately leading to the eradication of cancer as a life-threatening disease. This chapter details the computational methods and software combined with experimental validation methods to successfully identify molecular targets of any phytochemical or nutrient, and also provides citations of examples for the reader's reference.

Key words Computational biology, In silico screening, Molecular target, Nutrient, Dietary factor, Phytochemical

1 Introduction

Cancer development is a multifaceted process that involves thousands of cellular molecules, including genes and proteins, which are essential in the regulation of a vast assortment of cellular functions. Our work over the last decade has focused on a clearer understanding of molecular and cellular mechanisms and identification of cellular targets central in cancer prevention.

Ann M. Bode and Zigang Dong (eds.), *Cancer Prevention: Dietary Factors and Pharmacology*, Methods in Pharmacology and Toxicology, DOI 10.1007/978-1-4614-9227-6_1, © Springer Science+Business Media New York 2014

An important outcome of these investigations has been the identification and elucidation of signal transduction pathways induced by a variety of tumor promoters in cancer development. The predominant idea today is that cancer might be prevented [1] or treated by using small molecules directed at specific and, perhaps, multiple cancer genes, signaling proteins, and transcription factors. In particular, natural nutritional or dietary factors have emerged as modulators of important cellular signaling pathways and thus could be some of the most promising small-molecule inhibitors. Molecules of this type are professed as being generally safe and might have the capability to prevent or reverse premalignant lesions and/or reduce secondary primary tumor incidence [2]. Many of these compounds appear to act on multiple tumor promoter-stimulated cellular pathways with potent anticancer activity, low toxicity, and limited adverse side effects (reviewed in [1, 3–13]. This activity at the tumor promotion stage is highly significant because even though each stage of cancer development could provide potential targets for anticancer agents, the promotion stage is probably the most ideal target because of its long time span.

Historically, research efforts have focused heavily on early detection and treatment with little emphasis on environmental or lifestyle causes. Unfortunately, the efficacy of cancer therapies, especially for late-stage disease, remains dismal. Anticancer agent discovery is long and expensive process, and cancer prevention research per se has seemingly never been a major health research emphasis until very recently [1]. Thus, powerful cutting-edge technologies are indispensable in the quest for accelerating the process of drug discovery, especially to identify molecules that can suppress multiple cellular signaling pathways and to understand how these chemicals perturb these pathways by modeling their interactions with their target proteins.

Combining supercomputer technologies, including in silico screening, molecular docking, and protein simulation and modeling, with determination of protein crystal structure and validation through cell- and animal-based experimental laboratory assays to identify multiple protein targets of natural anticancer compounds is an example of the type of technologies needed. The supercomputer has been indispensable in the progress made in mapping protein interaction networks in cancer cells and, in particular, the network of protein kinase interactions with substrates and regulatory molecules [14–16]. High-speed calculating methods have increased our ability to use computational virtual screening of the ever-increasing number of available chemical and natural compound libraries against specific target proteins based on crystal structure or homology screening. In addition, reverse docking or shape similarity screening has been effective in the identification of a specific chemical's molecular target(s). This chapter details the computational methods and software combined with experimental validation methods we have used to successfully identify molecular targets of numerous phytochemicals or nutrients, and also provides citations of examples the readers may refer.

2 Materials

2.1 Computer Hardware

Our high performance computing (HPC) has been developed to provide state-of-the-art tools specifically to be used in biomedical (e.g., cancer) research. Drug discovery is increasingly dependent upon high-throughput biotechnological advances that are limited by inadequate access to high-end supercomputing power. Typically, cancer researchers struggle for computer time at large academic computer centers or even resort to creating their own clusters using a large number of desktop PCs. For successful drug development, researchers must systematically screen millions of small molecules to find a successful match between a chemical and its protein target—a process that can take years and requires a picture of the 3D structure of the protein.

The Hormel Institute's High Performance Computing facility consists of two supercomputers completely dedicated to molecular modeling and docking experiments. The computational power of the two systems together clocks in at approximately 35 TFLOPS (teraflops). The original system installed in 2008 is a single rack IBM BlueGene/L with 1,024 dual core Power PC CPUs. System management and storage are implemented with five Linux servers and a DS4200 storage system. The system installed in 2011 is an IBM supercomputing Linux GPU (Graphics Processing Unit) cluster optimized for molecular modeling and simulation applications. A total of 37 extremely fast computational nodes using iDataplex dx360 M3 servers form the computational building blocks of the HPC cluster. The cluster consists of computation, storage and management building blocks tightly coupled into an integrated HPC cluster by a high-performance network, a global parallel file system, and management software. Each of the 37 computational nodes has two Intel hex core Westmere X5650 CPUs, 48GB of RAM, 500GB hard drive, and two NVidia Tesla M2050 Fermi GPUs. Storage and management is handled with three dedicated servers using GPFS for a parallel storage system directly accessible by all the nodes. An open-source cluster management software tool from IBM, XCAT, provides management and system control. The entire system is interconnected with Quad-data-rate (QDR) Infiniband technology. This configuration has proven to be powerful and flexible enough for the most demanding molecular biology simulations. Supporting our supercomputers, we have eight Dual Quad core workstations running the visualization software, including two 3D projection systems. The supercomputer chemical screening uses data from our protein crystallography facility and protein modeling and simulation with 3D projection to create and analyze many proteins associated with diseases like cancer. The long-term goal is to develop new technologies to accelerate discovery and facilitate comprehensive study of human disease by combining analyses of protein structure/function with advanced methods of data management and drug screening. These tools for studying proteins and pathways provide the foundation for even more complex future projects.

2.2 Software Ported to the Supercomputers

2.2.1 Dock6 (Version 6.4)

DOCK6 (http://dock.compbio.ucsf.edu/) addresses the problem of "docking" or fitting molecules to a specific protein site. In general, "docking" is the identification of the low-energy binding modes of a small molecule, or ligand, within the active or other biological relevant site of a macromolecule, or receptor, whose structure is known. A compound that interacts strongly with, or binds, a receptor, which is associated with a disease such as cancer, may inhibit its function and thus act as a drug.

2.2.2 Amber (Version 11)

Amber (http://ambermd/org) refers to a set of molecular mechanical force fields for the simulation of biomolecules, which are in the public domain and are used in a variety of simulation programs, and to a package of molecular simulation programs, which includes source code and demos.

2.2.3 AutoDock 4.2.3

Autodock (http://autodock.scripps.edu/) is a suite of automated docking tools designed to predict the means by which small molecules, such as substrates or drug candidates, bind to a receptor with a known 3D structure.

2.2.4 NAMD 2.8

NAMD (http://www.ks.uiuc.edu/Research/namd/) is a parallel molecular dynamics program for UNIX platforms designed for high-performance simulations in structural biology.

2.2.5 Rosetta 3.3

Rosetta (https://www.rosettacommons.org/) comprises a software suite used for predicting and designing protein structures, protein folding mechanisms, and protein–protein interactions. Rosetta has been consistently successful in CASP (Critical Assessment of protein Structure Prediction) and CAPRI (Critical Assessment of Prediction of Interactions) competitions.

2.2.6 CHARMM (Chemistry at HARvard Macromolecular Mechanics)

CHARMM (http://www.charmm.org/) is a versatile and widely used molecular simulation program that has broad application to many-particle systems. It was developed with a primary focus on the study of molecules of biological interest, including peptides, proteins, prosthetic groups, small-molecule ligands, nucleic acids, lipids, and carbohydrates, as they occur in solution, crystals, and membrane environments.

2.3 The Linux Workstation Applications

These applications include those ported to the supercomputer and several others.

2.3.1 Schrödinger Suite

The Schrödinger Suite (http://www.schrodinger.com) is a commercially available software suite used for modeling and simulation as well as visualization and automation. This suite covers the entire molecular mechanics, molecular dynamics, protein modeling and bioinformatics, structural biology-crystallography, and molecular visualization.

2.3.2 Haddock-2.0

Haddock (http://www.nmr.chem.uu.nl/haddock/) refers to High Ambiguity Driven biomolecular DOCKing and the docking is based on biochemical and/or biophysical information.

2.3.3 Openeye

OpenEye (http://www.eyesopen.com) has provided software to the pharmaceutical industry for molecular modeling and cheminformatics since 1997. Its mission is to provide novel software, new science, and better business practices to the industry. Central to their approach is the importance of shape and electrostatics as primary variables of molecular description, platform-independent code for high-throughput 2D and 3D modeling, and a preference for the rigorous rather than the ad hoc.

2.3.4 Amsol Version 7.1

Amsol (http://comp.chem.umn.edu/amsol/ or http://www.license.umn.edu/Products/AMSOL-71--Software-to-Calculate-Free-Energies-of-Solvation__Z05201.aspx) is a computational chemistry software program that calculates the free energy of a solvated molecule. The software application calculates the change in energy when molecules are dissolved in water or an organic solvent. The results may also be used to calculate partition coefficients and their logarithms (Log P). The SM1-SM5.42R solvation models are used to calculate the free energies of solvation in water. The SM4 solvation model is used to calculate the free energies of solvation in alkanes, and the SM5.0-SM5.42R solvation models are used for general organic solvents.

2.3.5 Chimera

UCSF Chimera (http://www.cgl.ucsf.edu/chimera/) is a highly extensible program for interactive visualization and analysis of molecular structures and related data, including density maps, supramolecular assemblies, sequence alignments, docking results, trajectories, and conformational ensembles. High-quality images and animations can be generated.

2.3.6 Ligplot

Ligplot (http://www.ebi.ac.uk/thorton-srv/software/LIGPLOT/) is a program that automatically generates schematic diagrams of protein–ligand interactions for a given PDB file.

2.3.7 Gromacs 4.6.2

Gromacs (http://www.gromacs.org/) is a versatile package to perform molecular dynamics (i.e., simulate the Newtonian equations of motion for systems with hundreds to millions of particles) and is primarily designed for biochemical molecules like proteins, lipids, and nucleic acids that have many complicated bonded interactions. However, because Gromacs is extremely fast at calculating nonbonded interactions, which usually dominate simulations, many groups are also using it for research on nonbiological systems, e.g., polymers.

2.3.8 Modeller 9.12

The Modeller (http://salilab.org/modeller/) program is used for homology or comparative modeling of protein 3D structures. The user provides an alignment of a sequence to be modeled with known related structures and Modeller automatically calculates a model containing all non-hydrogen atoms. Modeller implements comparative protein structure modeling by satisfaction of spatial restraints. This program can perform many additional tasks, including *de novo* modeling of loops in protein structures, optimization of various models of protein structure with respect to a flexibly defined objective function, multiple alignment of protein sequences and/or structures, clustering, searching of sequence databases, and comparison of protein structures.

2.3.9 VMD

VMD (Visual Molecular Dynamics; http://www.ks.uiuc.edu/Research/vmd) is designed for modeling, visualization, and analysis of biological systems such as proteins, nucleic acids, and lipid bilayer assemblies. It may be used to view more general molecules because VMD can read standard Protein Data Bank (PDB) files and display the contained structure. VMD provides a wide variety of methods for rendering and coloring a molecule, including simple points and lines, CPK (**Note 1**) spheres and cylinders, licorice bonds, backbone tubes and ribbons, cartoon drawings, and others. VMD can be used to animate and analyze the trajectory of a molecular dynamics simulation. In particular, VMD can act as a graphical front end for an external molecular dynamics program by displaying and animating a molecule undergoing simulation on a remote computer.

2.4 Laboratory Validation Materials

2.4.1 Standard Laboratory Equipment

Researchers should have access to standard laboratory equipment including centrifuges, scintillation counter, gel scanners with data acquisition, refrigerators, freezers, rotators, temperature-controlled water baths, western blot and electrophoretic transfer boxes, power supplies, culture hoods and incubators, computers, and gel photography system as examples.

2.4.2 Reagents

1. Many compounds can be purchased from Sigma-Aldrich (St. Louis, MO).

2. Active proteins and peptide substrates may be purchased from Millipore (Temecula, CA) or Signal Chem (Richmond, BC).
3. Antibodies against selected targets can be purchased from a variety of companies, including Cell Signaling Biotechnology (Beverly, MA), Santa Cruz Biotechnology (Santa Cruz, CA), R&D Systems (Minneapolis, MN), Cayman Chemical (Ann Arbor, MI), Pharmingen, Becton Dickinson Co. (Franklin Lakes, NJ), Zymed Laboratory (San Francisco, CA), and BD Biosciences (Sparks, MD).
4. Fetal bovine serum can be purchased from Atlanta Biologicals (Lawrenceville, GA) or Invitrogen (GIBCO, Grand Island, NY).
5. CNBr-Sepharose 4B beads are purchased from Amersham Pharmacia Biotech (Piscataway, NJ).
6. Small-hairpin RNA (shRNA) constructs against *various genes* can be obtained from the BioMedical Genomics Center at the University of Minnesota (Minneapolis, MN) or from Open Biosystems, Inc. (Huntsville, AL).
7. G418, the luciferase assay substrate and the Cell Titer 96 Aqueous One Solution Reagent [3-(4,5-dimethylthiazol-2-yl)-5-(3-carboxymethoxyphenyl)-2-(4-sulfophenyl)-2H-tetrazolium, inner salt (MTS)] kit for the cell proliferation assay is purchased from Promega (Madison, WI).
8. Cell lines can be purchased from the American Type Culture Collection (ATCC, Manassas, VA).
9. Cells can be transfected with plasmids using the jetPEI poly transfection reagent (Qbiogene, Inc., Montreal, Quebec, Canada), following the manufacturer's suggested protocols.

3 Methods

3.1 Computational Strategies

Computer modeling combined with biological simulation are progressively being used as highly effective tools in cancer-related research. The overall scheme for identifying specific molecular or cellular targets of small molecules involves several different approaches. The approach taken will depend on whether the initial frame of reference is a protein with a proven role in cancer development or a small natural or synthetic molecule with proven anticancer activity. Proteins or small molecules identified using computational strategies must then be validated through intensive laboratory experimentation (For workflow scheme, *see* Fig. 1).

An X-ray crystallographic structure of a protein of interest either alone or bound to an inhibitor or ligand is particularly important in the process of elucidating the interactions between proteins and small molecules and in the design and development of

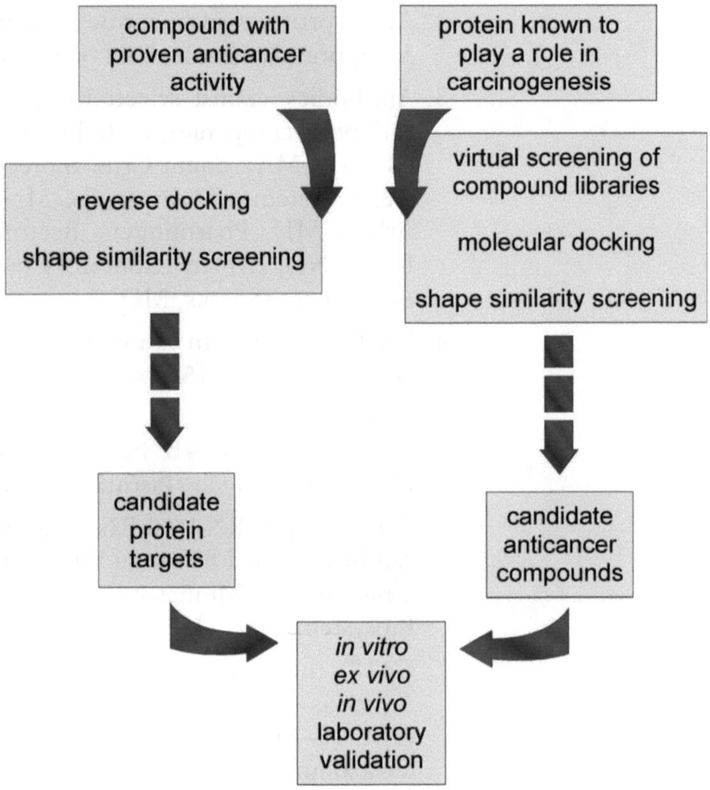

Fig. 1 Workflow for identifying potential anticancer compounds. The starting point can be a compound with proven anticancer activity but with an unknown molecular target or a protein known to play a role in carcinogenesis. Reverse docking and shape similarity screening can be used to find potential protein targets for a known compound. Virtual screening of compound libraries, molecular docking, and shape similarity screening can be used to identify candidate compounds to affect the activity of a protein known to have a role in carcinogenesis. All candidate proteins and compounds must be validated in in vitro, ex vivo, and in vivo laboratory experiments

additional specific inhibitors. Solved protein crystal structures can be found in the RCSB Protein Data Bank [17] (http://www.rcsb.org/pdb/home/home.do). Homology modeling methods can be used to create a suitable structure with which to work if a protein crystal structure with a resolution of about 2.0 Å does not exist or if the structure has not been solved. This type of modeling between proteins requires that the two proteins possess a minimum protein sequence identity of 30 % [18]. The European Bioinformatics Institute (http://www.ebi.ac.uk/) Web service provides a variety of the tools needed for protein sequence searching and alignment [19]. The National Center for Biotechnology Information (http://www.ncbi.nlm.nih.gov/) also provides protein structure and sequence databases.

3.1.1 Virtual Screening

The computational process referred to as "virtual screening" utilizes the crystal structure or homology modeling to search for potential drug candidates [20]. Virtual screening is commonly used in drug discovery and involves the rapid in silico (**Note 2**) assessment of large libraries of compound structures. From these libraries, virtual screening is used to identify the most promising compound structures that are likely to bind to a protein target. The protein target is usually a protein receptor or an enzyme that has been identified experimentally or by computer. Coupled with databases of virtual chemical compounds, the computational processes of "docking" and "scoring" are implemented using known and hypothetical drug targets on a protein. In docking, various computational methods (i.e., algorithms) are used to position (or dock) a chemical from a virtual library into a specified target site or sites on the protein of interest. The objective of molecular docking is to elucidate the binding interactions between two proteins or a protein and ligand. Mathematical models are used to score the interaction once a compound is docked. Scoring approximates the chemical interactions such as energy state or binding strength between the protein and ligand, which assists in ranking the efficacy of the compound being scored. Evaluation of the docked and scored complexes leads to the selection of compounds to be moved into the laboratory for in vitro, ex vivo, and in vivo testing.

Schrödinger's Suite [21] is used by many laboratories for virtual screening because this platform provides a variety of computational tools in one package (http://www.schrodinger.com/). Virtual screening is the major computational method utilized in drug discovery for "hit" (**Note 3**) identification [22]. The primary procedure used is structure-based virtual screening, which involves docking of thousands to millions of candidate ligands into a protein target followed by scoring the protein–ligand binding interaction to approximate the binding energy of the ligand [23]. Structure-based virtual screening requires a three-dimensional (3D) structure of the ligand. The ZINC (i.e., an acronym for "ZINC is not commercial") Database (http://zinc.docking.org/) contains over 21 million compounds in "ready to dock, 3D formats," which are freely available to use for virtual screening [24]. From this huge database, smaller and more specific high-quality libraries can be built for targeted virtual screening [25]. For example, we have built a specific flavonoid database [26]. The National Institute of Health's PubChem online database contains over 27 million unique 2D structures (http://pubchem.ncbi.nlm.nih.gov/). The National Cancer Institute (NCI) Database (Enhanced NCI Database Browser; http://cactus.nci.nih.gov/ncidb2.2/) contains over 250,000 compounds and the Human Metabolome Database (http://www.hmdb.ca/) comprises about 2,500 metabolites linked to over 5,500 protein and DNA sequences to which they correspond. The Asinex Database (http://www.asinex.com/)

is a large library of searchable natural compounds that are also available for purchase from the site. The Available Chemicals Directory (ACD) http://accelrys.com/products/databases/sourcing/available-chemicals-directory.html), which is a proprietary chemical database containing over 480,000 chemical compounds, is available on a pay-per-use basis. The Drugbank Database (www.drugbank.ca) contains 6,711 drug entries including 85 nutraceuticals, 131 FDA-approved biotech (protein/peptide) drug, 1,447 FDA-approved small-molecule drugs, and 5,080 experimental drugs with 4,227 nonredundant protein (i.e., drug target/enzyme/transporter/carrier) sequences are linked to these drug entries. A supercomputer can screen these libraries against a target protein in a relatively short period of time.

3.1.2 Molecular Docking [26]

Molecular docking has become a standard tool in computational biology and, in combination with virtual screening, is used to envisage the binding orientation of target proteins with small-molecule drug candidates in order to assess the affinity and activity of the small molecule. Thus, molecular docking plays an important role in the rational design of drugs. The GLIDE module from the Schrödinger Suite [21] provides a range of speed versus accuracy options and a variety of docking protocols. GLIDE can automate calculations for huge compound libraries and provides detailed reports and summaries of docking results. Various protocols for docking are usually attempted before finalizing the most accurate set of parameters to be utilized for docking. The correct re-docking of the ligand that was crystallized with a target protein is commonly used to validate the parameters chosen. When more than one crystal structure of a target protein is available, cross-docking (**Note 4**) is performed to determine which crystal structure is most suitable for docking [27].

When more detail is needed, molecular docking is used to study the binding of a specific molecule with a target protein. The X-ray crystal structure of a protein of interest bound with its ligand is downloaded from the PDB and prepared for docking using the Protein Preparation Wizard in the Schrödinger Suite. All crystallographic waters are removed and a grid is generated based on the ATP-competitive or -noncompetitive ligand-binding site on the protein receptor. MacroModel from the Schrödinger Suite is used to build and energetically minimize the compound of interest to create the most energetically favorable conformation needed for docking studies. Finally, docking with high-throughput virtual screening (HTVS), standard precision (SP), and extra precision (XP) are three of the standard procedures from Schrödinger's GLIDE docking protocols (**Note 5**). Induced-Fit Docking (IFD) is a more CPU (central processing unit)-intensive method that can be used with SP and XP docking. All these docking procedures allow ligand-docking flexibility (**Note 6**).

3.1.3 Reverse Docking

Another approach is a compound-based method that begins with the selection of potential cancer preventive candidates based on previous research studies. These compounds have been shown to exert anticancer activity but their molecular target is unknown. From the selected compounds, the most effective candidates are moved forward as lead compounds using laboratory experimental methods such as anchorage-independent growth, cell proliferation, kinase or reporter gene assays and animal studies. After selecting one or more lead compounds, candidate target proteins that directly interact with the compounds can be identified by "reverse docking" the compound onto available protein crystal structures [28, 29]. Reverse docking involves flexible molecular receptors around rigid transition state models of the catalyst-free asymmetric reaction (referred to as "TS-models"), whereas normal docking explores the configuration of a small molecule in the confines of a large receptor [30]. To identify potential target proteins of the lead candidate compounds, protein databases (e.g., DrugBank http://www.drugbank.ca/databases; Potential Drug Target Database (PDTD); http://www.dddc.ac.cn/pdtd/index.php) that contain structural information, such as the position and conformation of the active site, for known or potential protein drug targets, are commonly used [30]. However, the number of available predicted potential protein targets is quite low compared to the number of known genes limiting the widespread use of this strategy. The selected database is screened against the compound of interest with the reverse docking tool referred to as Target Fishing Dock or TarFisDock [31]. TarFisDock (http://www.dddc.ac.cn/tarfisdock/) is a Web-based tool used to search for potential binding proteins for a known ligand. It uses a ligand–protein reverse docking strategy to dock the ligand into possible binding sites of all potential protein targets from the selected database. For validation of the protein target, proteomic tools can include the lead compound being chemically immobilized onto an affinity resin or attached to a biotin molecule. Protein extracts are applied to these resins and liquid chromatography analysis is used to separate the proteins bound to the compound of interest. The natural product–protein adducts can then be identified using 2D gel electrophoresis and mass spectroscopy (MS)/MS analysis. We have used this method to identify leukotriene A4 hydrolase as a direct target of [6]-gingerol in colon cancer [32].

3.1.4 Shape-Similarity Screening Method [26]

Shape-based virtual screening of chemical libraries can also be used to search for compounds in a library that are structurally similar to known inhibitors of a given protein. Shape-similarity screening is based on the idea that molecules having similar shapes and electrostatic properties might exhibit comparable biological activity. For shape similarity screening, the PHASE [33, 34] module from the Schrödinger Suite is used to search for 3D-shape similarity and to examine the shared elements of ligands with a reference molecule. The atom type information is included for consideration of not only shape similarity but also to align potential pharmacophore points between the queries and targets. A pharmacophore involves the steric and electronic features, such as hydrophobic centroids, aromatic rings, hydrogen bond donors or acceptors, anions, and cations, that are necessary to guarantee optimal molecular interactions with a specific biological target and to trigger (or block) its biological response [35]. The pharmacophore and physical features of a molecule are quantitatively compared with a library of compounds for more molecules that share the same features arranged in an identical relative orientation. The endpoint to be used for the results selects the best aligned structure for each molecule identified, and all conformers possessing a Tanimoto similarity coefficient (**Note 7**) less than 0.7 are omitted [36]. Compounds having a Tanimoto similarity coefficient greater than 0.7 are selected. Each chemical is then "docked" into the target protein by computational methods, which enables the acquisition of detailed protein–ligand interactions. When searching for potential target proteins, the compound library used should comprise crystallized ligands extracted from the most recent version of the PDB [37]. The ligand conformation in the crystal structure is used because the atoms should be oriented in a manner optimized for binding to the protein. Any available database such as those indicated earlier can be used when searching for similar compounds.

3.2 Summary of Computational Strategies

Each of these computational strategies requires the methods of docking and scoring using known and hypothetical drug binding sites on a protein and is coupled with databases of virtual chemical compounds. In docking, numerous algorithms are used to position a chemical from a virtual library into a specified target site or sites on the protein of interest. The goal of molecular docking is to elucidate the binding interactions between two molecules—either protein to protein or protein to ligand. Once a compound is docked, mathematical models are used to score its ability to bind. Scoring approximates the chemical interactions such as binding strength and energy state between the ligand and protein to facilitate in ranking the efficacy of the compound being scored [38, 39]. From these strategies, candidate small natural or synthetic compounds that directly interact with target proteins can be identified. The cancer preventive effects and interactions of selected molecules with protein targets must then be validated using laboratory experiments. To further confirm the specific interaction and binding site of a selected phytochemical and its target protein, X-ray crystallography, nuclear magnetic resonance (NMR), and protein point mutation methods can be used. Finally, modulation of the selected pathway and target protein should be validated in animal models and humans, with tissue analysis before and after exposure to the agent, ideally in preneoplastic lesions. Promising candidate chemopreventive compounds can then be fully evaluated in clinical trials to determine their suitability for use as cancer preventive or therapeutic agents.

3.3 Laboratory Validation Methods

The results of the computational screening must be validated in the laboratory.

3.3.1 Cell Culture

Standard culture conditions are utilized. In general, cells are cultured in Minimum Essential Medium (MEM), DMEM (Dulbecco's Modified Eagle Medium), or a specific medium required. The medium is supplemented with a specific percentage of fetal bovine serum or calf serum and antibiotics. Most journals now require verification that cells have been cytogenetically tested and authenticated before being frozen. Each vial of frozen cells is thawed and maintained for a maximum of 8–20 passages depending on the cell line. Enough frozen vials should be available to ensure that all cell-based experiments are performed on cells that have been tested and in culture for 8–20 weeks, depending on the cell line. The reader is referred to ATCC or other cell sources for specific culture details.

3.3.2 Cytotoxicity Assay

Compounds should generally be nontoxic in their effective range of anticancer activity. To estimate cytotoxicity, cells are seeded (~2×10^4 cells/well) in 96-well plates with appropriate percentage of FBS and required medium at 37 °C in a 5 % CO_2 incubator. The cells are fed with fresh medium after 4 h and treated with the compound or vehicle (**Note 8**) at various concentrations (e.g., 0, 1, 10, 25, or 50 μM). After culturing for the desired times, 20 μl of Cell Titer 96 Aqueous One Solution (Promega) is added to each well, and the cells are then incubated for 1 h at 37 °C in a 5 % CO_2 incubator. Absorbance is measured at 490 and (690 nm background) using a 96-well plate reader (Labsystem Multiskan MS, Labsystem, Finland).

3.3.3 Cell Proliferation Assay (Anchorage-Dependent Growth)

Effective compounds should inhibit cancer cell proliferation at low concentrations. Cells are seeded (~1×10^3 cells per well) in 96-well plates and incubated for 24 h and then treated with vehicle or different doses of each compound (**Note 9**). After incubation for various times (e.g., 1, 2, 6, 12, 24, 48 up to 72 h), 20 μl of CellTiter96 Aqueous One Solution (Promega) is added and then the cells are incubated for 1 h at 37 °C in a 5 % CO_2 incubator. Absorbance is measured at 492 nm (690 nm background) using a 96-well plate reader (Labsystem Multiskan).

3.3.4 Anchorage-Independent Neoplastic Transformation Assay

The ability of a compound to prevent neoplastic transformation is a good indication of its potential as an anticancer agent. This assay is commonly referred to as the "soft-agar assay." Different cell lines (e.g., human skin HaCaT or mouse epidermal JB6 P+ or promotion positive; **Note 10**) are seeded in a 6-well plate (8,000 cells/well) and exposed or not exposed to epidermal growth factor (EGF, 10 ng/ml) or another tumor promoter and various concentrations of desired compound in 1 ml of 0.33 % BME (Eagle's basal medium) agar containing for example 10 % FBS over 3.5 ml of 0.5 % BME agar containing for example 10 % FBS and the same doses of tumor promoter and desired compound. The cultures are maintained in a 37 °C, 5 % CO_2 incubator for 10–21 days, and the cell colonies are counted under a microscope with the aid of the Image-Pro Plus software program (version 6; Media Cybernetics).

3.3.5 Anchorage-Independent Growth Assay

The ability to grow in soft-agar under anchorage-independent conditions is a hallmark of cancer. This assay is identical to the anchorage-independent neoplastic transformation assay except that tumor promoters (e.g., EGF) are not required because cancer cells are already transformed. Cancer cells (8×10^3 per well) suspended in complete growth medium (supplemented with appropriate percentage of FBS and 1 % antibiotics) are added to 0.33 % agar along with various doses of compounds (or not treated as a control). This is then added onto a base layer of 0.5 % agar containing complete growth medium and FBS with the same doses of compounds. The cell colonies are counted under a microscope with the aid of the Image-Pro Plus software program (version 6; Media Cybernetics).

3.3.6 Focus-Forming Assay

Another method to assess the effectiveness of phytochemicals is the focus-forming assay. Transformation of NIH3T3 cells is conducted according to a standard protocol. Cells are transiently transfected with various combinations of pcDNA3-H-RasG12V (100 ng), e.g., pcDNA4-gene of interest-wild type (200 ng) or pcDNA4-gene of interest-mutant (200 ng), and pcDNA3-mock (to achieve equal amounts of DNA), cultured in for example 5 % calf bovine serum-DMEM. After 14 days, foci are fixed by methanol and stained with 0.5 % crystal violet and foci are counted in a manner similar to that for the anchorage-independent assays.

3.3.7 Lentiviral Infection

To confirm a compound's target, transfection experiments are commonly performed in which the targeted gene of interest can be silenced with small or short hairpin RNA (**Note 11**). The lentiviral expression vectors, including *pLKO.1-shgene of interest* and packaging vectors, including *pMD2.0G* and *psPAX*, are purchased from Addgene Inc. (Cambridge, MA). To prepare viral particles expressing the gene of interest, each viral vector and packaging vectors (*pMD2.0G and psPAX*) are transfected into for example HEK293T cells using jetPEI (Polyplus Transfection, New York, NY) following the manufacturers' suggested protocols. The transfection medium is changed at 4 h after transfection and then the cells are cultured for 36 h. The viral particles are harvested by filtration using a 0.45 mm sodium acetate syringe filter and then combined with 8 mg/ml of polybrene (Millipore, Billerica, MA) for infection overnight into 60 % confluent, for example, colon cancer cells. The cell culture medium is replaced with fresh complete growth medium for 24 h and then cells selected with 1.5 mg/ml of puromycin for 36 h. If the compound targets the transfected gene (i.e., gene product or protein target) of interest, the compound should have little or no effect on characteristics (e.g., growth) of the transfected cancer cells.

3.3.8 Luciferase Assay to Determine Effect of Compound on Reporter Gene Activity

Confluent monolayers of cells of interest that have been stably transfected with the gene of interest *luciferase* reporter plasmid are trypsinized (**Note 12**). Viable cells (4×10^4) suspended in 1 ml of the appropriate percentage FBS and medium are added to each well of a 24-well plate. Plates are incubated overnight at 37 C in a humidified atmosphere of 5 % CO_2. The cells are usually starved in serum-free medium (to reduce background) for another 24 h. The cells are treated for the appropriate time with various concentrations of the compound of interest (e.g., 0–50 μM) and harvested after the appropriate time. Cells are then disrupted with 100 μl of lysis buffer (0.1 M potassium phosphate pH 7.8, 1 % Triton X-100, 1 mM dithiothreitol (DTT), and 2 mM EDTA), and luciferase activity is measured using a luminometer (Luminoskan Ascent, Thermo Electro, Helsinki, Finland).

3.3.9 Apoptosis Assay

Many compounds exert their anticancer activity by inducing controlled cell death or apoptosis. Cells are plated into 60-mm culture dishes (1×10^5 cells/dish) and incubated for 1 day in medium containing the appropriate amount of FBS. The culture medium is then replaced with a 0.1–1 % serum medium and cultured for 1–4 days with various doses of each compound. The cells are collected by trypsinization and washed with phosphate buffered saline (PBS) and then resuspended in 200 μl of binding buffer (contained in the apoptosis detection kit). Apoptosis is assessed using an annexin V or annexin V-FITC (fluorescein isothiocyanate) apoptosis detection kit as recommended by the manufacturer (e.g., MBL International Corp., Watertown, MA). The cells are observed under a fluorescence microscope using a dual filter set for FITC and propidium iodide and then analyzed by flow cytometry (FACS Calibur flow cytometer, BD Biosciences, Franklin Lakes, NJ).

3.3.10 Cell Cycle Assay

Many compounds act by causing changes in cell cycle progression such as G1 arrest, inhibition of the G1 to S transition, or G2–M arrest. Cells are seeded (~2×10^5 cells/well) in 60-mm dishes with appropriate percentage FBS and medium at 37 °C in a 5 % CO_2 incubator overnight. Then cells are usually starved in a serum-free medium for 24 h followed by treatment with the compound of interest (e.g., 0, 1, 10, or 25 μM) for 12 or 24 h in medium containing the appropriate amount of FBS. The cells are trypsinized, washed twice with cold PBS, and fixed with ice-cold 70 % ethanol at −20 °C overnight. Cells are then washed twice with PBS, incubated with 20 mg/ml RNase A and 200 mg/ml propidium iodide in PBS at room temperature for 30 min in the dark, and subjected to flow cytometry using for example the FACSCalibur flow cytometer. Data can be analyzed using ModFit LT (Verity Software House, Inc., Topsham, ME).

3.3.11 Western Blot Analysis

The most common method to assess a compound's effect on protein expression is western blot analysis (also referred to as immunoblot analysis). Cells (1×10^6) are cultured in 10-cm dishes for 24 h and then starved in serum-free medium for 24–48 h. The cells are then treated with various concentrations (e.g., 0, 20, 40, or 80 μM) of the desired compound for 24 h. Cells are harvested and disrupted with NP-40 lysis buffer [150 mM NaCl, 50 mM Tris–HCl pH 7.5, 1 % Nonidet P-40, and Complete Protease Inhibitor Cocktail Tablets (Roche, Indianapolis, IN)]. Equal amounts of protein are determined using the bicinchoninic acid (BCA) assay kit (Pierce, Rockford, IL) or dye-binding protein assay kit (Bio-Rad Laboratories, Hercules, CA). Equal amounts of lysate proteins (e.g., 30–100 μg) are boiled for 5 min and then subjected to 6–12 % (depending on the size of the protein) sodium dodecyl sulfate–polyacrylamide gel electrophoresis (SDS-PAGE) and electrophoretically transferred to a polyvinylidene difluoride (PVDF) membrane. After blocking the membrane with 5 % nonfat dry milk for 1 h, the membrane is incubated with a specific primary antibody at 4 °C overnight. Protein bands are visualized by a chemifluorescent detection (e.g., ECL system, GE Healthcare) after washing with PBS containing 0.1 % Tween 20 and hybridization with a horseradish peroxidase-conjugated or alkaline phosphatase secondary antibody.

3.3.12 Preparation of Compound of Interest—Sepharose 4B Beads and Pull-Down Assay

Many compounds can be conjugated to Sepharose 4B beads if they contain a hydroxyl group to verify their direct interaction or binding with a target protein. CNBr-activated Sepharose 4B beads (GE Healthcare; 0.5 g) are washed 3 times with 1 mM HCl and then rotated with the compound of interest (~2.5 mg) in coupling buffer (0.1 M $NaHCO_3$ and 0.5 mM NaCl) at 4 °C overnight. The solution is transferred to 0.1 M Tris–HCl buffer (pH 8.0) and again rotated end-over-end at 4 °C overnight. The beads are washed 3 times with 0.1 M acetate buffer (pH 4.0) containing 0.5 M NaCl followed by a wash with 0.1 M Tris–HCl (pH 8.0) containing 0.5 M NaCl. Compound-conjugated beads are then suspended in 1.5 ml of PBS containing 0.05 % sodium azide and kept at 4 °C. Active proteins (0.2 μg) or cell lysates (500 μg) containing the protein of interest are individually incubated with

100 μl of the compound conjugated—Sepharose 4B (or Sepharose 4B only as a control; 100 μl, 50 % slurry) in a reaction buffer (50 mM Tris–HCl pH 7.5, 5 mM EDTA, 150 mM NaCl, 1 mM DTT, 0.01 % Nonidet P-40, 2 μg/ml bovine serum albumin, 0.02 mM PMSF, and 1× protease inhibitor mixture). After incubation with gentle rocking overnight at 4 °C, the beads are washed 5 times with reaction buffer excluding the protease inhibitor mixture. The proteins bound to the beads are analyzed by western blotting using an antibody to detect the protein of interest.

3.3.13 In Vitro Kinase Assay

Because of their proven critical role in carcinogenesis, most of the targeted proteins are kinases. The influence of a compound on a kinases activity can be assessed using a kinase assay both in vitro and in cells (i.e., ex vivo). Cells are cultured to 80 % confluence and then treated with various concentrations of each compound of interest for various times. The cells are then harvested and kinase assays are performed in accordance with instructions provided by Upstate Biotechnology (Billerica, MA). Briefly, the reaction is carried out in the presence of 10 μCi of [γ-^{32}P] ATP with each compound in 40 μl of reaction buffer containing 20 mM HEPES (pH 7.4), 10 mM $MgCl_2$, 10 mM $MnCl_2$, and 1 mM dithiothreitol. After incubation at room temperature for 30 min, the reaction is stopped by adding 10 μl of protein loading buffer and the mixture is separated by SDS-PAGE. Each experiment is repeated 2–3 times. The relative amounts of incorporated radioactivity are assessed using a scintillation counter (LS6500; Beckman Coulter, Brea, CA, USA). For in vitro assessment of kinase activity, the active kinase can be purchased and then incubated (100 ng) with 10 μCi [γ-^{32}P] ATP, the compound of interest and reaction buffer. The activity is measured by the scintillation counter.

3.3.14 In Vitro PI3-K Kinase Assay

The Akt (or protein kinase B; PKB)/phosphatidylinositol 3-kinase (PI3-K) pathway is one of the most important targeted pathways in cancer prevention or therapeutics. Measuring PI3-K kinase activity differs from the traditional kinase assay. Active PI3-K (100 ng) or cell lysates (500 μg) are incubated with the compound of interest at various concentrations (e.g., 0, 20, 40, or 80 μM) or LY294002 (10 μM; **Note 13**) in buffer [10 mM Tris–HCl (pH 7.6), 100 mM NaCl, 1 mM DTT, and 0.1 mM Na_3VO_4] for 10 min at 30 °C. LY 294002, a well-known PI3-K inhibitor, is used as a positive control. The mixtures are incubated with 20 μl of 0.5 mg/ml phosphatidylinositol (MP Biomedicals, Solon, OH) in substrate buffer [50 mM HEPES buffer, 1 mM EGTA and 1 mM NaH_2PO_4] for 5 min at room temperature, and then incubated with 10 μl [γ-^{32}P] ATP buffer [10 mM Tris–HCl (pH 7.6), 60 mM $MgCl_2$ and 0.25 mM ATP containing 10 μCi [γ-^{32}P] ATP] for 10 min at 30 °C. The reaction is stopped by adding 15 μl of 4 N HCl and then 130 μl of chloroform–methanol (1:1) is added.

After mixing, 30 μl of the lower chloroform phase are spotted onto a thin layer chromatography plate (TLC Silica Gel $60F^{254}$, Merck KGaA, Darmstadt, Germany) previously activated for 1 h at 110 °C. The resulting [γ-^{32}P]-labeled phosphatidylinositol-3-phosphate (PI3P) is separated by thin layer chromatography with developing solvent [chloroform–methanol–NH_4OH–H_2O (60:47:2:11.3)] and radiolabeled spots are visualized by autoradiography.

3.3.15 ATP and Compound of Interest Competition Assay

Many compounds act by competing with ATP by binding in the same active site as ATP. To determine whether a compound inhibits a kinase by competing with ATP, ATP (1, 10, or 100 μM) is mixed with the active protein (0.2 μg) of interest to a final volume of 500 μl for 30 min. Then 100 μl of compound conjugated–Sepharose 4B (or Sepharose 4B for control) is added and the mixture is incubated for 12 h at 4 °C. The samples are washed, and proteins of interest are then detected by western blotting.

3.4 Animal Studies to Validate the Effectiveness of Compounds of Interest

Several types of animal studies can be utilized to study the effectiveness of anticancer compounds identified by in silico methods and verified in experimental laboratory assays. The animal model selected depends on the target organ. Models can include the solar UV-induced 2 stage skin carcinogenesis model, genetic knockout, overexpressing or other transgenic mouse models, and the xenograft model.

3.4.1 Solar UV-Induced 2 Stage Skin Carcinogenesis Model

In this model, skin carcinogenesis is induced by a solar ultraviolet (UV) irradiation system (SUV-340, Q-LAB, Cleveland, OH) with peak emission at 340 nm. We chose solar-simulated light because the optimal source for skin photobiology is the sun with wavelengths ranging from a spectrum of 290–400 nm. Solar UV is more relevant to the human condition and the spectrum comprises a majority of UVA, which is highly similar to natural sunlight. The dorsal skin of mice will be exposed to solar UV irradiation, using a bank of 4 UVA-340 sunlamps (Q-Panel Lab Products, Cleveland, OH). UVA-340 sunlamps emit UV between 295 and 390 nm, which closely resembles the UV spectrum of sunshine through the mid-UVA range. Lamp output is measured using the IL1700 Research Radiometer/Photometer (International Light Technologies, Peabody, MA). The mice are exposed to UV at a distance of 15 inches because the heat produced by the lamp is negligible under these conditions. Mice are not restrained during UV exposure. Total dose is calculated using the measured value and the length of exposure. Doses are environmentally relevant, being equivalent to 60 min of noonday summer sun in Minneapolis, Minnesota. Degradation of bulbs must be measured after every 12 h of use and dose calibration calculated and verified.

Method Using SKH-1 Hairless Mice

SKH-1 hairless mice are the most common model used for studying the effectiveness of compounds to prevent UV-induced skin carcinogenesis. Mice are generally divided into 5 age-matched groups: (a) a vehicle (usually acetone)-only treated group ($n = 10$); (b) compound-treated group (e.g., 1.0 mg in vehicle) with no solar UV ($n = 10$); (c) vehicle treated plus solar UV treated group ($n = 20$); (d) compound-treated (e.g., 0.5 mg) plus solar UV group ($n = 20$); and (e) compound-treated (e.g., 1.0 mg) plus solar UV group ($n = 20$, **Note 14**). In the vehicle-treated group, the dorsal skin is topically treated with 200 μl of acetone only. In the 1.0 mg compound of interest group, for example, the dorsal skin is topically treated with 1.0 mg compound in 200 μl of acetone and mice are not exposed to SUV. In the vehicle/solar UV group, the dorsal skin is topically treated with 200 μl of acetone 30–60 min before solar UV irradiation (**Note 15**). The mice in the 0.5 mg compound/solar UV or 1.0 mg compound/solar UV groups receive topical application of the compound of interest (e.g., 0.5 or 1.0 mg) in 200 μl of acetone before solar UV irradiation. Solar UV irradiation is given 3 times a week for 15 weeks as described below (**Notes 16, 17**). At week 1, the mice are irradiated with solar UV at a dose of 30 kJ/m^2 UVA and 1.8 kJ/m^2 UVB 3 times a week. The dose of solar UV is progressively increased (10 % each week) due to the ensuing hyperplasia that can occur with solar UV irradiation of the skin. At week 6, the dose of solar UV is 48 kJ/m^2 UVA and 2.9 kJ/m^2 UVB, this dose is maintained for weeks 6–15. At week 15, solar irradiation is stopped and mice are observed for another 15 weeks (**Note 18**). The mice are weighed and tumors are measured by caliper once a week until week 30 or tumors reach 1 cm^3 total volume (**Note 19**), at which time mice are euthanized and then the tumors and skins are collected (**Notes 20–23**).

Sample Experimental Design

For study design for a long-term exposure experiment, see Table 1.

Acute Solar UV Experiments

This type of experiment is designed to determine if the compound of interest hits its target in the early stages of solar UV exposure. The acute experiments will be conducted using a single dose response of solar UV. A small pilot study should be first conducted to determine the optimal dose and time points for harvesting skin. Based on the results of our pilot studies, we found that using 60 kJ/m^{2}UVA/3.6 kJ UVB was sufficient to induce various signaling molecules in dorsal mouse skin. One of two doses of compound is applied 30 min prior to solar UV exposure and the post-irradiation time points to be studied could include 0, 0.5, 3, 6, 12, and 24 h after exposure (5 mice each time point/total of 30 mice each group). Vehicle control (acetone but no solar UV) mice (3 mice each time point/total of 18 mice each group) are also sacrificed at each time point (Table 2). Mice are sacrificed at desired

Table 1
Experimental design for testing the effect of a candidate compound on solar UV-induced skin carcinogenesis

Group	Treatment	Amount of compound	No. of mice
SKH-1 hairless	Acetone	None	10–20
SKH-1 hairless	Solar UV	None	20–30
SKH-1 hairless	Solar UV + low dose compound	10 μmol	20–30
SKH-1 hairless	Solar UV + high dose compound	20 μmol	20–30
SKH-1 hairless	High dose compound (no solar UV)	20 μmol	20–30
		Total	90–140

Table 2
Experimental design for testing the acute (1 dose solar UV at 60 kJ/m² UVA/3.6 kJ/m² UVB and 6 time points/group) effect of a compound of interest

Groups	Treatment	Number of mice (acute study)
SKH-1 hairless	Acetone (vehicle control)	18
SKH-1 hairless	Solar UV + low dose compound	30
SKH-1 hairless	Solar UV + high dose compound	30
SKH-1 hairless	High dose compound-No solar UV	30
		Total = 96

time points and dorsal skin is divided into 2 portions. One part is snap frozen for western blotting and the other is suspended in 10 % buffered formalin for immunohistochemistry (IHC) analysis. The number of mice to be used in the experiments should be based on a power calculation and previous experience in order to achieve statistically significant differences.

3.4.2 In Vivo Xenograft Mouse Model

The xenograft mouse model is a powerful, although not perfect model, to study the effect of newly identified compounds on human tumor growth. Athymic nude mice (Cr:NIH(S), NIH Swiss nude, 6–8 weeks old) are purchased from Charles River (Wilmington, MA), Jackson Laboratories (Bar Harbor, ME) or other sources. Animals are maintained under "Specific Pathogen Free (SPF)" conditions and all animal studies are performed according to guidelines approved by the respective Institution's Institutional Animal Care and Use Committee (IACUC). New animals are acclimated to the facility for 1–2 weeks before the study

Table 3
A pilot study to determine the optimal dose of a compound

Group	Treatment	No. of mice
1	Control	5
2	Compound	5
3	Compound	5
4	Compound	5
Total		20

and have free access to food and water. The animals are housed in climate-controlled quarters with a 12-h light–12-h dark cycle.

General Procedures

The mice to be used are a hairless nude phenotype that results from an inherited developmental defect. In addition to being virtually hairless, homozygous mutant nude mice also suffer from a congenital failure to develop a normal thymus gland. Thus these mice are deficient in thymus-dependent (T-cell) immunological functions. Because the nude mouse is unable to reject implanted cells or tissues from a genetically nonidentical donor, they have become an extremely useful model for tumor studies in which they can serve as host for human or animal tumor cells to study tumor development and progression. Tumor growth can occur over a relatively short period of time. All mice have free access to food and water and the overall health of the mice and tumor size is monitored closely. Mice are weighed each week and tumors measured (cm^3) 2–3×/week and size recorded. When tumors reach a maximum size of 1–2 cm^3 (**Note 24**), mice are euthanized and tumors removed. Other organs (e.g., lung, liver, kidney, brain, heart) are also collected to analyze for metastases and the activities of proteins of interest.

General Methods

Animals are randomly assigned to the following groups: (a) Vehicle group ($n=15$); (b) e.g., 10 mg/kg body weight (B.W.) compound group ($n=15$); (c) e.g., 25 mg/kg B.W. compound group ($n=15$); (d) e.g., 50 mg/kg B.W. compound group ($n=15$); and (e) e.g., 50 mg/kg B.W. compound control group ($n=15$; no cells; **Note 25**). Each mouse is administrated the appropriate dose of compound in 100 μl of the proper vehicle or only vehicle 5×/week by oral gavage or 3×/week by intraperitoneal injection. A sample study design for a pilot study is shown in Table 3 and a sample study design for a full study is shown in Table 4. After 2 weeks of treatment, the desired human cancer cells (1×10^6 cells) are injected subcutaneously (s.c.) into the right flank of mice in the respective groups. Following injection, the mice continue to be administered

Table 4
A full experimental design for testing the effect of a compound of interest in a xenograft mouse model

Group	Treatment	Amount of compound	No. of mice
1	No treatment	None	20
2	Positive control	For example 50 mg/kg B.W.	20
3	Compound	Optimized lowest concentration of compound	20
4	Compound	Optimized midrange concentration of compound	20
4	Compound	Optimized highest concentration of compound	20
Total			100

the appropriate dose of compound or vehicle. The mice in one of the highest dose control group are not injected with cells, but maintained for comparison of body weight and tumor development. The mice are weighed and tumors measured by caliper 3×/week. Tumor volume is calculated from measurements of 2 diameters of the individual tumor according to the formula: tumor volume (mm^3) = [length × width × height × 0.52]. The mice are monitored until the tumors reach 1–2 cm^3 total volume (**Note 24**) at which time the mice are euthanized and the tumors extracted.

Injection of Tumor Cells

Cells are harvested from culture vessels and counted. The cells are washed in serum free culture medium and resuspended to a final concentration of 10^7 cells/ml. For each injection point, 0.2 ml of the suspension is injected using a sterile 1-ml-capacity tuberculin syringe fitted with a 21-gauge needle. The injection of cells into the mouse will require one person to hold the mouse, by firmly grasping at the base of the tail and at the back of the head behind the ears, thus keeping the mouse gently stretched out. The person holding the syringe then lifts the fold of the skin on the flank of the mouse midway between the front and the hind legs and using the other hand for injection. No anesthetization is needed or desirable for this purpose. The cells are deposited subcutaneously at a single point, as far away as possible from the point of penetration in order to prevent the cells from oozing out when the needle is withdrawn. Immediately after removal of the needle, the needle opening is held open briefly between 2 fingers. The fact that the cells are injected subcutaneously can be observed during the injection process due to the transparency of the mouse's skin. Injections can be made bilaterally to increase the assay points per nude mouse and about 1–3 million cells can be injected at each site. Following injection, the mice are checked every day thereafter both visually and by manual palpation. The latency period between the injection of cells and the first appearance of a palpable nodule at the site of injection varies and depends on the malignancy and the number of cells injected. Palpable nodules can occur 1–2 weeks following injection of 1 million viable cells, depending on the cell line. Formalin fixed tumor tissues can be processed for histopathology and analyzed for cell proliferation index, apoptotic index, and angiogenesis. Some frozen tumor samples and blood samples can be used to determine the levels of the compound of interest. Tumor growth is an endpoint and it serves as a basis for mechanistic studies (**Note 26**).

3.4.3 The APC^{Min+} Mouse Model for Studying the Effectiveness of Chemopreventive Compounds Against Colon Cancer

The C57BL/6J-*Apc*$^{Min+}$ strain is highly susceptible to spontaneous intestinal adenoma formation but homozygous mice are not viable. An initial report showed that 100 % of the C57BL/6J-*Apc*Min heterozygous mice raised on a high-fat diet developed more than 30 adenomas throughout the intestinal tract and most die by 120 days of age. Heterozygotes also develop anemia [40, 41]. A small number of C57BL/6J-*Apc*^{Min} heterozygous female mice develop mammary tumors. The *Min* mutation was discovered in the progeny of a C57BL/6J male mutagenized by ethylnitrosourea. The founding (AKR × C57BL/6J)F1 female displayed circling behavior and was mated to a C57BL/6J male. Some progeny from this backcross developed adult onset anemia and intestinal adenomas. The circling behavior was determined to be a separate heritable trait and was eliminated through subsequent crosses to C57BL/6J. This strain was imported into The Jackson Laboratory in 1992 and is a well-accepted model to study colon carcinogenesis [42–44].

General Procedures

Male and female heterozygous APC^{Min+} mice (5 weeks old) are used for these experiments. Male C57BL/6J$^{(Min/+)}$ mice are obtained from Jackson Laboratory and are bred with C57BL/6J APC wild type female mice. The progeny are genotyped by PCR assay to determine whether they were heterozygous for the *min* allele or are homozygous wild type. These mice will develop colon cancer and die by about 120 days old unless an intervention with chemopreventive agents is administered. The length of the study proposed is 10 weeks and therefore mice should still be viable at 105 days when euthanized at the end of the study. At the end of the study, the bowel is cleaned prior to euthanization of mice and removal of the colon to examine for colon cancer. To do this, solid food is removed from the cage 18 h before euthanizaation and drinking water is replaced with a solution of 20 % glucose (W/V) and then at 18 h later, mice are euthanized and the colon is removed for analysis.

General Methods

The potential toxicity of the compound of interest may not be known and therefore the potential toxicity of the compound should be tested in a pilot study using wild type mice. In this case, mice are divided into four groups and fed vehicle or 1 of 3 amounts of the compound of interest in vehicle. The mice are monitored by investigators and animal care staff for potential signs of toxicity. Because the compound might be novel, the optimal dose will need to be determined in vivo. The doses could include 0, 10, 50, or 100 mg/kg B.W. compound fed by gavage ($n = 20$ total, 5 per group; Table 3). APC^{Min} mice should be 5 weeks old at the beginning of the study and should receive the compound for 10 weeks 5 days/week. The mice should be monitored closely for any signs of toxicity. Once the optimal dose is determined, the full experiment can be performed (Table 4). Age-matched male and female heterozygous APC-Min mice (5 week) are divided into 4 groups of 20 mice each. They are fed 1 of 3 doses of compound by gavage 5 days week for 10 weeks. At the end of 10 weeks, mice are euthanized by tanked CO_2 (according to IACUC guidelines) and the colon is removed, washed and examined for polyp formation and appropriate protein activity. If possible, a known inhibitor of colon carcinogenesis should be used as a positive control (**Note 27**).

4 Notes

1. CPK models are space-filling models, also known as a calotte model. CPK model was named after the chemists Robert Corey, Linus Pauling, and Walter Koltun, who were the first to use them.
2. In silico is an expression used to mean "performed on computer or by computer simulation" (http://en.wikipedia.org/wiki/in_silico).
3. A "hit" is the stage in early drug discovery where small-molecule "hits" from a computational screen for example are identified to be evaluated as eventual "lead" compounds.
4. Cross docking refers to docking a ligand into each of two or more superimposed protein structures originally bound with other ligands in an ensemble of protein structures [45].
5. Glide offers the full range of speed versus accuracy options, from the HTVS (high-throughput virtual screening) mode for efficiently enriching million-compound libraries, to the SP (standard precision) mode for reliably docking tens to hundreds of thousands of ligands with high accuracy, to the XP (extra precision) mode where further elimination of false positives is accomplished by more extensive sampling and advanced scoring, resulting in even higher enrichment (See http://isp.ncifcrf.gov/files/isp/uploads/2010/07/glide.pdf).
6. Various conformations of a ligand can be generated in the absence of the protein target and subsequently docked or

conformations can be created in the presence of the protein-binding site.

7. A measure of shared features. For example, in comparing molecule A and B, N_A is the number of features in A and N_B is the number of features in B, and N_{AB} is the number of features common to both A and B. Therefore, the Tanimoto coefficient is: $T = N_{AB}/N_A + N_B - N_{AB}$. A ratio higher than 0.7 is an indication of good similarity.
8. Vehicle is the reagent in which the compound is dissolved and should be nontoxic and not interfere with the compound's activity or cell viability or growth.
9. Some cells may need to be serum starved for 24 h (to eliminate nonspecific background activity, including the influence of FBS on the activation of kinases such as the mitogen-activated protein kinases, or synchronize cells at G0) and then treated with various doses of compound or vehicle followed by incubation for various times.
10. HaCaT cells are human keratinocytes that are commonly used to study transformation. They require EGF in order to be transformed. The mouse epidermal skin JB6 P+ cell line is a well-established [46] cell model to study the effectiveness of potential anticancer agents to suppress neoplastic transformation induced by EGF or 12-*O*-tetradecanoylphorbol-13-acetate (TPA).
11. A small hairpin RNA or short hairpin RNA (shRNA) is an RNA sequence that makes a tight hairpin turn, which can be used to silence a specific gene's expression by RNA interference. Expression of shRNA in cells is commonly achieved by delivering a plasmid containing the desired gene sequence using viral or bacterial vectors.
12. Adherent cells attach themselves to surface of tissue culture flasks or dishes because they contain proteins, which they secrete to form a bridge between the cell and the surface. In order to disassociate the protein from the surface, a proteolytic (protein degrading) enzyme like trypsin is used to digest the proteins. EDTA (a metal chelator) is often included in the trypsin solution to facilitate trypsin's activity. Trypsin should never be left on cells longer than 5 min and should be in solution over the cells.
13. LY294002 is a morpholine derivative of quercetin and a potent inhibitor of PI3-K.
14. In a power calculation, assuming a standard deviation of 40 % in tumor volume, using 20 mice per experimental group will allow one to detect a 30 % (25 %) reduction in tumor volume with a power of 0.91 at a significance level of 5 % based on a two-tailed test.

15. Mice should be housed under yellow lighting to prevent degradation of selected compounds.
16. A minimum of two amounts or concentrations of the compound of interest should be administered to determine whether the compound works through the proposed target protein to inhibit carcinogenesis in this model.
17. The doses of compound are based on information from cell culture studies and the literature, if available.
18. Tumors might not be apparent at this time but should begin to develop by week 18.
19. Total volume or size of tumor allowed will depend upon the respective institution's IACUC guidelines.
20. Depending on the strain of mice used, DMBA (200 nmol; dimethylbenz(a)anthracene) may be needed to applied as a tumor initiator 2 weeks before beginning solar UV treatment and mice may need to be treated with solar UV for the entire 30 weeks. For example, some mouse strains (e.g., C57BL/6 and BALB-c background mice are less sensitive to solar UV-induced carcinogenesis).
21. This protocol can also be adapted to the two stage DMBA/TPA (12-O-tetradecanoylphorbol-13-acetate). In this case, one topical application of DMBA (200 nmol) is applied 2 weeks before TPA (17 nmol) treatment is begun. TPA is applied twice weekly.
22. If haired mice are used, the dorsal surface must be carefully shaved 2 days prior to treatment with DMBA, solar UV or TPA.
23. We have used this protocol in LTA4H wild type and knockout mice to show that resveratrol specifically targets LTA4H [47]. We have also shown that taxifolin can suppress solar UV-induced skin carcinogenesis by directly targeting the epidermal growth factor receptor (EGFR) and PI3-K [39].
24. Size depends on IACUC guidelines.
25. Dose of compound is extrapolated from cell culture studies, research literature or pilot studies (Table 3).
26. For prevention studies, the mice are treated with compound for 1–3 weeks before cells are injected. For therapeutic studies, the mice are injected with cells and tumor growth is monitored until the tumor reaches 50–100 cm^3 at which time treatment with the compound is initiated.
27. For examples of successful natural compound identification through a combination of computational screening, in vitro and ex vivo cell-based laboratory validation studies, and animal studies, please refer to references [26, 32, 34, 39, 47–81].

5 Conclusions

A tremendous volume of scientific data has accrued elucidating the molecular mechanisms of carcinogenesis and the action of anticancer agents in cancer prevention and therapy. These research findings are the basis for clarifying the molecular mechanisms for cancer prevention and treatment. Importantly, these innovations have resulted in the elucidation of key molecular targets for screening and testing novel natural anticancer agents, which have fewer unwanted side effects. However, even with the cumulative advances in drug discovery and preclinical testing, anticancer drug development remains a laborious, time-consuming process with only partial success. This indicates an important need to discriminate at an earlier stage of development between promising candidates and those less likely to be effective. Although advancement has been made in identifying principal molecular targets and potential nontoxic anticancer agents, transitioning preclinical results into the clinic has been enormously challenging. Regrettably, only a few compounds have shown tangible promise in clinical trials. Using individual agents that target multiple pathways or combining agents at lower doses are strategies that are rapidly acquiring general acceptance. Some investigators suggest that several pathways should be pursued for a controlled period of time and certain cancers might require a customized combination of prevention strategies for successful intervention [82, 83]. Some have indicated that combinations of drugs could act through a variety of inhibitory mechanisms that could result in a synergistic increase in efficacy mainly because single agents are not likely to impede heterogeneous cancers, which has clearly been shown in numerous clinical trials [84, 85]. Furthermore, combining agents, and in particular, natural compounds, most likely would require a lower dose of each compound, which could result in substantially lower toxicity and fewer unfavorable side effects.

In silico screening uses molecular docking programs that "place" molecules non-covalently into the active site, a protein-interaction site, a regulatory site, or another biologically relevant site of a protein and then ranks aspirant molecules by their ability to interact with the target protein. These drug targets identified in silico can be validated in vitro, ex vivo, and in vivo using cell-based biochemical assays, site mutagenesis, and animal studies. Finally, on a cellular or organ level, modeling cancer development to study cancer promotion, progression, and therapeutic effectiveness or the potential for drug resistance is highly promising.

Acknowledgements

This work is supported by The Hormel Foundation, the Rochester Eagle's Telethon, Hormel Foods, Pediatric Pharmaceuticals, University of Minnesota Office Vice President of Research and grants from the American Institute for Cancer Research and NIH grants CA027502, CA081064, CA077646, CA088961, CA111356, CA074916, CA111536, CA120388, ES016548, and CA077451.

References

1. Bode AM, Dong Z (2009) Cancer prevention research—then and now. Nat Rev Cancer 9(7):508–516. doi:10.1038/nrc2646, pii: nrc2646
2. Hong WK (2003) General keynote: the impact of cancer chemoprevention. Gynecol Oncol 88(1 Pt 2):S56–S58
3. Bode AM, Dong Z (2004) Targeting signal transduction pathways by chemopreventive agents. Mutat Res 555(1–2):33–51
4. Bode AM, Dong Z (2004) Beneficial effects of resveratrol. In: Bao Y, Fenwick R (eds) Phytochemicals in health and disease, vol 12, Oxidative stress and disease. Marcel Dekker Inc, New York, pp 257–284
5. Bode AM, Dong Z (2004) Cancer prevention by food factors through targeting signal transduction pathways. Nutrition 20(1): 89–94
6. Bode AM, Dong Z (2005) Signal transduction pathways in cancer development and as targets for cancer prevention. Prog Nucleic Acid Res Mol Biol 79:237–297
7. Bode AM, Dong Z (2006) Molecular and cellular targets. Mol Carcinog 45(6):422–430
8. Bode AM, Dong Z (2007) The enigmatic effects of caffeine in cell cycle and cancer. Cancer Lett 247(1):26–39
9. Bode AM, Dong Z (2009) Modulation of cell signal transduction by tea and ginger. In: Surh Y-J, Cadenas E, Dong Z, Packer L (eds) Dietary modulation of cell signaling pathways. Oxidative stress and disease. CRC Press–Taylor & Francis Group, New York, pp 45–74
10. Bode AM, Dong Z (2009) Signal transduction molecules as targets for cancer prevention. Sci Signal 2(59):mr2. doi:10.1126/scisignal.259mr2, pii: scisignal.259mr2
11. Bode AM, Dong Z (2011) The amazing and mighty ginger. In: Benzie IFF, Wachtel-Galor S (eds) Herbal medicine—biomolecular and clinical aspects. Oxidative stress and disease, 2nd edn. CRC Press–Taylor and Francis Group, New York, pp 131–156
12. Bode AM, Dong Z (2011) The two faces of capsaicin. Cancer Res 71(8):2809–2814. doi:10.1158/0008-5472.CAN-10-3756, pii: 0008-5472.CAN-10-3756
13. Bode AM, Dong Z (2012) Effects of dietary effectors on signal transduction pathways related to cancer prevention. In: Bidlack WR, Rodriguez RL (eds) Nutritional genomics—the impact of dietary regulation of gene function on human disease. CRC Press, New York, pp 243–268
14. Blume-Jensen P, Hunter T (2001) Oncogenic kinase signalling. Nature 411(6835):355–365. doi:10.1038/35077225
15. Manning G, Whyte DB, Martinez R, Hunter T, Sudarsanam S (2002) The protein kinase complement of the human genome. Science 298(5600):1912–1934. doi:10.1126/science.1075762
16. Venter JC, Adams MD, Myers EW, Li PW, Mural RJ, Sutton GG, Smith HO, Yandell M, Evans CA, Holt RA, Gocayne JD, Amanatides P, Ballew RM, Huson DH, Wortman JR, Zhang Q, Kodira CD, Zheng XH, Chen L, Skupski M, Subramanian G, Thomas PD, Zhang J, Gabor Miklos GL, Nelson C, Broder S, Clark AG, Nadeau J, McKusick VA, Zinder N, Levine AJ, Roberts RJ, Simon M, Slayman C, Hunkapiller M, Bolanos R, Delcher A, Dew I, Fasulo D, Flanigan M, Florea L, Halpern A, Hannenhalli S, Kravitz S, Levy S, Mobarry C, Reinert K, Remington K, Abu-Threideh J, Beasley E, Biddick K, Bonazzi V, Brandon R, Cargill M, Chandramouliswaran I, Charlab R, Chaturvedi K, Deng Z, Di Francesco V, Dunn P, Eilbeck K, Evangelista C, Gabrielian AE, Gan W, Ge W, Gong F, Gu Z, Guan P, Heiman TJ, Higgins ME, Ji RR, Ke Z, Ketchum KA, Lai Z, Lei Y, Li Z, Li J, Liang Y, Lin X, Lu F, Merkulov GV, Milshina N, Moore HM, Naik AK, Narayan VA, Neelam B, Nusskern D, Rusch DB, Salzberg S, Shao W, Shue B, Sun J, Wang Z, Wang A, Wang X, Wang J, Wei M, Wides R, Xiao C, Yan C, Yao A, Ye J, Zhan M, Zhang W, Zhang H, Zhao Q,

Zheng L, Zhong F, Zhong W, Zhu S, Zhao S, Gilbert D, Baumhueter S, Spier G, Carter C, Cravchik A, Woodage T, Ali F, An H, Awe A, Baldwin D, Baden H, Barnstead M, Barrow I, Beeson K, Busam D, Carver A, Center A, Cheng ML, Curry L, Danaher S, Davenport L, Desilets R, Dietz S, Dodson K, Doup L, Ferriera S, Garg N, Gluecksmann A, Hart B, Haynes J, Haynes C, Heiner C, Hladun S, Hostin D, Houck J, Howland T, Ibegwam C, Johnson J, Kalush F, Kline L, Koduru S, Love A, Mann F, May D, McCawley S, McIntosh T, McMullen I, Moy M, Moy L, Murphy B, Nelson K, Pfannkoch C, Pratts E, Puri V, Qureshi H, Reardon M, Rodriguez R, Rogers YH, Romblad D, Ruhfel B, Scott R, Sitter C, Smallwood M, Stewart E, Strong R, Suh E, Thomas R, Tint NN, Tse S, Vech C, Wang G, Wetter J, Williams S, Williams M, Windsor S, Winn-Deen E, Wolfe K, Zaveri J, Zaveri K, Abril JF, Guigo R, Campbell MJ, Sjolander KV, Karlak B, Kejariwal A, Mi H, Lazareva B, Hatton T, Narechania A, Diemer K, Muruganujan A, Guo N, Sato S, Bafna V, Istrail S, Lippert R, Schwartz R, Walenz B, Yooseph S, Allen D, Basu A, Baxendale J, Blick L, Caminha M, Carnes-Stine J, Caulk P, Chiang YH, Coyne M, Dahlke C, Mays A, Dombroski M, Donnelly M, Ely D, Esparham S, Fosler C, Gire H, Glanowski S, Glasser K, Glodek A, Gorokhov M, Graham K, Gropman B, Harris M, Heil J, Henderson S, Hoover J, Jennings D, Jordan C, Jordan J, Kasha J, Kagan L, Kraft C, Levitsky A, Lewis M, Liu X, Lopez J, Ma D, Majoros W, McDaniel J, Murphy S, Newman M, Nguyen T, Nguyen N, Nodell M, Pan S, Peck J, Peterson M, Rowe W, Sanders R, Scott J, Simpson M, Smith T, Sprague A, Stockwell T, Turner R, Venter E, Wang M, Wen M, Wu D, Wu M, Xia A, Zandieh A, Zhu X (2001) The sequence of the human genome. Science 291(5507):1304–1351. doi:10.1126/science.1058040

17. Bernstein FC, Koetzle TF, Williams GJ, Meyer EF Jr, Brice MD, Rodgers JR, Kennard O, Shimanouchi T, Tasumi M (1977) The Protein Data Bank: a computer-based archival file for macromolecular structures. J Mol Biol 112(3):535–542
18. Xiang Z (2006) Advances in homology protein structure modeling. Curr Protein Pept Sci 7(3):217–227
19. McWilliam H, Valentin F, Goujon M, Li W, Narayanasamy M, Martin J, Miyar T, Lopez R (2009) Web services at the European Bioinformatics Institute-2009. Nucleic Acids Res 37(Web Server):W6–W10. doi:10.1093/nar/gkp302
20. McInnes C (2007) Virtual screening strategies in drug discovery. Curr Opin Chem Biol 11(5):494–502. doi:10.1016/j.cbpa.2007.08.033, pii: S1367-5931(07)00117-2
21. Friesner RA, Banks JL, Murphy RB, Halgren TA, Klicic JJ, Mainz DT, Repasky MP, Knoll EH, Shelley M, Perry JK, Shaw DE, Francis P, Shenkin PS (2004) Glide: a new approach for rapid, accurate docking and scoring. 1. Method and assessment of docking accuracy. J Med Chem 47(7):1739–1749. doi:10.1021/jm0306430
22. Rester U (2008) From virtuality to reality—virtual screening in lead discovery and lead optimization: a medicinal chemistry perspective. Curr Opin Drug Discov Dev 11(4):559–568
23. Lyne PD (2002) Structure-based virtual screening: an overview. Drug Discov Today 7(20):1047–1055, pii: S1359644602024832
24. Irwin JJ, Shoichet BK (2005) ZINC—a free database of commercially available compounds for virtual screening. J Chem Inf Model 45(1):177–182. doi:10.1021/ci049714+
25. Hartshorn MJ, Verdonk ML, Chessari G, Brewerton SC, Mooij WT, Mortenson PN, Murray CW (2007) Diverse, high-quality test set for the validation of protein–ligand docking performance. J Med Chem 50(4):726–741. doi:10.1021/jm061277y
26. Chen H, Yao K, Nadas J, Bode AM, Malakhova M, Oi N, Li H, Lubet RA, Dong Z (2012) Prediction of molecular targets of cancer preventing flavonoid compounds using computational methods. PLoS One 7(5):e38261. doi:10.1371/journal.pone.0038261
27. Cavasotto CN, Abagyan RA (2004) Protein flexibility in ligand docking and virtual screening to protein kinases. J Mol Biol 337(1):209–225. doi:10.1016/j.jmb.2004.01.003, pii: S0022283604000324
28. Cheng KW, Wong CC, Wang M, He QY, Chen F (2010) Identification and characterization of molecular targets of natural products by mass spectrometry. Mass Spectrom Rev 29(1):126–155. doi:10.1002/mas.20235
29. Rix U, Superti-Furga G (2009) Target profiling of small molecules by chemical proteomics. Nat Chem Biol 5(9):616–624. doi:10.1038/nchembio.216, pii:nchembio.216
30. Harriman DJ, Deslongchamps G (2006) Reverse-docking study of the TADDOL-catalyzed asymmetric hetero-Diels-Alder reaction. J Mol Model 12(6):793–797. doi:10.1007/s00894-006-0097-z
31. Li H, Gao Z, Kang L, Zhang H, Yang K, Yu K, Luo X, Zhu W, Chen K, Shen J, Wang X, Jiang H (2006) TarFisDock: a web server for identifying drug targets with docking approach. Nucleic Acids Res 34(Web Server):W219–W224. doi:10.1093/nar/gkl114
32. Jeong CH, Bode AM, Pugliese A, Cho YY, Kim HG, Shim JH, Jeon YJ, Li H, Jiang H,

Dong Z (2009) [6]-Gingerol suppresses colon cancer growth by targeting leukotriene A4 hydrolase. Cancer Res 69(13):5584–5591. doi:10.1158/0008-5472.CAN-09-0491, pii: 0008-5472.CAN-09-0491
33. Dixon SL, Smondyrev AM, Knoll EH, Rao SN, Shaw DE, Friesner RA (2006) PHASE: a new engine for pharmacophore perception, 3D QSAR model development, and 3D database screening: 1. Methodology and preliminary results. J Comput Aided Mol Des 20(10–11):647–671. doi:10.1007/s10822-006-9087-6
34. Kang NJ, Lee KW, Kim BH, Bode AM, Lee HJ, Heo YS, Boardman L, Limburg P, Dong Z (2011) Coffee phenolic phytochemicals suppress colon cancer metastasis by targeting MEK and TOPK. Carcinogenesis 32(6):921–928. doi:10.1093/carcin/bgr022, bgr022
35. Wermuth CG, Ganellin CR, Lindberg P, Mitscher LA (1998) Glossary of terms used in medicinal chemistry (IUPAC Recommendations 1998). Pure Appl Chem 70(5):1129–1143
36. Willett P, Barnard JM, Downs GM (1998) Chemical similarity searching. J Chem Inf Comput Sci 38:983–996
37. Berman HM, Westbrook J, Feng Z, Gilliland G, Bhat TN, Weissig H, Shindyalov IN, Bourne PE (2000) The Protein Data Bank. Nucleic Acids Res 28(1):235–242
38. Nagarajan S, Doddareddy M, Choo H, Cho YS, Oh KS, Lee BH, Pae AN (2009) IKKbeta inhibitors identification part I: homology model assisted structure based virtual screening. Bioorg Med Chem 17(7):2759–2766. doi:10.1016/j.bmc.2009.02.041, pii: S0968-0896(09)00191-6
39. Oi N, Chen H, Ok Kim M, Lubet RA, Bode AM, Dong Z (2012) Taxifolin suppresses UV-induced skin carcinogenesis by targeting EGFR and PI3K. Cancer Prev Res (Phila) 5(9):1103–1114. doi:10.1158/1940-6207.CAPR-11-0397
40. Moser AR, Pitot HC, Dove WF (1990) A dominant mutation that predisposes to multiple intestinal neoplasia in the mouse. Science 247(4940):322–324
41. Su LK, Kinzler KW, Vogelstein B, Preisinger AC, Moser AR, Luongo C, Gould KA, Dove WF (1992) Multiple intestinal neoplasia caused by a mutation in the murine homolog of the APC gene. Science 256(5057):668–670
42. Ignatenko NA, Besselsen DG, Stringer DE, Blohm-Mangone KA, Cui H, Gerner EW (2008) Combination chemoprevention of intestinal carcinogenesis in a murine model of familial adenomatous polyposis. Nutr Cancer 60(Suppl 1):30–35. doi:10.1080/01635580802401317
43. Khor TO, Cheung WK, Prawan A, Reddy BS, Kong AN (2008) Chemoprevention of familial adenomatous polyposis in Apc(Min/+) mice by phenethyl isothiocyanate (PEITC). Mol Carcinog 47(5):321–325. doi:10.1002/mc.20390
44. Mandir N, Goodlad RA (2008) Conjugated linoleic acids differentially alter polyp number and diameter in the Apc(min/+) mouse model of intestinal cancer. Cell Prolif 41(2):279–291. doi:10.1111/j.1365-2184.2008.00524.x
45. Huang SY, Zou X (2007) Ensemble docking of multiple protein structures: considering protein structural variations in molecular docking. Proteins 66(2):399–421. doi:10.1002/prot.21214
46. Dong Z, Birrer MJ, Watts RG, Matrisian LM, Colburn NH (1994) Blocking of tumor promoter-induced AP-1 activity inhibits induced transformation in JB6 mouse epidermal cells. Proc Natl Acad Sci U S A 91(2): 609–613
47. Oi N, Jeong CH, Nadas J, Cho YY, Pugliese A, Bode AM, Dong Z (2010) Resveratrol, a red wine polyphenol, suppresses pancreatic cancer by inhibiting leukotriene a4 hydrolase. Cancer Res 70(23):9755–9764. doi:10.1158/0008-5472.CAN-10-2858, pii: 0008-5472.CAN-10-2858
48. Xie H, Lee MH, Zhu F, Reddy K, Peng C, Li Y, Lim do Y, Kim DJ, Li X, Kang S, Li H, Ma W, Lubet RA, Ding J, Bode AM, Dong Z (2013) Identification of an Aurora kinase inhibitor specific for the Aurora B isoform. Cancer Res 73(2):716–724. doi:10.1158/0008-5472.CAN-12-2784
49. Xie H, Lee MH, Zhu F, Reddy K, Huang Z, Kim DJ, Li Y, Peng C, Lim DY, Kang S, Jung SK, Li X, Li H, Ma W, Lubet RA, Ding J, Bode AM, Dong Z (2013) Discovery of the novel mTOR inhibitor and its antitumor activities in vitro and in vivo. Mol Cancer Ther. doi:10.1158/1535-7163.MCT-12-1241
50. Lee MH, Huang Z, Kim DJ, Kim SH, Kim MO, Lee SY, Xie H, Park SJ, Kim JY, Kundu JK, Bode AM, Surh YJ, Dong Z (2013) Direct targeting of MEK1/2 and RSK2 by silybin induces cell-cycle arrest and inhibits melanoma cell growth. Cancer Prev Res (Phila) 6(5):455–465. doi:10.1158/1940-6207.CAPR-12-0425
51. Kim DJ, Lee MH, Reddy K, Li Y, Lim do Y, Xie H, Lee SY, Yeom YI, Bode AM, Dong Z (2013) CInQ-03, a novel allosteric MEK inhibitor, suppresses cancer growth in vitro and in vivo. Carcinogenesis 34(5):1134–1143. doi:10.1093/carcin/bgt015
52. Xie H, Zhu F, Huang Z, Lee MH, Kim DJ, Li X, Lim do Y, Jung SK, Kang S, Li H, Reddy K, Wang L, Ma W, Lubet RA, Bode AM, Dong Z (2012) Identification of mammalian target of rapamycin as a direct target of fenretinide both in vitro and in vivo. Carcinogenesis 33(9):1814–1821. doi:10.1093/carcin/bgs234

53. Liu K, Park C, Li S, Lee KW, Liu H, He L, Soung NK, Ahn JS, Bode AM, Dong Z, Kim BY (2012) Aloe-emodin suppresses prostate cancer by targeting the mTOR complex 2. Carcinogenesis 33(7):1406–1411. doi:10.1093/carcin/bgs156
54. Li X, Li H, Li S, Zhu F, Kim DJ, Xie H, Li Y, Nadas J, Oi N, Zykova TA, Yu DH, Lee MH, Kim MO, Wang L, Ma W, Lubet RA, Bode AM, Dong Z (2012) Ceftriaxone, an FDA-approved cephalosporin antibiotic, suppresses lung cancer growth by targeting Aurora B. Carcinogenesis 33(12):2548–2557. doi:10.1093/carcin/bgs283
55. Li J, Mottamal M, Li H, Liu K, Zhu F, Cho YY, Sosa CP, Zhou K, Bowden GT, Bode AM, Dong Z (2012) Quercetin-3-methyl ether suppresses proliferation of mouse epidermal JB6 P+ cells by targeting ERKs. Carcinogenesis 33(2):459–465. doi:10.1093/carcin/bgr281
56. Li J, Malakhova M, Mottamal M, Reddy K, Kurinov I, Carper A, Langfald A, Oi N, Kim MO, Zhu F, Sosa CP, Zhou K, Bode AM, Dong Z (2012) Norathyriol suppresses skin cancers induced by solar ultraviolet radiation by targeting ERK kinases. Cancer Res 72(1):260–270. doi:10.1158/0008-5472.CAN-11-2596
57. Kim DJ, Li Y, Reddy K, Lee MH, Kim MO, Cho YY, Lee SY, Kim JE, Bode AM, Dong Z (2012) Novel TOPK inhibitor HI-TOPK-032 effectively suppresses colon cancer growth. Cancer Res 72(12):3060–3068. doi:10.1158/0008-5472.CAN-11-3851
58. Urusova DV, Shim JH, Kim DJ, Jung SK, Zykova TA, Carper A, Bode AM, Dong Z (2011) Epigallocatechin-gallate suppresses tumorigenesis by directly targeting Pin1. Cancer Prev Res (Phila) 4(9):1366–1377. doi:10.1158/1940-6207.CAPR-11-0301
59. Liu K, Cho YY, Yao K, Nadas J, Kim DJ, Cho EJ, Lee MH, Pugliese A, Zhang J, Bode AM, Dong Z (2011) Eriodictyol inhibits RSK2-ATF1 signaling and suppresses EGF-induced neoplastic cell transformation. J Biol Chem 286(3):2057–2066. doi:10.1074/jbc.M110.147306, pii: M110.147306
60. Li Y, Kim DJ, Ma W, Lubet RA, Bode AM, Dong Z (2011) Discovery of novel checkpoint kinase 1 inhibitors by virtual screening based on multiple crystal structures. J Chem Inf Model 51(11):2904–2914. doi:10.1021/ci200257b
61. Lee KW, Bode AM, Dong Z (2011) Molecular targets of phytochemicals for cancer prevention. Nat Rev Cancer 11(3):211–218. doi:10.1038/nrc3017, pii: nrc3017
62. Lee DE, Lee KW, Jung SK, Lee EJ, Hwang JA, Lim TG, Kim BY, Bode AM, Lee HJ, Dong Z (2011) 6,7,4′-Trihydroxyisoflavone inhibits HCT-116 human colon cancer cell proliferation by targeting CDK1 and CDK2. Carcinogenesis 32(4):629–635. doi:10.1093/carcin/bgr008, pii: bgr008
63. Lee DE, Lee KW, Byun S, Jung SK, Song N, Lim SH, Heo YS, Kim JE, Kang NJ, Kim BY, Bowden GT, Bode AM, Lee HJ, Dong Z (2011) 7,3′,4′-Trihydroxyisoflavone, a metabolite of the soy isoflavone daidzein, suppresses ultraviolet B-induced skin cancer by targeting Cot and MKK4. J Biol Chem 286(16):14246–14256. doi:10.1074/jbc.M110.147348, pii: M110.147348
64. Kim JE, Lee DE, Lee KW, Son JE, Seo SK, Li J, Jung SK, Heo YS, Mottamal M, Bode AM, Dong Z, Lee HJ (2011) Isorhamnetin suppresses skin cancer through direct inhibition of MEK1 and PI3-K. Cancer Prev Res (Phila) 4(4):582–591. doi:10.1158/1940-6207.CAPR-11-0032, pii: 1940-6207.CAPR-11-0032
65. Kim DJ, Reddy K, Kim MO, Li Y, Nadas J, Cho YY, Kim JE, Shim JH, Song NR, Carper A, Lubet RA, Bode AM, Dong Z (2011) (3-Chloroacetyl)-indole, a novel allosteric AKT inhibitor, suppresses colon cancer growth in vitro and in vivo. Cancer Prev Res (Phila) 4(11):1842–1851. doi:10.1158/1940-6207.CAPR-11-0158
66. Shim JH, Su ZY, Chae JI, Kim DJ, Zhu F, Ma WY, Bode AM, Yang CS, Dong Z (2010) Epigallocatechin gallate suppresses lung cancer cell growth through Ras-GTPase-activating protein SH3 domain-binding protein 1. Cancer Prev Res (Phila) 3(5):670–679. doi:10.1158/1940-6207.CAPR-09-0185, pii: 1940-6207.CAPR-09-0185
67. Lee KM, Lee KW, Jung SK, Lee EJ, Heo YS, Bode AM, Lubet RA, Lee HJ, Dong Z (2010) Kaempferol inhibits UVB-induced COX-2 expression by suppressing Src kinase activity. Biochem Pharmacol 80(12):2042–2049. doi:10.1016/j.bcp.2010.06.042, pii: S0006-2952(10)00476-4
68. Lee KM, Lee KW, Byun S, Jung SK, Seo SK, Heo YS, Bode AM, Lee HJ, Dong Z (2010) 5-Deoxykaempferol plays a potential therapeutic role by targeting multiple signaling pathways in skin cancer. Cancer Prev Res (Phila) 3(4):454–465. doi:10.1158/1940-6207.CAPR-09-0137, pii: 1940-6207.CAPR-09-0137
69. Lee DE, Lee KW, Song NR, Seo SK, Heo YS, Kang NJ, Bode AM, Lee HJ, Dong Z (2010) 7,3′,4′-Trihydroxyisoflavone inhibits epidermal growth factor-induced proliferation and transformation of JB6 P+ mouse epidermal cells by suppressing cyclin-dependent kinases and phosphatidylinositol 3-kinase. J Biol Chem 285(28):21458–21466. doi:10.1074/jbc.M109.094797, pii: M109.094797
70. Jung SK, Lee KW, Kim HY, Oh MH, Byun S, Lim SH, Heo YS, Kang NJ, Bode AM, Dong Z, Lee HJ (2010) Myricetin suppresses UVB-

induced wrinkle formation and MMP-9 expression by inhibiting Raf. Biochem Pharmacol 79(10):1455–1461. doi:10.1016/j.bcp.2010.01.004, pii:S0006-2952(10)00015-8
71. Jung SK, Lee KW, Byun S, Lee EJ, Kim JE, Bode AM, Dong Z, Lee HJ (2010) Myricetin inhibits UVB-induced angiogenesis by regulating PI-3 kinase in vivo. Carcinogenesis 31(5):911–917. doi:10.1093/carcin/bgp221, pii: bgp221
72. Byun S, Lee KW, Jung SK, Lee EJ, Hwang MK, Lim SH, Bode AM, Lee HJ, Dong Z (2010) Luteolin inhibits protein kinase C(epsilon) and c-Src activities and UVB-induced skin cancer. Cancer Res 70(6):2415–2423. doi:10.1158/0008-5472.CAN-09-4093, pii: 0008-5472.CAN-09-4093
73. Kwon JY, Lee KW, Kim JE, Jung SK, Kang NJ, Hwang MK, Heo YS, Bode AM, Dong Z, Lee HJ (2009) Delphinidin suppresses ultraviolet B-induced cyclooxygenases-2 expression through inhibition of MAPKK4 and PI-3 kinase. Carcinogenesis 30(11):1932–1940. doi:10.1093/carcin/bgp216, pii: bgp216
74. Kang NJ, Lee KW, Shin BJ, Jung SK, Hwang MK, Bode AM, Heo YS, Lee HJ, Dong Z (2009) Caffeic acid, a phenolic phytochemical in coffee, directly inhibits Fyn kinase activity and UVB-induced COX-2 expression. Carcinogenesis 30(2):321–330. doi:10.1093/carcin/bgn282, pii: bgn282
75. Zykova TA, Zhu F, Zhai X, Ma WY, Ermakova SP, Lee KW, Bode AM, Dong Z (2008) Resveratrol directly targets COX-2 to inhibit carcinogenesis. Mol Carcinog 47(10):797–805. doi:10.1002/mc.20437
76. Shim JH, Choi HS, Pugliese A, Lee SY, Chae JI, Choi BY, Bode AM, Dong Z (2008) (−)-Epigallocatechin gallate regulates CD3-mediated T cell receptor signaling in leukemia through the inhibition of ZAP-70 kinase. J Biol Chem 283(42):28370–28379. doi:10.1074/jbc.M802200200, pii: M802200200
77. Lee KW, Kang NJ, Heo YS, Rogozin EA, Pugliese A, Hwang MK, Bowden GT, Bode AM, Lee HJ, Dong Z (2008) Raf and MEK protein kinases are direct molecular targets for the chemopreventive effect of quercetin, a major flavonol in red wine. Cancer Res 68(3):946–955
78. Kang NJ, Lee KW, Lee DE, Rogozin EA, Bode AM, Lee HJ, Dong Z (2008) Cocoa procyanidins suppress transformation by inhibiting mitogen-activated protein kinase kinase. J Biol Chem 283(30):20664–20673. doi:10.1074/jbc. M800263200
79. Kang NJ, Lee KW, Kwon JY, Hwang MK, Rogozin EA, Heo YS, Bode AM, Lee HJ, Dong Z (2008) Delphinidin attenuates neoplastic transformation in JB6 Cl41 mouse epidermal cells by blocking Raf/mitogen-activated protein kinase kinase/extracellular signal-regulated kinase signaling. Cancer Prev Res (Phila) 1(7):522–531. doi:10.1158/1940-6207.CAPR-08-0071, pii: 1/7/522
80. Jung SK, Lee KW, Byun S, Kang NJ, Lim SH, Heo YS, Bode AM, Bowden GT, Lee HJ, Dong Z (2008) Myricetin suppresses UVB-induced skin cancer by targeting Fyn. Cancer Res 68(14):6021–6029. doi:10.1158/0008-5472.CAN-08-0899, pii: 68/14/6021
81. He Z, Tang F, Ermakova S, Li M, Zhao Q, Cho YY, Ma WY, Choi HS, Bode AM, Yang CS, Dong Z (2008) Fyn is a novel target of (−)-epigallocatechin gallate in the inhibition of JB6 Cl41 cell transformation. Mol Carcinog 47(3):172–183
82. Steele VE (2003) Current mechanistic approaches to the chemoprevention of cancer. J Biochem Mol Biol 36(1):78–81
83. Steele VE, Kelloff GJ (2005) Development of cancer chemopreventive drugs based on mechanistic approaches. Mutat Res 591(1–2):16–23. doi:10.1016/j.mrfmmm. 2005.04.018
84. Aggarwal BB, Sethi G, Baladandayuthapani V, Krishnan S, Shishodia S (2007) Targeting cell signaling pathways for drug discovery: an old lock needs a new key. J Cell Biochem 102(3):580–592. doi:10.1002/jcb.21500
85. Aggarwal BB, Shishodia S (2006) Molecular targets of dietary agents for prevention and therapy of cancer. Biochem Pharmacol 71(10):1397–1421. doi:10.1016/j.bcp.2006.02.009

Chapter 2

Common Methods Used for the Discovery of Natural Anticancer Compounds

Min Tang, Xinfang Yu, Yiqun Jiang, Ying Shi, Xiaolan Liu, Wei Li, and Ya Cao

Abstract

Carcinogenesis is a long-term, multifactorial, and multistep process. Dietary phytochemicals can play a significant role in cancer prevention. In this chapter, we describe common protocols to study the role of phytochemicals in chemoprevention and divide the protocols into two types. In the first part of the chapter, the methods including cell proliferation, cell cycle, and cell apoptosis assays are related to the analysis of the effect of a compound on cellular phenotype. In the second part, the methods focus on the discovery of molecular targets and mechanisms for chemopreventive and therapeutic compounds, and include descriptions for an immunoassay for kinase inhibitor discovery, immunofluorescence, co-immunoprecipitation, and chromatin immunoprecipitation (ChIP).

Key words Cell proliferation, Cell cycle, Apoptosis, Protein kinase, Small molecular compound, ELISA, Confocal microscopy, Immunoprecipitation, Protein–protein interaction, Chromatin immunoprecipitation

1 Introduction

1.1 The Use of Cellular Phenotype Analysis for Discovery of Natural Anticancer Compounds

Phenotypic screens are used as the mainstay for drug development in the laboratory. Through comparative analysis of the effects of potential compounds on cell proliferation, cell cycle arrest, and induction of apoptosis, leading candidate anticancer or chemopreventive compounds can be identified. In this portion of the chapter, we describe the cell proliferation assay, FACS analysis, Annexin V/FITC detection, TUNEL assay, and caspase detection methods.

1.1.1 Cell Proliferation or Viability Assay

The colorimetric method is a routine assay for determining the number of viable cells and evaluating the effect of anticancer compounds in vitro. The tetrazolium compound [3-(4,5-dimethylthiazol-2-yl)-5-(3-carboxy methoxy phenyl)-2-(4-sulfophenyl)-2H-tetrazolium, inner salt; MTS] is bio-reduced by viable cells into a

Ann M. Bode and Zigang Dong (eds.), *Cancer Prevention: Dietary Factors and Pharmacology*, Methods in Pharmacology and Toxicology, DOI 10.1007/978-1-4614-9227-6_2, © Springer Science+Business Media New York 2014

colored formazan product that is soluble in tissue culture medium. This transformation is presumably accomplished by the conversion of NADPH or NADH to NADP+ or NAD+ by dehydrogenases in metabolically active cells (1). The quantity of formazan product is measured by its absorbance at 490 nm and is directly proportional to the number of living cells in culture. Assays are performed by adding a small amount of the MTS reagent directly to culture wells, incubating for 1–4 h and then recording the absorbance at 490 nm with a 96-well plate reader. Typically, in MTS-based assays, toxicity is determined by the IC_{50} value, which is calculated using a dose–response curve and represents the concentration of the tested substance required to reduce the light absorbance capacity of exposed cell cultures by 50 % [1].

1.1.2 Cell Cycle Analysis by FACS

The cell cycle is made up of four phases: G1, S, G2, and M. Analysis of a population of a cell's replication state can be achieved by fluorescence labeling of the nuclei of cells in suspension and then analyzing the fluorescence properties of each cell in the population. Nucleic acid dyes like propidium iodide (PI) are applied for DNA assays [2]. Quiescent and G1 phase cells with only one DNA copy will have 1× fluorescence intensity. Cells in G2–M phase of the cell cycle have two DNA copies and accordingly have 2× intensity. Because cells in S phase are synthesizing DNA, they populate in a range between 1× and 2× fluorescence intensity. The cell cycle can be arrested at restriction points or checkpoints, such as G1–S and G2–M checkpoints, by the activation of cell cycle inhibitors, like Rb and p53 [3]. Also, many chemopreventive compounds act by blocking or arresting cells in G1–S phase or G2–M phase.

1.1.3 Cellular Apoptosis Analysis Using Annexin V/FITC

Besides being able to cause cell cycle arrest, chemopreventive compounds can also induce apoptosis. Thus another method to determine whether a compound has good chemopreventive or therapeutic activity is to evaluate its ability to induce apoptosis. The apoptotic program is characterized by certain morphological features, including loss of plasma membrane asymmetry and attachment, condensation of the cytoplasm and nucleus, and internucleosomal cleavage of DNA. In apoptotic cells, the membranous phospholipid phosphatidylserine (PS) is translocated from the inner leaflet to the outer leaflet of the plasma membrane [4], thereby exposing the PS to the external cellular environment. Annexin V, a 35–36 kDa Ca^{2+} dependent phospholipid-binding protein has a high affinity for PS and thus is able to bind to apoptotic cells with exposed PS [5]. When conjugated to fluorochromes including FITC, Annexin V can serve as a sensitive probe for analysis of apoptotic cells by flow cytometry. Because externalization of PS occurs in the earlier stages of apoptosis, FITC-Annexin V staining can detect apoptosis at an earlier stage than assays based on nuclear changes such as DNA fragmentation. In this way, FITC-Annexin V is typically used in conjunction with nucleic acid dye such as propidium iodide (PI) to allow the investigator to identify early apoptotic cells (i.e., PI negative, FITC-Annexin V positive) from the late apoptotic cells (i.e., both PI and FITC-Annexin V positive), because only membranes of dead and damaged cells (late apoptotic cells) are permeable to PI, whereas viable cells with intact membranes exclude PI.

1.1.4 Cellular Apoptosis Analysis by TUNEL Assay

Cleavage of genomic DNA during apoptosis yields double-stranded, low molecular weight DNA fragments as well as single-strand breaks in high molecular weight DNA. These DNA strand breaks can be identified by labeling the free 3′-OH termini with modified nucleotides in an enzymatic reaction [6]. The terminal deoxynucleotidyl transferase (Tdt) enzyme will add nucleotides to the 5′ ends of DNA fragments in apoptotic cells. A labeled nucleotide is used, which can subsequently be visualized. Before fixation in ethanol, the cells are fixed in formaldehyde (typically 1 % *para-formaldehyde*), in order to cross-link the DNA fragments into the cell and to maximize the number of broken DNA ends. The TUNEL reaction is a precise, fast, and nonradioactive technique to detect and quantify apoptotic cell death at a single cell level in cells and tissues. By preferentially labeling DNA strand breaks generated during apoptosis, the TUNEL assay allows one to distinguish apoptosis from necrosis and from primary DNA strand breaks induced by potential chemopreventive compounds.

1.1.5 Cellular Apoptosis Analysis by Detection of Caspase Activities and Levels of Cleaved Caspases

One of the key mediators in apoptosis is a family of cysteine-dependent aspartate-directed proteases, referred to as caspases. In mammalian cells, the apoptosis-related caspases are generally divided into two classes: the initiator caspases, which include caspase-2, -8, -9, and -10; and the effector caspases, which include caspase-3, -6, and -7. The initiator caspases control the activation of the effectors by cleaving the pro-forms of the effector caspases. Subsequently, the cleaved effectors will cleave protein substrates containing aspartic acid in the cell death pathway at specific sites triggering the apoptotic process [7].

Caspase activity assays in multiwell plate format represent powerful tools for understanding experimental modulation of the apoptotic response. The Caspase-Glo Assays are homogeneous luminescent assays that measure caspase activities. These members of the cysteine aspartic acid-specific protease (caspase) family play key effector roles in apoptosis in mammalian cells. The assays provide a luminogenic caspase substrate in a buffer system optimized for caspase activity, luciferase activity and cell disruption. Following caspase cleavage, a substrate for luciferase (aminoluciferin) is released, resulting in the luciferase reaction and the production of light. The assay provides a luminogenic caspase substrate, which contains the tetrapeptide sequence, in a reagent optimized for caspase activity, luciferase activity, and cell disruption [8].

The precursor form of all caspases is composed of a prodomain, and large or small catalytic subunits. The active forms of caspases are generated by several stimuli including ligand receptor interactions, growth factor deprivation, and inhibitors of cellular functions. All known caspases require cleavage adjacent to aspartates to liberate one large and one small subunit, which associate into a 2b2 tetramer to form the active enzyme.

1.2 Discovering the Target and Molecular Mechanism(s) of Action for Chemopreventive and Therapeutic Compounds

In this portion of our chapter, we describe the immunoassay, immunofluorescence analysis, co-immunoprecipitation, and chromatin immunoprecipitation for use in the discovery of chemopreventive or therapeutic natural compounds.

1.2.1 The Use of Immunoassays for Kinase Inhibitor Discovery

Protein kinases are enzymes that add a phosphate group to a protein or other organic molecules, usually on the serine, threonine, or tyrosine amino acid of the protein [9]. Hence, protein kinase inhibitors can be subdivided or characterized by the amino acids whose phosphorylation is inhibited. Many kinases (i.e., serine/threonine kinases) phosphorylate both serine and threonine residues, whereas tyrosine kinases act on tyrosine, and a number of other kinases (dual-specificity kinases) act on all three.

The ELISA assay system utilizes a monoclonal antibody directly against a distinct antigenic determinant on the target molecule and is used for solid phase immobilization [10]. A target antibody is conjugated to horseradish peroxidase (HRP) in the antibody–enzyme conjugate solution. The sample being tested is allowed to react simultaneously with the two antibodies, resulting in the target molecule being sandwiched between the solid phase and enzyme-linked antibodies. After incubation at room temperature, the wells are washed with water to remove unbound labeled antibodies. A solution of tetramethylbenzidine (TMB) reagent is added and incubated at room temperature, resulting in the development of a blue color. The activity of the kinase is directly proportional to the color intensity of the test sample. Absorbance is measured spectrophotometrically at 450 nm. This method is a simple but effective means to assess the effectiveness of compounds for kinase inhibition.

1.2.2 Immunofluorescence Analysis

Proteins can interact with each other in vivo when they are co-localized or display overlapping distributions within the cell. The intracellular localization of two or more proteins can be identified and visualized directly by immunofluorescence analysis. In this assay, cells are fixed, permeated, and incubated with primary antibodies against the interacting proteins (note that 2 or more primary antibodies must always be generated from different species). After incubation with primary antibodies, cells are incubated with secondary antibodies conjugated with different fluorophores, such as Cy2 or Cy3, which exhibit different emission maxima. The intracellular localization of the proteins is then monitored by confocal microscopy [11].

Immunofluorescence is only limited to fixed (i.e., dead) cells when structures within the cell are to be visualized because antibodies cannot cross the membrane of unfixed cells. Proteins in the supernatant fraction or on the outside of the cell membrane can be bound by the antibodies, which allows for staining of living cells. Depending on the fixative that is being used, proteins of interest might become cross-linked and this could result in either false positive or false negative signals due to nonspecific binding.

As powerful methods to visualize protein–protein interactions, immunofluorescence and confocal microscopy are commonly used in cancer research, especially for biomarker detection [12], determination of molecule relocation after drug treatment, and signal pathway detection [11]. A quantum dot technique has now been developed as a new fluorophore, which has a wider optical spectrum and is more sensitive than traditional Cy2 or Cy3. Therefore, the quantum dot technique is now used a novel immunofluorescence staining method [13].

1.2.3 Co-immunoprecipitation (Co-IP) Analysis

Co-IP is an extension of the immunoprecipitation (IP) assay based on the fundamental principle of a specific antigen–antibody reaction that is quite straightforward: an antibody (against a specific primary target called the "bait" protein as well as other molecules called "prey" proteins) binds to the primary target by native interaction and forms an immune complex [14]. The immune complex is then precipitated by agarose or magnetic beads that are coated with antibody-binding proteins such as Protein A or G, and the other nonprecipitated antibody or proteins are washed away. Then, the precipitated complex is disassociated from the beads by boiling or elution buffer and analyzed by sodium dodecyl sulfate–polyacrylamide gel electrophoresis (SDS-PAGE), usually followed by Western Blot analysis to verify the presence of the prey protein. Co-IP has been routinely used over the past several decades to study protein–protein interactions and thereby elucidate cellular signaling pathways and the effect of anticancer compounds on protein–protein interaction.

1.2.4 Chromatin Immunoprecipitation (ChIP) Assay

ChIP is an invaluable method for studying interactions between specific proteins or modified forms of proteins and a region of genomic DNA. The procedure involves the cross-linking of the chromatin protein–DNA complex by formaldehyde and the generation of short random fragments of this chromatin by sonication.

Using antibodies directed against the protein of interest, cross-linked chromatin fragments are immunoprecipitated. The isolated antibody–chromatin complexes and the input or non-immunoprecipitated materials are treated to remove the cross-link and the DNA is purified. Both control and immunoprecipitated samples are amplified by quantitative PCR using primers specific for the genomic region of interest [15]. With different antibody combinations, ChIP allows for profiling chromatin-associated factors, histone modifications, and histone variants, as well as local nucleosome density. When ChIP is combined with DNA microarray technology (ChIP-chip), it can be applied to the identification of DNA binding sites for transcription factors. Combining ChIP with genomic tiling array hybridization or massive-parallel sequencing (ChIP-seq) allows whole genome studies, including global methylome analysis [16].

2 Materials

2.1 Equipment

2.1.1 Cell Proliferation Assay

1. 96-Well plates suitable for cell culture.
2. BioTek ELX800 96-well plate reader for measuring absorbance at 490 nm.

2.1.2 Cell Cycle Analysis

BD FACSDiva™ flow cytometer for detection of the fluorescent agent signal.

2.1.3 Cellular Apoptosis Analysis by Annexin V/FITC

BD FACSDiva™ flow cytometer for detection of the fluorescent agent signal.

2.1.4 Cellular Apoptosis Analysis by TUNEL Assay

Leica MDI3000 fluorescent microscope for detection of the cellular fluorescent signal.

2.1.5 Immunoassay for Discovering Kinase Inhibitors

1. Pipettors: 2–20, 20–200, and 100–1,000 μL precision pipettors with disposable tips (Eppendorf, Hamburg, Germany).
2. Wash bottle or multichannel dispenser for plate washing.
3. Microcentrifuge and tubes for sample preparation (Eppendorf AG, Hamburg, Germany).
4. Vortex mixer (Eppendorf, Hamburg, Germany).
5. Plate reader capable of measuring absorbance in 96-well plates at dual wavelengths of 450 nm/540 nm (BIO-TEK ELX800, USA).

2.1.6 Chromatin Immunoprecipitation Assay

1. Descriptions of specific equipment used in this experiment are given, however any model of comparable capability can easily be substituted.
2. Sonicator 3000, Misonix.

2.2 Reagents and Solutions

2.2.1 Cell Proliferation Assay

CellTiter 96 AQueous One Solution Cell Proliferation Assay (Promega).

2.2.2 Cell Cycle Analysis

Propidium Iodide (PI): Prepare a 50 μg/mL stock solution of PI in 1× PBS buffer, store at 4 °C.

2.2.3 Cellular Apoptosis Analysis by Annexin V/FITC

1. Fluorescein-conjugated Annexin V (Annexin V–FITC).
2. 1× Binding buffer: 10 mM Hepes/NaOH, pH 7.4, 140 mM NaCl, 2.5 mM $CaCl_2$, store at 4 °C.

2.2.4 Cellular Apoptosis Analysis by TUNEL Assay

1. Fixation solution: paraformaldehyde (4 % in PBS, pH 7.4), freshly prepared.
2. Permeabilization solution: 0.1 % Triton X-100 in 0.1 % sodium citrate, freshly prepared.
3. TUNEL reaction mixture: add total volume (5 μL) of enzyme solution to the remaining 45 μL label solution to obtain 50 μL TUNEL reaction mixture.

2.2.5 Apoptosis Analysis by Caspase Activity Assay

This assay kit is the products from Caspase-Glo® 6 Assay (Cat.#s G0970, Promega Corporation, USA).

1. White multiwell plates (black plates may be used, but RLU will be reduced).
2. Multichannel pipette or automated pipetting station.
3. Plate shaker or other device for mixing multiwell plates.
4. Luminometer capable of reading multiwell plates.
5. Caspase-6 enzyme (e.g., BIOMOL International Cat.# SE-170 or Calbiochem Cat.# 218799).
6. Optional: Prionex® carrier (Centerchem, Inc. Norwalk, CT).

2.2.6 Immunoassay for Discovering Kinase Inhibitors

This assay kit is a product from CycLex (CY1180, Japan) or Takara (MK410).

1. Kinase substrate immobilized microplate (store at 4 °C).
2. Kinase buffer (store at 4 °C).
3. 20× ATP (lyophilized, ATP-Na2 salt) (store at 4 °C).
4. Anti-target kinase substrate antibody (store at 4 °C).
5. Kinase positive control (store at −80 °C).
6. HRP conjugated Ab IgG (store at 4 °C).
7. Blocking solution (store at 4 °C).
8. HRP substrate solution (TMBZ) (store at 4 °C).
9. Stop solution: 1 N H_2SO_4 (store at 4 °C; Strong acid).
10. 10× Washing buffer: PBS including 0.05 % (v/v) Tween-20.

2.2.7 Immunofluorescence Analysis

1. PBS (NaCl 137 mM, KCl 2.7 mM, Na_2HPO_4 10 mM, KH_2PO_4 2 mM.
2. –20 °C Precooled methanol.
3. 5 % Normal donkey serum (Millipore, Cat. # S30-100ML) in PBS.
4. BSA-PBS = PBS containing 1 % BSA.
5. ProLong® Gold Antifade Reagent with DAPI Reagents (Invitrogen, Catalog #P36931).

2.2.8 Co-immunoprecipitation Analysis

1. High Salt Lysis Buffer: 400 mM NaCl; 25 mM HEPES; 1.5 mM $MgCl_2$; 0.2 mM EDTA; 1 % NP-40.
2. Low salt lysis buffer: 150 mM NaCl; 50 mM HEPES; 1.5 mM $MgCl_2$; 1 mM EDTA; 1 % Triton X-100; 10 % glycerol.
3. Proteinase inhibitor (or phosphatase inhibitor if necessary): 40× cocktail stock solution, dissolve 1 tablet in 250 μL distilled H_2O; will be stable at least for 12 weeks at –15 to –25 °C, (Roche Catalog #04693124001).
4. Protein G Sepharose, (Sigma, Cat. P3296).
5. Dynabeads® Protein G (Invitrogen, Cat. 10004D).
6. Pierce BCA Protein Assay Kit (Thermo Scientific Cat. #23228).

2.2.9 Chromatin Immunoprecipitation Assay

1. Fixation solution: Add 0.81 mL of 37 % formaldehyde to 30 mL minimal cell culture medium and mix thoroughly. Leave at room temperature.
2. Cell lysis buffer: 50 mM Tris–HCl, pH 7.4, 150 mM NaCl, 1 mM EDTA, 1 mM EGTA, 5 mM $MgCl_2$, 0.5 % Triton X-100, proteinase, and phosphorylation inhibitors.
3. SDS lysis buffer: 1 % SDS, 10 mM EDTA, 50 mM Tris–HCl, pH 8.0.
4. Protein G agarose/salmon sperm DNA beads (Cat#16-201, Upstate).
5. Dynabeads Protein G (Cat# 100.03D, Invitrogen).
6. Sol I: 0.1 % SDS, 1 % Triton X-100, 2 mM EDTA, 20 mM Tris pH 8.0, 150 mM NaCl.
7. Sol II: 0.1 % SDS, 1 % Triton X-100, 2 mM EDTA, 20 mM Tris pH 8.0, 0.5 M NaCl.
8. Sol III: 0.25 M LiCl, 1 % NP40, 1 % NaDOC, 1 mM EDTA, 10 mM Tris pH 8.0.
9. Chelex-100 (Cat# 142-1253, Bio-Rad).

3 Methods

3.1 Cell Proliferation Assay

1. Determine cell number and viability by trypan blue exclusion, and resuspend the cells to a final concentration of 1×10^5 cells/mL in RPMI 1640 supplemented with 10 % FBS.
2. Dispense 50 μL of the cell suspension (5,000 cells) into all wells of the plate. The total volume in each well should be 100 μL (**Note 1**).
3. Five separate serial dilutions of each test compound in culture medium are prepared for addition to cells.
4. Add test compound to cells and incubate the plate at 37 °C for 24–72 h in a humidified, 5 % CO_2 atmosphere.
5. Pipet 20 μL of Cell Titer ^{96}AQueous One Solution Reagent (see Sect. 2.2) into each well of the 96-well assay plate containing the samples in 100 μL of culture medium.
6. Incubate the plate at 37 °C for 1–4 h in a humidified, 5 % CO_2 atmosphere.
7. Record the absorbance at 490 nm using a 96-well plate reader (**Note 2**).
8. Plot the corrected absorbance at 490 nm (Y axis) versus concentration of growth factor (X axis; **Note 3**). Determine the X-axis value corresponding to one-half the difference between the maximum (plateau) and minimum (no growth factor control) absorbance values; this is the ED_{50} value (ED_{50} = the concentration of growth factor necessary to give one-half the maximum response).
9. To determine the IC_{50} value using the dose–response curve method, a reading of the absorbance representing five separate serial dilutions of each test compound (50 % of the total population in each well) is specified. To calculate IC_{50}, you will need a series of dose–response data (e.g., drug concentrations x_1, $x_2,\ldots,x_n$ and growth inhibition rate y_1, $y_2,\ldots,y_n$). The values of y are in the range of 0–1. The simplest estimate of IC_{50} is to plot $x-y$ and fit the data with a straight line (linear regression). The IC_{50} value is then estimated using the fitted line,

   $Y = a \times (X + b)$,

   $IC_{50} = (0.5 - b)/a$.

   Frequently, the response-curve fits better to a straight line if the X-axis is logarithm-transformed.

3.2 Cell Cycle Analysis

1. Add test compound to cells and incubate the plate at 37 °C for 24–72 h in a humidified, 5 % CO_2 atmosphere.
2. Cells are trypsinized and washed with PBS, resuspended in 70 % ethanol, and stored at 4 °C overnight.

3. Cells are then centrifuged, washed with PBS, resuspended in 450 μL PBS and 10 μL 10 μg/mL DNase-free RNase, and incubated at 37 °C for 45 min.
4. Following RNase treatment, 50 μL of propidium iodide is added and cells are incubated at room temperature for 10 min protected from light.
5. Cell aggregates are removed by filtration prior to analysis.
6. Cell cycle analysis is carried out using the BD FACSDiva™ flow cytometer. The population of cells in each of the G1, S, M, and G2 phases is determined for at least 250,000 cells with doublet discrimination. Analysis of cell cycle position is performed using the BD FACSDiva software (**Note 4**).

3.3 Cellular Apoptosis Analysis with Annexin V/FITC

1. Add test compound to cells and incubate the plate at 37 °C for 24–72 h in a humidified, 5 % CO_2 atmosphere (**Note 5**).
2. Cells are trypsinized and washed twice with cold PBS and then resuspended in 1× binding buffer at a concentration of 1×10^6 cells/mL.
3. Transfer 100 μL of the solution (1×10^5 cells) to a 5 mL culture tube.
4. Add 5 μL of Annexin V–FITC and 10 μL of PI.
5. Gently vortex the cells and incubate for 15 min at room temperature (20–25 °C) in the dark.
6. Add 400 μL of 1× Binding Buffer to each tube. Analyze by flow cytometry as soon as possible (within 1 h).

3.4 Cellular Apoptosis Analysis by TUNEL Assay

1. Cells are trypsinized and seeded onto slides and incubated at 37 °C, 5 % CO_2 overnight.
2. Add test compound to cells and incubate the slide at 37 °C for 24–72 h in a humidified, 5 % CO_2 atmosphere.
3. Fix air-dried cell samples with a freshly prepared fixation solution for 1 h at 15–25 °C.
4. Incubate in permeabilization solution for 2 min on ice (2–8 °C).
5. Rinse slide twice with PBS and dry the area around the sample.
6. Add 50 μL TUNEL reaction mixture to the sample slide and incubate the slide in a humidified atmosphere for 1 h at 37 °C in the dark (**Note 6**).
7. Rinse slide twice with PBS and stain the slide with DAPI (1 μg/μL) and observe under a fluorescent microscope.

3.5 Analysis of Apoptosis by Caspase Assay

1. Prepare the following reactions to detect activity (or inhibition of activity) in purified enzyme preparations:
   (a) Blank: Caspase-Glo® 6 Reagent + vehicle control for test compound or inhibitor (no test compound or inhibitor included).

Table 1
Preparation of kinase reaction buffer

	1 Assay (μL)	10 Assays (μL)
Kinase buffer (provided)	95	950
20× ATP solution (provided)	5	50
Total	100	1,000

(b) Positive Control: Caspase-Glo® 6 Reagent + vehicle control + purified caspase-6 enzyme.

(c) Assay: Caspase-Glo® 6 Reagent + treatment agent + purified caspase-6 enzyme.

2. Add 50 μL of Caspase-Glo® 6 Reagent to each well of a white or black 96-well plate containing 50 μL of blank, positive control or assay treatment.
3. Gently mix the contents of the wells using a plate shaker at 300–500 rpm for 30 s. Incubate at room temperature for 30 min to 3 h.
4. Record luminescence with a plate-reading luminometer.

3.6 Immunoassay for Discovering Kinase Inhibitors

3.6.1 Summary and Introduction

Many methods are used for kinase inhibitor discovery, such as biochemical assays for high-throughput screening. This protocol generally is used for quantitative measurement of kinase activity in the presence of Mg^{2+} and ^{32}P-labeled ATP. While sensitive, this method is labor-intensive, generates hazardous radioactive waste, and depends on a radioisotope with a short half-life. This method uses a phospho-antibody and peroxidase coupled anti-rabbit IgG antibody as a reporter molecule in a 96-well enzyme-linked immunosorbent assay (ELISA) format. This assay provides a non-isotopic, sensitive, and specific method to measure the kinase activities.

3.6.2 Preparation of Solutions

1. Prepare a working solution of wash buffer by adding 100 mL of the stock wash buffer to 900 mL of ddH_2O. Mix well.
2. Prepare a 20× ATP solution by adding 1.6 mL of ddH_2O to the vial of 20× ATP. Mix gently until dissolved.
3. Prepare kinase reaction buffer (plus ATP) by mixing the reagents shown in Table 1.

3.6.3 Assay Procedure

1. Remove the appropriate number of microtiter wells from the foil pouch and place them onto the well holder. Return any unused wells to the foil pouch, then seal with tape and store at 4 °C.
2. Prepare all samples (diluted with kinase buffer as needed). All samples should be assayed in duplicate.
3. Following Table 2, add the reagents to each well and initiate the reaction by adding 10 μL of a kinase positive control to

Table 2
Preparation of kinase reaction systems

Assay reagents	Test sample (μL)	Solvent control (μL)	Inhibitor control (μL)
Kinase reaction buffer	80	80	80
10× inhibitor or equivalent	10	–	–
Solvent for inhibitor	–	10	–
Purified kinase sample	10	10	10

each well and mix thoroughly at room temperature. Cover with plate sealer or lid, and incubate at 30 °C for 30 min (Table 2).

4. Wash wells 5 times with wash buffer making sure each well is filled completely. Remove residual wash buffer by gentle tapping or aspiration (**Note** 7).
5. Add 100 μL of anti-phospho-target substrate–HRP solution into each well, cover with plate sealer or lid, and incubate for 30 min at room temperature (25 °C).
6. Wash wells 5 times as in **step 4**.
7. Pipette 100 μL of HRP-conjugated secondary IgG into each well, cover with plate sealer or lid, and incubate for 30 min at room temperature (25 °C). Discard any unused conjugate after use.
8. Wash wells 5 times as in **step 4**.
9. Substrate reaction: fully empty washing buffer on a paper towel. Add 100 μL of HRP substrate solution (TMBZ) into each well. Incubate for 5–15 min at 25 °C.
10. Stop color development by adding 100 μL of stop solution into each well in the same order as the previously added substrate reagent.
11. Measure the absorbance with a plate reader at dual wavelengths of 450/540 nm. Dual wavelengths of 450/540 or 450/595 nm can also be used. Read the plate at 450 nm if only a single wavelength can be used. Wells must be read within 30 min of adding the stop solution.

3.7 Immunofluorescence Analysis

3.7.1 Summary and Introduction

Immunofluorescence is a technique built on immunology, biochemistry and microscopy, allowing the visualization of a specific protein or antigen in cells or tissue sections by binding a specific antibody chemically conjugated with a fluorescent dye such as fluorescein isothiocyanate (FITC). Immunofluorescence staining can be performed on cells fixed on slides and tissue sections then examined under a fluorescence microscope or confocal microscope. Two main kinds of immunofluorescence staining methods are used: (1) direct immunofluorescence staining in which the primary antibody is labeled with fluorescence dye; and (2) indirect immunofluorescence staining in which a secondary antibody labeled with a fluorochrome is used to recognize a primary antibody. Although direct staining can reduce the number of steps and nonspecificity in the staining procedure, the number of fluorescent dyes that can bind to the primary antibody is limited, thus direct staining is less sensitive than indirect staining. In this part, we will focus on indirect staining.

3.7.2 Fixing Cells in Methanol

1. Cells are seeded directly into a MillicelloR EZ Slide and the confluence should be 70–80 % by the next day.
2. Wash cells briefly 3× with PBS.
3. Fix cells 10 min at −20 °C with 500 μL pre-cooled (−20 °C) methanol.
4. Wash 2 times, 5 min each time with PBS.
5. Block cells with 500 μL 5 % normal donkey serum in PBS for 1 h at room temperature with shaking.
6. Wash 3 times, 5 min each time with PBS.

3.7.3 Staining Cells

1. Dilute primary antibody in BSA-PBS. Additional primary antibodies raised in different species can be added in the same BSA-PBS if two or more proteins need to be labeled (**Note 8**).
2. Incubate with primary antibodies overnight at 4 °C with shaking.
3. Wash 3 times, 5 min each time with PBS at room temperature.
4. Dilute secondary antibodies in BSA-PBS; incubate at room temperature for 45–60 min and keep under lucifugal (i.e., avoiding light) conditions (**Note 9**).
5. Wash 3 times, 5 min each time with PBS at room temperature under lucifugal conditions.
6. Carefully mount the slide with 10 μL ProLong® Gold Antifade Reagent with DAPI and avoid bubble formation (**Note 10**).
7. Store slides at 4 °C in the dark or observe with a laser scanning confocal microscope immediately.

3.8 Co-immunoprecipitation Analysis

3.8.1 Summary and Introduction

Co-immunoprecipitation (Co-IP) is a popular technique to demonstrate physiologically relevant protein–protein interactions [17]. Utilizing target protein-specific antibodies allows us to indirectly capture protein complexes that contain the target protein and its interacting proteins from a whole cell extract where proteins are present in their native conformation. These protein complexes can

Table 3
Preparation of diluted albumin (BSA) standards

Vial	Volume of diluent (μL)	Volume and source of BSA (μL)	Final BSA concentration (μg/μL)
A	0	300 of stock	2,000
B	125	375 of stock	1,500
C	325	325 of stock	1,000
D	175	175 of vial B dilution	750
E	325	325 of vial C dilution	500
F	325	325 of vial E dilution	250
G	325	325 of vial F dilution	125
H	400	100 of vial G dilution	25
I	400	0	0 = Blank

Dilution scheme for standard test tube protocol and microplate procedure (working range = 20–20,000 μg/mL)

then be analyzed to identify new binding partners, binding affinities, the kinetics of binding and the function of the target protein (**Note 11**).

3.8.2 Prepare Cell Lysates

1. Remove the media, rinse cells briefly with ice-cold PBS.
2. Add 1 mL ice-cold PBS with proteinase inhibitor and then harvest by scraping the cells from the 100 mm dishes.
3. Collect cell suspension into a new 1.5 mL EP tube.
4. Spin down the cells at 500 × *g* for 5 min, 4 °C.
5. Remove the supernatant fraction, resuspend cells with 500 μL ice-cold high salt lysis buffer (with proteinase inhibitor).
6. Pipet up and down to create a suspension; then keep the suspension on ice for at least 30 min. Mix the suspension several times during the ice incubation.
7. Spin down the DNA and cellular debris at 16,000 × *g* for 5 min at 4 °C.
8. Transfer the supernatant fraction to a new 1.5 mL EP tube.
9. Aliquot and store the cell lysates at −80 °C or directly go to IP step (**Note 12**).

3.8.3 Determining the Protein Concentration (BCA Method)

Pierce BCA Protein Assay Kit, Thermo, Cat. #23228.

1. Create standard curve (Table 3).
2. Dilute 3 μL protein sample in 27 μL ddH_2O; use 10 μL protein sample dilution for each reaction, and run duplicate assays.

3. Add 200 μL dye mixture (Reagent A:B = 50:1) and incubate at 37 °C for 30 min.
4. Read absorbance at 562 nm.

3.8.4 Immunoprecipitation

1. For 1 reaction (Rxn): to 200 μg total cell lysate, add low salt lysis buffer (with proteinase inhibitor) to a final volume of 600 μL.
2. Pre-clear: for 1 Rxn, to 200 μg cell lysate, add 30 μL protein G-Sepharose and rotate at 4 °C for 1 h.
3. Centrifuge at 500 rpm for 1 min, and then remove the supernatant fraction to a new 1.5 mL EP tube.
4. Add 1 μg antibody and rotate at 4 °C overnight (**Note 13**).
5. Add 30 μL PBS pre-washed Protein G dynabeads (Invitrogen Cat. # 100-04D) and rotate at 4 °C for 30 min.
6. Precipitate the dynabeads with the included magnet and discard the supernatant fraction.
7. Wash dynabeads with 1 mL low salt lysis buffer 4 times and discard the supernatant fraction.
8. Add 30 μL SDS-loading buffer, boil for 5 min, and then analyzed by Western blot.

3.9 Chromatin Immunoprecipitation Assay

3.9.1 Summary and Introduction

Chromatin immunoprecipitation (ChIP) is an invaluable method for studying interactions between specific proteins or modified forms of proteins and a genomic DNA region. Understanding how various factors regulate transcription elongation in cells has been greatly aided by ChIP studies. ChIP can be used to determine whether a transcription factor interacts with a candidate target gene and is used with equal frequency to monitor the presence of histones with post-translational modifications at specific genomic locations.

3.9.2 Cell Fixation, Chromatin Isolation, and Sonication Shearing

This section describes preparation of chromatin from 3 15-cm plates (i.e., this corresponds to approximately 4.5×10^7 cells). Note: several of the buffers used below require the addition of PMSF and/or protease inhibitors. Thaw these reagents before starting the protocol and add to the buffers immediately before use.

1. Grow cells to 70–80 % confluence on 3 15-cm plates.
2. Pour medium off the 3 plates and add 10 mL fixation solution to each plate. Incubate on a shaking platform for 10 min at room temperature.
3. Stop the fixation reaction by adding 1/10 volume of 1.25 M glycine for 5 min with gentle shaking.
4. Discard the medium, and rinse the cells with 10 mL ice-cold PBS with proteinase inhibitors and collect the cells by scraping.
5. Centrifuge at ~500 × g for 5 min at 4 °C.

Table 4
Preparation of ChIP assay reaction system

Reagent	μL for one ChIP rxn
Chromatin	100 μL
Resuspended protein G beads	40 μL
Cell lysis buffer	860 μL
Total volume	1,000 μL

6. Remove the supernatant fraction. At this point, the protocol can be continued or the pellet can be frozen. If freezing the pellet, add 1 μL 100 mM PMSF and protease inhibitors and freeze at −80 °C. When you are ready, continue with **step 7**.
7. Loosen cell pellets by gently vortexing for 5 s and resuspend cells in 5 mL cell lysis buffer. After lysis buffer is completely added, vortex cells 10 s at half of high maximal speed.
8. Incubate the lysed cells on ice for 5 min. Centrifuge at ~500 × *g* for 5 min at 4 °C.
9. Carefully remove the supernatant fraction. Resuspend the nuclei pellet in 1 mL cell lysis buffer (this time switch to 1.5 mL tube).
10. Centrifuge at ~500 × *g* for 5 min at 4 °C.
11. Discard the supernatant fraction and resuspend the nuclei in 300 μL SDS lysis buffer by gently vortexing. Keep the lysed cells on ice for at least 10 min.
12. Sonication on ice: 20 s on, 20 s off, total 2 min, at 25 % power (**Note 14**).
13. Centrifuge the sheared chromatin samples at 13,000 × *g* for 10 min at 4 °C.
14. Take the supernatant fraction and determine the protein concentration with the Bradford assay.

3.9.3 Pre-clearing of Chromatin

1. Use Table 4 to calculate the amount of chromatin, resuspended Protein G beads and cell lysis buffer for pre-clearing reactions. Combine reagents in a 1.5 mL microcentrifuge tube (**Note 15**).
2. Rotate the tube at 4 °C for 1 h.
3. Centrifuge at 5,000 × *g* for 5 min at 4 °C.
4. Transfer the supernatant fraction (chromatin) to a fresh tube. Do not disturb the beads.

3.9.4 Addition of Antibodies to Pre-cleared Chromatin

1. Transfer 10 μL of the pre-cleared chromatin to a tube and store at −20 °C. This sample is the "Input DNA" and will be used in the PCR analysis.

2. Add the appropriate antibody to each of the pre-cleared chromatin fractions. We recommend using between 1 and 3 μg of antibody for each ChIP reaction (**Note 16**).
3. Incubate the tubes for 4 h to overnight on a rotator at 4 °C.

3.9.5 Addition of Protein G to Antibody/Chromatin Mixture

1. Centrifuge at 13,000 rpm for 1 min at 4 °C.
2. Pipette 30 μL of Dynabeads Protein G and wash the beads with cell lysis buffer.
3. Remove the supernatant fraction of the antibody/chromatin incubations and mix with the Dynabeads.
4. Incubate the tubes on a rotator for 1 h at 4 °C.

3.9.6 Washing ChIP Reactions

1. Spin down with a microcentrifuge and then use the magnetic separation stand to wash the beads with Sol I, Sol II, Sol III, and 1× TE.
2. Repeat the above **step 3** times with 10 min for each washing.

3.9.7 Reverse Cross-Link and Purify the Eluted DNA

1. Add 100 μL 10 % Chelex-100 and place tubes in a 99 °C incubator for 10 min to reverse cross-link.
2. Remove the supernatant fraction after centrifugation at 13,000 rpm for 2 min at 4 °C.
3. Wash the resin with 125 μL H_2O, remove the supernatant fraction, and combine with the first supernatant fraction. Purify the DNA with the Qiagen PCR purification kit if necessary.

3.9.8 PCR Analysis

1. Program the thermocycler (**Note 17**).
2. Dilute the eluted input DNA 1:10 by adding 20–180 μL ddH_2O.
3. Analysis of PCR products.

4 Notes

1. Proliferation assays require cells to grow over a period of time. Therefore, choose an initial number of cells per well that produces an assay signal near the low end of the linear range of the assay. For most tumor cells, hybridomas and fibroblast cell lines, 5,000 cells per well are recommended to initiate proliferation studies, although fewer than 1,000 cells can usually be detected.
2. To measure the amount of soluble formazan produced by cellular reduction of MTS, read the plate immediately. Alternatively, to measure the absorbance later, add 25 μL of 10 % SDS to each well to stop the reaction. Store SDS-treated plates protected from light in a humidified chamber at room temperature for up to 18 h and then read the plate.

3. Background 490 nm absorbance can be corrected as follows: Prepare a triplicate set of control wells (without cells) containing the same volumes of culture medium and CellTiter 96 AQueous One Solution Reagent as in the experimental wells. Subtract the average 490 nm absorbance acquired from the "no cell" control wells from all other absorbance values to yield corrected absorbances.
4. The quality of a DNA histogram is estimated from the width of the peak of DNA from cells in the G1 phase of the cell cycle. This is measured by the coefficient of variation (CV) across the peak and is calculated from the standard deviation (SD). The smaller the CV of the peaks in the DNA histogram, the more accurate is the measurement of ploidy and the better the estimation of the percentage of cells in the different phases of the cell cycle.
5. The following controls are used to set up compensation and quadrants: Unstained cells, cells stained with Annexin V-FITC (no PI) and cells stained with PI (no Annexin V-FITC).
6. The TUNEL reaction mixture should be prepared immediately before use and should not be stored. Keep the TUNEL reaction mixture on ice until use. TUNEL assay negative control: incubate fixed and permeabilized cells in 50 μL/well labeling solution (without terminal transferase) instead of TUNEL reaction mixture. Positive control: incubate fixed and permeabilized cells with DNase for 10 min at 15–25 °C to induce DNA strand breaks prior to labeling procedures.
7. Complete removal of liquid at each step is essential to obtain good results. After the last wash, remove any remaining wash buffer by aspirating or decanting. Invert the plate and blot with clean paper towels.
8. Choose primary/secondary antibodies from different species to conduct double immunofluorescence staining.
9. Immunofluorescence causes photobleaching and therefore keep samples under lucifugal conditions.
10. Carefully mount the slide and avoid bubble formation.
11. The signals of low-affinity protein interactions might not be detected. To choose an appropriate antibody, the target protein needs to be properly predicted or positive co-immunoprecipitation results cannot be obtained.
12. Lysates for co-immunoprecipitation analysis should be kept in ice to avoid degradation.
13. Proper normal IgG without specific antigen affinity should be used as a negative control.
14. 200–1,500 bp-sheared chromatin is required for performing ChIP experiments.

15. Be sure to include the appropriate control ChIP reactions in your calculations. Also, note that if you wish to analyze the effect of particular compounds or culturing conditions on transcription factor–DNA interactions, you should prepare chromatin from control cells as an un-induced reference sample.
16. Antibodies to be used for the chromatin immunoprecipitation assay must be suitable for ChIP. ChIP performed with an unproven antibody must include appropriate controls (such as the included RNA pol II antibody) to demonstrate that the antibody and the prepared chromatin are appropriate for ChIP.
17. The PCR primers should efficiently and specifically amplify the desired target.

References

1. Tsuiji K, Takeda T, Li B, Wakabayashi A, Kondo A, Kimura T, Yaegashi N (2011) Inhibitory effect of curcumin on uterine leiomyoma cell proliferation. Gynecol Endocrinol 27(7):512–517. doi:10.3109/09513590 .2010.507287
2. Nunez R (2001) DNA measurement and cell cycle analysis by flow cytometry. Curr Issues Mol Biol 3(3):67–70
3. Colin D, Gimazane A, Lizard G, Izard JC, Solary E, Latruffe N, Delmas D (2009) Effects of resveratrol analogs on cell cycle progression, cell cycle associated proteins and 5fluoro-uracil sensitivity in human derived colon cancer cells. Int J Cancer 124(12):2780–2788. doi:10.1002/ijc.24264
4. Williamson P, van den Eijnde S, Schlegel RA (2001) Phosphatidylserine exposure and phagocytosis of apoptotic cells. Methods Cell Biol 66:339–364
5. Boersma HH, Kietselaer BL, Stolk LM, Bennaghmouch A, Hofstra L, Narula J, Heidendal GA, Reutelingsperger CP (2005) Past, present, and future of annexin A5: from protein discovery to clinical applications. J Nucl Med 46(12):2035–2050
6. Hengartner MO (2000) The biochemistry of apoptosis. Nature 407(6805):770–776. doi:10.1038/35037710
7. Kurokawa M, Kornbluth S (2009) Caspases and kinases in a death grip. Cell 138(5):838–854. doi:10.1016/j.cell.2009.08.021
8. Su H, Yang JR, Xu T, Huang J, Xu L, Yuan Y, Zhuang SM (2009) MicroRNA-101, down-regulated in hepatocellular carcinoma, promotes apoptosis and suppresses tumorigenicity. Cancer Res 69(3):1135–1142. doi:10.1158/0008-5472.CAN-08-2886
9. Toker A, Newton AC (2000) Cellular signaling: pivoting around PDK-1. Cell 103(2):185–188
10. Hoshino T, Sakai Y, Yamashita K, Shirahase Y, Sakaguchi K, Asaeda A, Kishi K, Schlattner U, Wallimann T, Yanai M, Kumasaka K (2009) Development and performance of an enzyme immunoassay to detect creatine kinase isoenzyme MB activity using anti-mitochondrial creatine kinase monoclonal antibodies. Scand J Clin Lab Invest 69(6):687–695. doi:10.3109/00365510902981171
11. Shi Y, Tao Y, Jiang Y, Xu Y, Yan B, Chen X, Xiao L, Cao Y (2012) Nuclear epidermal growth factor receptor interacts with transcriptional intermediary factor 2 to activate cyclin D1 gene expression triggered by the oncoprotein latent membrane protein 1. Carcinogenesis 33(8):1468–1478. doi:10.1093/carcin/bgs171
12. Zigangirova NA, Rumyantseva YP, Morgunova EY, Kapotina LN, Didenko LV, Kost EA, Koroleva EA, Bashmakov YK, Petyaev IM (2013) Detection of C. trachomatis in the serum of the patients with urogenital chlamydiosis. Biomed Res Int 2013:489489. doi:10.1155/2013/489489
13. Killingsworth MC, Lai K, Wu X, Yong JL, Lee CS (2012) Quantum dot immunocytochemical localization of somatostatin in somatostatinoma by Widefield Epifluorescence, super-resolution light, and immunoelectron microscopy. J Histochem Cytochem 60(11):832–843. doi:10.1369/0022155412459856
14. Poetz O, Luckert K, Herget T, Joos TO (2009) Microsphere-based co-immunoprecipitation in multiplex. Anal Biochem 395(2):244–248. doi:10.1016/j.ab.2009.08.002

15. Kus-Liskiewicz M, Widlak W (2011) Finding targets of transcriptional regulators—chromatin immunoprecipitation assay (ChIP). Postepy Biochem 57(4):418–424
16. Collas P (2010) The current state of chromatin immunoprecipitation. Mol Biotechnol 45(1): 87–100. doi:10.1007/s12033-009-9239-8
17. Riss TL, Moravec RA (2004) Use of multiple assay endpoints to investigate the effects of incubation time, dose of toxin, and plating density in cell-based cytotoxicity assays. Assay Drug Dev Technol 2(1):51–62. doi:10.1089/154065804322966315

Chapter 3

Nrf2-Target Approaches in Cancer Chemoprevention Mediated by Dietary Phytochemicals

Francisco Fuentes, Limin Shu, Jong Hun Lee, Zheng-Yuan Su, Kyeong-Ryoon Lee, and Ah-Ng Tony Kong

Abstract

Cancer chemoprevention with natural phytochemical compounds is an emerging strategy to prevent, impede, delay, or cure cancer. This chapter reviews the basic methods used to study the cancer chemopreventive potential of dietary phytochemicals acting by activating the transcriptional factor, nuclear factor-erythroid 2-related factor 2 (Nrf2 or NFE2L2), a basic-region leucine zipper (bZIP) transcription factor that regulates the expression of many phase II detoxifying/antioxidant enzymes. The Nrf2-target approaches in cancer chemoprevention comprise different methods including examining the Nrf2 signaling pathway, Nrf2-deficient tumor mouse models, pharmacokinetics (PK)/pharmacodynamics (PD) assessment, and epigenetic regulation.

Key words Nrf2, Cancer chemoprevention, Nrf2-deficient mouse models, Pharmacokinetics, Pharmacodynamics, Epigenetics

1 Introduction

Cancer chemoprevention involves the use of natural dietary and synthetic compounds to inhibit malignant transformation of initiated cells at either the promotion or the progression stages [1]. Thus, chemoprevention can involve preventing carcinogens from reaching the target sites, from undergoing metabolic activation, or from subsequently interacting with crucial cellular macromolecules (e.g., DNA, RNA, and proteins) at the initiation stage [2, 3]. In this context, the induction of phase II/detoxifying enzymes can neutralize reactive electrophiles and act as indirect antioxidants, which appears to be an effective means for achieving protection against a variety of carcinogens in animals and humans [4].

The antioxidant response element (ARE) is a critical regulatory element for the expression of many phase II drug metabolizing enzymes (DME), phase III transporters, and antioxidant enzymes. Xenobiotic detoxification, for example, NQO1 (NAD(P)

Ann M. Bode and Zigang Dong (eds.), *Cancer Prevention: Dietary Factors and Pharmacology*, Methods in Pharmacology and Toxicology, DOI 10.1007/978-1-4614-9227-6_3, © Springer Science+Business Media New York 2014

H:quinone oxidoreductase 1) and GST (glutathione S-transferase) may be activated through the stress- or antioxidant-response elements [5]. These *cis*-elements can be recognized by quite a few nuclear factors, including Nrf2, small Mafs (MafG and MafK), large Maf (c-Maf), c-Fos, Fra1 [6], and c-Myc which was reported to be able to bind with some electrophile response elements (EpRE) to regulate the expression of some phase II genes [7]. The stress response elements of the *heme oxygnesase-1 (HO-1)* gene are able to resemble the binding site for the activator protein-1 (Jun/Fos), Maf, and Cap'n'Collar/basic leucine zipper (CNC-bZIP) families of proteins [8]. Among the CNC-bZip protein, Nrf2 has been identified as a master regulator of cellular redox homeostasis and defense response. By cooperating with some small Maf proteins, Nrf2 activates the transcription of a battery of genes encoding antioxidants, detoxification enzymes, and xenobiotic transporters by binding to their ARE *cis* elements [9–11].

Several in vitro and in vivo studies involving natural dietary compounds have revealed that Nrf2 controls the expression of ARE-mediated gene expression and dramatically influences susceptibility to carcinogenesis [12]. Some examples of dietary compounds activating Nrf2 include curcumin from turmeric [13]; indole-3-carbinol (I3C), 3,30-diindolylmethane (DIM), phenethyl isothiocyanate (PEITC), and sulforaphane (SFN) from cruciferous vegetables [14, 15]; epigallocatechin-3-gallate (EGCG) from green tea [16]; resveratrol from grapes [17]; and gamma-tocopherol-enriched mixed tocopherols from soybeans and corn oil [18], among others. Most recently, the expression of Nrf2 has been found to be controlled epigenetically by CpG methylation of the promoter region associated with MBD2 (Methyl-CpG binding domain protein 2) and histone modifications in the prostate tumors of TRAMP (Transgenic adenocarcinoma of the mouse prostate) mice [19]. Interestingly, the treatment of TRAMP C1 cells with the DNMTs (DNA methyltransferases) inhibitor 5-aza-2′-deoxycytidine (5-aza) and HDACs (Histone deacetylases) inhibitor Trichostatin A (TSA), curcumin, and recently SFN has revealed a decreasing methylation level of the first five CpGs at the *Nrf2* gene and binding of anti-mecyt antibody to the *Nrf2* promoter [13, 15, 19]. Thus, our findings demonstrate that Nrf2 expression appears to be controlled by epigenetic alterations, such as DNA methylation and histone modifications, and that dietary phytochemicals can block or reverse these epigenetic alterations, which results in the prevention of carcinogenesis in the TRAMP prostate cancer model [12].

In this chapter, we provide the basic step-by-step methods used to study the cancer chemopreventive potential of dietary phytochemicals in in vitro and in vivo model systems targeting on Nrf2.

2 Phytochemical Selection Based on NRF2 Activation

Nrf2 is an important transcription factor in regulating the expression of phase II detoxifying/antioxidant enzymes against oxidative stress or electrophiles caused by toxicants and carcinogens. Many cellular functions, including cellular redox homeostasis, inflammatory responses, cell growth and apoptosis, and the ubiquitin-mediated degradation pathways, have been demonstrated to be related to Nrf2 downstream genes [20–24]. Negative regulator Keap1 can repress Nrf2-dependent transcription under normal conditions by the formation of an Nrf2-Keap1 complex, which promotes Nrf2 proteasomal degradation and decreases its translocation into the nucleus. Antioxidant response elements (AREs) containing a functional consensus sequence of 5′-RTGAYnnnGCR-3′ (where R = A or G and Y = C or T) are located upstream of most of the antioxidant genes [25]. When cells are exposed to oxidants or cancer chemopreventive compounds, the dissociation of Nrf2 from Keap1 occurs due to the oxidation of thiol-sensitive amino acids causing conformational changes in the Nrf2-Keap1 complex, which results in increased Nrf2 translocation into the nucleus. In the nucleus, Nrf2 binds to ARE and enhances gene expression of ARE-target phase II detoxifying/antioxidant enzymes [26, 27].

The stably transfected human hepatoma HepG2-C8-ARE-luciferase cell model was established many years ago [28]. This model has been well validated in the evaluation of the efficacy of many active compounds through the Nrf2-ARE-mediated up-regulation of Phase II drug metabolizing enzymes and antioxidative stress enzymes, which play a critical role in cancer chemoprevention [3, 29–35]. Utilizing this HepG2-C8 cell model, several studies focusing on the effects of many active phytochemicals on Nrf2-ARE signaling pathway have been published and correspond well with in vivo Nrf2$^{-/-}$ mice studies with regard to Nrf2-mediated phase II metabolism and antioxidative stress responses [3, 29–35]. Additionally, Nrf2-mediated anti-inflammatory activity of chemopreventive agents in macrophages has also been evaluated [31].

2.1 NRF2 Signaling Pathway

2.1.1 Materials

Equipment

1. Luminometer such as the SIRIUS luminometer (Berthold Detection System GmbH, Pforzheim, Germany).
2. 96-Well plate reader such as the μQuant Biomolecular Spectrophotometer (Bio-Tek Instruments Inc., Winooski, VT).
3. Electrophoresis tank (Bio-Rad, Hercules, CA).
4. Semi-dry transfer system (Bio-Rad, Hercules, CA).
5. Power supply (Thermo Fisher Scientific, Waltham, MA).
6. Bio-Rad ChemiDoc XRS system (Hercules, CA, USA).

7. MicroAmp® Optical 384-Well Reaction Plate (Applied Biosystems, Foster City, CA).
8. ABI 7900HT Real-Time PCR System (Applied Biosystems, Foster City, CA).
9. FLx-800 microplate fluorescence reader (Bio-Tek Instruments Inc., Winooski, VT).

Reagents and Solutions

1. Dulbecco's Modified Eagle Medium (DMEM) (Gibco, Grand Island, NY).
2. Penicillin/Streptomycin (Gibco, Grand Island, NY).
3. Fetal Bovine Serum (FBS) (Gibco, Grand Island, NY).
4. 0.25 % Trypsin-EDTA (1×) (Gibco, Grand Island, NY).
5. Phosphate buffered saline pH 7.2 (PBS) (Gibco, Grand Island, NY).
6. CellTiter 96® AQueous One Solution Cell Proliferation Assay (Promega, Madison, WI).
7. Luciferase Reporter System (Promega, Madison, WI) containing Lysis Buffers, Luciferase Assay Buffer, and Luciferase Assay Substrate.
8. 10× RIPA buffer (Cell Signaling Technology, Danvers, MA).
9. Protein inhibitor cocktail (Sigma-Aldrich, St. Louis, MO).
10. Bicinchoninic acid (BCA) kit (Pierce, Rockford, IL).
11. Laemmli's SDS-Sample Buffer (4×) (Boston BioProducts, Ashland, MA).
12. Protein standard (Bio-Rad, Hercules, CA).
13. 4–15 % SDS polyacrylamide gel (Criterion Tris–HCl gel, Bio-Rad Lab, Hercules, CA).
14. Tris-Glycine-SDS Running Buffer (10×) (Boston BioProducts, Ashland, MA).
15. Transfer Buffer (10×) (Boston BioProducts, Ashland, MA).
16. TBS-Tween-20 buffer (20×) (Boston BioProducts, Ashland, MA).
17. Bovine Serum Albumin (BSA) (Fraction V) (Thermo Fisher Scientific, Waltham, MA).
18. Primary antibodies such as anti-β-actin, anti-Nrf2, anti-NQO1, anti-HO-1, anti-UGT1A1, anti-SOD1, anti-GSTm2, etc. (Santa Cruz Biotechnology, Inc., CA).
19. Secondary antibodies (Santa Cruz Biotechnology, Inc., CA).
20. SuperSignal West Femto Chemiluminescent Substrate (Thermo Scientific, Rockford, IL).
21. RNeasy® Mini kit (Qiagen, Valencia, CA).

22. SuperScript III First-Strand Synthesis System (Invitrogen, Grand Island, NY).
23. Power SYBR Green PCR Master Mix (Applied Biosystem, Carlsbads, CA).
24. 2,3-Diaminonapthalene (Sigma-Aldrich, St. Louis, MO).
25. Nitrate sodium (Sigma-Aldrich, St. Louis, MO).

2.1.2 Methods

MTS Assay

1. Seed HepG2-C8 cells in a 96-well plate at a density of 1.0×10^5 cells per well in 100 μL of DMEM containing 10 % FBS.
2. After incubation at 37 °C in a humidified and 5 % CO_2 atmosphere for 24 h, the medium is replaced with DMEM containing 1 % FBS and various concentrations of phytochemical compound.
3. After 24 h treatment, discard DMEM containing phytochemical compound and add 100 μL DMEM containing 1 % FBS without samples and 20 μL of CellTiter 96® AQueous One Solution Reagent (**Note 1**).
4. Incubate the plate at 37 °C for 1–4 h and then record the absorbance at 490 nm using a 96-well plate reader (**Note 2**).
5. Calculate cell viability using the following equation: $[(OD_{sample} - OD_{blank})/(OD_{control} - OD_{blank})] \times 100\ \%$.

ARE-Luciferase Activity Induction in HepG2-C8 Cells

1. Seed and culture HepG2-C8 cells (1.0×10^6 cells/well) in 1 mL of DMEM containing 10 % FBS in a 12-well plate at 37 °C in a humidified and 5 % CO_2 atmosphere for 24 h.
2. Treat cells with DMEM containing 1 % FBS and various concentrations of phytochemical compound for an additional 24 h.
3. Remove the growth medium and rinse cells with PBS, then add 1× lysis buffer (about 250 μL) to completely cover the cells (**Note 3**).
4. Scrape and harvest the attached cells from the dish to a microcentrifuge tube. Lay whole lysate on ice.
5. Vortex the microcentrifuge tube for 10–15 s and centrifuge at $12{,}000 \times g$ for 2 min at 4 °C. Transfer the supernatant fraction to a new microcentrifuge tube.
6. Pipette 100 μL of the Luciferase Assay Reagent and 20 μL of the supernatant fraction into luminometer tubes sequentially. Mix by vortex briefly or pipetting 2–3 times (**Note 4**).
7. Place the tube in the luminometer and record the reading.
8. Measure protein concentration of the supernatant fractions using the bicinchoninic acid (BCA) method (**Note 5**) and normalize the reading values with protein concentration.
9. Calculate relative induced ARE-luciferase activity using the following equation: $(Reading_{sample} - Reading_{blank})/(Reading_{control} - Reading_{blank})$.

Detoxifying/Antioxidant Enzymes Assay in HepG2-C8 Cells

HepG2-C8 cells (3.0×10^6 cells/6-cm dish) are incubated and treated with the compounds similarly as the MTS and ARE-luciferase assays described above in 3 mL DMED containing 1 % FBS medium for 24 h. The treated cells can be harvested for the determination of protein and/or mRNA expressions.

1. Determination of protein expression
   (a) Harvest cells in 200 μL of lysis buffer ice-cold 1× RIPA buffer containing protein inhibitors after washing with ice-cold PBS (pH 7.4).
   (b) Sonicate on ice for 10 s × 3 times and centrifuge at 12,000 × *g* for 15 min at 4 °C. Transfer the supernatant fraction to a new microcentrifuge tube.
   (c) Measure protein concentration of the supernatant fractions using the bicinchoninic acid (BCA) method (**Note 5**).
   (d) Mix the supernatant fractions containing 15–25 μg of protein concentration with 5× Laemmli's SDS-Sample Buffer and denatured at 95 °C for 5 min.
   (e) Load samples and protein standard onto a 4–15 % SDS polyacrylamide gel and run gel electrophoresis in 1× Tris-Glycine-SDS Running Buffer at 130 mA for 60 min.
   (f) Transfer proteins onto a polyvinylidene difluoride (PVDF) membrane (Immobilon-P, Millipore, Bedford, MA) in 1× Transfer Buffer 1.5–2.0 h.
   (g) Block the membrane with 1× TBS-Tween-20 buffer containing 5 % BSA for 1 h at room temperature and wash with 1× TBS-Tween-20 buffer for 10 min × 3 times.
   (h) Incubate the membrane with the primary antibody in 1× TBS-Tween-20 buffer containing 3 % BSA overnight at 4 °C.
   (i) Wash the membrane with 1× TBS-Tween-20 buffer for 10 min × 3 times. Incubate the membrane with secondary antibody in 1× TBS-Tween-20 buffer for 1 h at room temperature.
   (j) Wash the membrane with 1× TBS-Tween-20 buffer for 10 min × 3 times.
   (k) Examine the immunocomplexes using SuperSignal West Femto Chemiluminescent Substrate to detect the horseradish peroxidase on the immunoblots and visualize and capture the bands by Bio-Rad ChemiDoc XRS system.
2. Determination of mRNA expression
   (a) Extract total RNA from the treated cells using RNeasy® Mini kit.
   (b) Synthesize first-strand cDNA from total RNA (500 ng) according to the manufacturer's instructions of SuperScript III First-Strand Synthesis System.

(c) Mix 4 μL of first-strand cDNA with 5 μL of 2× Power SYBR Green PCR Master Mix and 1 μL of specific primer pairs (**Note 6**) in a 384-well plate.

(d) Determine mRNA expression levels using quantitative real time-PCR (qPCR) in ABI 7900HT Real-Time PCR System.

Inflammation Assay in Macrophages

RAW 264.7 cells (1.0×10^5 cells/well) are seeded in DMEM containing 10 % FBS in a 96-well plate for 24 h. After discarding the old medium, the cells are incubated with various concentrations of phytochemical compound in 50 μL of DMEM containing 1 % FBS for 1 h. The LPS (Lipopolysaccharide) control or sample-treated cells are further incubated for 24 h after adding an additional 50 μL of DMEM containing 1 % FBS with LPS (the final concentration of LPS is 10 μg/mL). For normal control cells, an additional 50 μL of DMEM (1 % FBS) without LPS is needed. The inflammation-related cytokines, such as interleukin 1-β (IL-1β), tumor necrosis factor alpha (TNF-α), can be further examined using ELISA kits from various companies according to the manufacturers' instructions; hence they are not discussed in detail here. We only discuss the method of "Measurement of nitric oxide (NO) production" [36] for an example of anti-inflammation assays as follows:

1. Mix the medium (50 μL) from each well with 10 μL of 2,3-diaminonapthalene (50 μg/mL in 0.62 M HCl). Nitrate sodium solution (0, 1.56, 3.125. 6.25, 12.5, and 25 μg/mL) is prepared as nitrite standards in deionized water. Incubate the mixture at room temperature in the dark for 10 min.
2. Terminate the reaction with 5 μL of 2.8 M NaOH.
3. Measure the formation of 2,3-diaminonaphthotriazole in black opaque 96-well plates at 360 nm excitation and 460 nm emission using a gain setting of 75 % in a FLx-800 microplate fluorescence reader.
4. Use the following equation to calculate the NO suppression potentials of the tested samples: NO inhibition (%) = [(nitrite content in LPS control − nitrite content in sample treatments)/(nitrite content in LPS control − nitrite content in normal control)] × 100 %.

Notes

1. A set of control wells without cells needs to yield corrected 490 nm absorbances as the background. The wells must contain the same volumes of DMEM and CellTiter 96® AQueous One Solution Reagent as in the experimental wells.
2. The absorbance of formazan produced from reduction of MTS in cells can be measured immediately. However, 25 μL of 10 % SDS can also be added to each well to stop the reaction, and the absorbance can be further measured after keeping the plates from light at room temperature in a humidified chamber

for up to 18 h. Additionally, the absorbance can be read at wavelengths of 450–540 nm if the 96-well plate reader does not have a 490 nm filter. Excess cell debris, fingerprints and other nonspecific absorbance may cause additional background; hence the absorbance at a wavelength of 630–700 nm may also be measured as a reference reading.

3. Lysis Buffers from Promega (Madison, WI) has two recommended lysis buffers, Reporter Lysis Buffer (RLB) and Passive Lysis Buffer (PLB), for the preparation of cell lysates. It needs a single freeze–thaw cycle to completely lyse the cells when using RLB. PLB will passively lyse cells without performing a freeze–thaw cycle.
4. The Luciferase Assay Reagent needs to be equilibrated to room temperature before use. Add 20 μL water or lysis buffer instead of cell lysates in the Luciferase Assay Reagent for measuring the reading of background.
5. Determine various protein concentrations (0, 125, 250, 500, 1,000, and 2,000 μg/mL) of BSA solution as a standard curve for calculating the protein concentrations of the supernatant fractions.
6. Some primer pairs designed using Primer Quest Oligo Design and Analysis Tool by Integrated DNA Technologies Inc. (Coralville, IA, USA) can be used as follows [29]: GAPDH: sense 5′-TCG ACA GTC AGC CGC ATC TTC TTT-3′ and anti-sense 5′-ACC AAA TCC GTT GAC TCC GAC CTT-3′; Nrf2: sense 5′-TGC TTT ATA GCG TGC AAA CCT CGC-3′ and anti-sense 5′-ATC CAT GTC CCT TGA CAG CAC AGA-3′; NQO1: sense 5′-AAG GAT GGA AGA AAC GCC TGG AGA-3′ and anti-sense 5′-GGC CCA CAG AAA GGC CAA ATT TCT-3′; HO-1: sense 5′-ACG CGT TGT AAT TAA GCC TCG CAC-3′ and anti-sense 5′-TTC CGC TGG TCA TTA AGG CTG AGT-3′; UGT1A1: sense 5′-ATG ACC CGT GCC TTT ATC ACC CAT-3′ and anti-sense 5′-AGT CTC CAT GCG CTT TGC ATT GTC-3′; SOD1: sense 5′-GCA GGG CAT CAT CAA TTT CGA GCA-3′ and anti-sense 5′-TGC AGG CCT TCA GTC AGT CCT TTA-3′; GSTm2: sense 5′-ACT AAA GCC AGC CTG ACC TTC CTT-3′ and anti-sense 5′-AAT GCT GCT CCT TCA TGC AAC ACG-3′.

3 Animal Model Approaches for Chemoprevention Studies Based on NRF2 Targeting

In in vivo systems, Nrf2 has been shown to be dispensable for mouse growth and development [37], although aged female Nrf2-deficient mice have been reported to display a shortened lifespan and develop severe glomerulonephritis and lupus-like autoimmune nephritis [38]. Nrf2-deficient mice, however, are impaired in oxidative stress defense. They exhibit reduced expression of Alpha and class Mu transferases, Gsta1, Gsta2, Gstm1, Gstm2, Gstm3, Gstm4, and Gstm6 subunits in the liver and mice that lack Nrf2 are more sensitive than wild type (WT) animals to the cytotoxic and genotoxic effects of foreign chemicals and oxidants [39]. In addition, hyperoxia-induced mRNA levels of NAD(P)H:quinone oxidoreductase 1 (NQO1), glutathione-S-transferase (GST)-Ya and -Yc subunits, UDP glycosyl transferase (UGT), glutathione peroxidase-2 (GPx2), and heme oxygenase-1 (HO-1) were significantly lower in Nrf2 deficient mice compared with wild type mice [40]. In some mouse models, Nrf2 deficiency showed more resistance against cancer development [41]. However, Nrf2-deficient mice are recognized to be a very useful model for in vivo analysis of chemical carcinogenesis and resistance to anticancer drugs [42] or as an in vivo model for toxicological studies [43]. In general, Nrf2 deficient mice are more predisposed to chemical-induced DNA damage and show higher susceptibility towards cancer development compared with wild type mice. Nrf2 deficiency also causes mice to be more refractory to the protective actions of some chemopreventive agents [44].

3.1 NRF2 Null Mice Approaches

3.1.1 Materials

Equipment

1. Eppendorf Centrifuge 5415 R (4 °C) (Hamburg, Germany).
2. Microcentrifuge tubes, RNase/DNase-free.
3. BD Falcon™ 14 mL polystyrene round-bottom tube.
4. Fisher animal water bottle with sipper cap (Pittsburgh, PA).

Reagents and Solutions

1. 7,12-Dimethylbenz[*a*]anthracene (DMBA) (Sigma, St. Louis, MO).
2. Phorbol 12-myristate 13-acetate (TPA) (Sigma, St. Louis, MO).
3. Azoxymethane (AOM) (Sigma, St. Louis, MO).
4. Dextran sulfate sodium salt (DSS) (Sigma, St. Louis, MO).
5. Dimethyl sulfoxide (DMSO) (Sigma, St. Louis, MO).

3.1.2 Methods

DMBA-TPA Induced Skin Carcinogenesis

The development of skin cancer is a multistep process including initiation, promotion, and progression. Animal models mimicking this process can be used as a strong tool for the study of carcinogenesis and chemoprevention. The two-step treatment with carcinogen and promoter on mouse skin has been used for many years. Particularly, treatment with 7,12-dimethylbenz(a)anthracene (DMBA) and 12-*O*-tetradecanoylphorbol-13-acetate (TPA) on dorsal mouse skin is reliable model for skin cancer studies. To determine the role of Nrf2 in the development of skin cancer, we can incorporate this two-step chemical-induced model on the skin of Nrf2 deficient mice [45]. Usually, the cancer prevention reagent is applied before/after DMBA/TPA induction on Nrf2 wild-type (+/+) and Nrf2 knockout (−/−) mice, which enable us to determine if Nrf2 is regulated by the reagent. We also can examine the chemoprevention mechanism of the cancer prevention reagents using this model [14].

1. House female Nrf2(−/−) (C57BL/SV129) and Nrf2(+/+) C57BL/6J mice (10–12 weeks of age) in a proper facility. All animal use procedures should be in accordance with the NIH Guide for the Care and Use for Laboratory Animals and approved by the Institutional Animal Care and Use Committee. All animals can be allowed water and food ad libitum.
2. Shave the dorsal region of each mouse 2 days prior to any application of DMBA or experimental chemopreventive phytochemical.
3. Apply 200–300 nmol of DMBA in 100 μL of acetone topically. The dosage, duration time of application of experimental chemopreventive phytochemical will vary depending on the experimental purpose.
4. 1 Week later, 8 or 16 nmol of TPA in 200 μL of acetone is applied to the same site.
5. Continue the TPA treatment twice weekly for 25 consecutive weeks.
6. Count and record the number of skin tumors >1 mm in diameter every week.

Dextran Sulfate Sodium (DSS)-Induced Experimental Colitis

Accumulating evidence from epidemiologic and clinical studies indicate that chronic inflammatory disorders can increase the risk of cancer development [46, 47]. Inflammation occurs in response to various stimuli such as microbial infection and noninfective physical or chemical irritants [14]. In chronic inflammation, activated inflammatory-immune cells such as eosinophiles, dendritic cells, leukocytes, macrophages, mast cells, monocytes, natural killer cells, neutrophils, and phagocytes, release pro-inflammatory molecules including cytokines, chemokines, matrix-remodeling proteases, reactive oxygen species (ROS), and reactive nitrogen species (RNS) to eliminate pathogens and to repair tissue damage. However, various pro-inflammatory cytokines, chemokines, ROS, and RNS can cause genetic changes or epigenetic alterations such as DNA methylation and post-translational modification in tumor suppressor genes [12, 48]. Inflammatory bowel diseases (IBD), such as ulcerative colitis and Crohn's disease, have been strongly linked with an increased risk of colorectal cancer [49]. The dextran sulfate sodium (DSS)—induced mouse model of colitis is one of the most widely used models that mimics ulcerative colitis–like disease in humans [50]. This model system has been used to reveal important events leading to IBD and colorectal carcinogenesis. Moreover, administration of DSS to Nrf2 KO mice becomes a very strong strategy to identify genes that could be important in maintaining the integrity of intestinal tissue [51].

1. House female Nrf2(−/−) (C57BL/SV129) and Nrf2(+/+) C57BL/6 J mice (10–12 weeks of age) in a proper facility. All animal use procedures should be in accordance with the NIH Guide for the Care and Use for Laboratory Animals and approved by the Institutional Animal Care and Use Committee. All animals can be allowed water and food ad libitum.
2. Divide mice into 4 groups: group I, wild type + 1 % DSS in drinking water; group II, Nrf2(−/−) + 1 % DSS in drinking water; group III, control wild type; group IV, control Nrf2(−/−).
3. Give 1 % DSS (w/v) in water as the sole source of drinking fluid for 1 week, after which the DSS is stopped and drinking fluid is shifted back to drinking water.
4. 1 Week after the DSS administration, sacrifice all mice by carbon dioxide asphyxiation. For autopsy, flush the large bowel with saline and excise. After measuring the length and weight of the large bowel, cut longitudinally and fix in 10 % formalin before being embedded in paraffin.

3.2 Pharmacokinetics (PK) and Pharmacodynamics (PD) Assessment

3.2.1 Materials

Equipment

1. Applied Biosystems® ViiA™ 7 Real-Time PCR System (Carlsbad, CA).
2. Vertical rotating mixer capable of holding 0.2-mL PCR tubes or strip wells.
3. Eppendorf Centrifuge 5415 R (4 °C) (Hamburg, Germany).
4. Microcentrifuge tubes, RNase/DNase-free.
5. Fisher Touch Mixer Model 231 (Pittsburgh, PA).

Reagents and Solutions

1. Dimethyl sulfoxide (DMSO) (St. Louis, MO).
2. Methanol (Fisher Scientific, Pittsburgh, PA).
3. Phosphate Buffered Saline (PBS), PH 7.4, 1× liquid (Gibco).
4. Ficoll-Paque PLUS density gradient centrifugation medium (GE Healthcare Life Sciences, Piscataway, NJ).
5. SYBR® Green Real-Time PCR Master Mixes (Applied Biosystems).
6. Qiagen RNeasy Mini Kit buffer RLT, a lysis buffer (Valencia, CA).
7. Quant-It reagents (Invitrogen, Carlsbad, CA).
8. qPCR primers for specific sequence of interest.

3.2.2 Methods

Animal Experiments

The purpose of this method is to assess the pharmacokinetics (PK) and pharmacodynamics (PD) of Nrf2-mediated increased expression of phase II drug metabolizing enzymes (DME) and antioxidant enzymes, which represents an important component of cancer chemoprevention in rat lymphocytes following intravenous (iv) administration of an chemopreventive phytochemical [52]. Male Sprague-Dawley rats weighing 250–300 g with jugular vein cannulae are prepared. One group is composed of 4 animals, due to the small amount of lymphocytes in the blood and the limited amount of blood that can be drawn at each time point from a rat. To determine the induction of mRNA in lymphocytes, all samples from each of the 4 rats should be pooled. For example, to perform a study in triplicate, a total of twelve rats are used.

1. Administer a compound solution into the each rat at an appropriate dose through the jugular vein cannulae.
2. Collect blood samples (~300 μL) for each rat at 0, 2, 5, 15, 30, 45 min, 1, 1.5, 2, 4, 6, 8, 12, 16, or 24 h after intravenous bolus administration of the compound.
3. Pool the blood samples within a group at each time point to be approximate 1.0 mL.
4. Separate plasma from half of the collected blood sample by centrifugation and store the plasma at −80 °C until analysis (*see* Sect. 4.1).
5. Extract lymphocytes from the remaining blood samples using Ficoll-Paque PLUS density gradient centrifugation medium (GE Healthcare Life Sciences, Piscataway, NJ).
6. Disrupt lymphocytes in Qiagen RNeasy Mini Kit buffer RLT, a lysis buffer (Valencia, CA).
7. Store the lysed lymphocytes at −80 °C until analysis (*see* Sect. 4.2).

Plasma and Bioanalytical Analysis

To characterize pharmacokinetics, the plasma concentration of each compound is determined using the plasma obtained from samples above by HPLC, LC-MS or GC-MS.

1. Thaw and then prepare 50 μL of the plasma samples.
2. Add the internal standard (if necessary).
3. Add methanol of 100 μL into the each sample.
4. Vortex the mixture and then centrifuge at 10,000 × *g* at 4 °C for 3–5 min.
5. Collect the supernatant fractions and dry on a stream of nitrogen.
6. Reconstitute with appropriate solvent.
7. Analyze the compound concentrations in the plasma samples.

Lymphocyte RNA and qRT-PCR

To characterize pharmacodynamics, induction of mRNA is determined in lymphocytes using quantitative real-time PCR (qRT-PCR). Expression of Nrf2-mediated mRNA including *NQO1, GSTT1, Nrf2, GPx, Maf,* and *HO-1* may serve as surrogate biomarkers. The house keeping gene *β-actin* is used for mRNA level normalization. The oligonucleotide primers used qRT-PCR are designed using Nucleotide (http://www.ncbi.nlm.nih.gov) and PrimerQuest from Integrated DNA Technologies (http://www.idtdna.com, Coralville, IA) with 120–200 bp in amplicon size.

1. Thaw the lymphocyte RLT buffer solutions obtained from animal experiments.
2. Extract total RNA following the Qiagen RNeasy Mini Kit protocol.
3. Measure the total RNA concentrations using Quant-It reagents (Invitrogen, Carlsbad, CA).
4. Verify the purity using the spectrophotometric A260/A280 method.
5. Perform reverse-transcription using the same amount of RNA (~250 ng) to obtain cDNA with Applied Biosystems Taqman Reagent and oligo DT.
6. Conduct qRT-PCR using Applied Biosystems SYBR Green Master Mix (Foster City, CA).
7. Perform the analyses on an Applied Biosystems PRISM 7900HT following the established protocol of the ΔΔCt method.
8. Estimate the relative mRNA expression at each time point against their respective expression at time zero with Applied Biosystems Sequence Detection System software and Relative Quantitation Manager software.

Pharmacokinetic/Pharmacodynamic (PK/PD) Model Development

Pharmacokinetic profiles (i.e., plasma concentration–time profiles) for the compound are usually fitted according to a two-compartment system (Fig. 1), where the plasma concentration declines bi-exponentially. Pharmacodynamic profiles (i.e., relative mRNA expression-time profiles) are fitted according to Jusko's [53] indirect response model (Fig. 1). All pharmacokinetic and pharmacodynamic parameters are estimated by nonlinear regression analysis with various modeling software.

1. Fit the plasma concentration–time profile to the two-compartment model.

$$\frac{\mathrm{d}A_{\mathrm{c}}(t)}{\mathrm{d}t} = k_{pc} \cdot A_{\mathrm{p}} - \left(k_{pc} + \frac{CL}{V_{\mathrm{c}}}\right) \cdot A_{\mathrm{c}}; \quad A_{\mathrm{c}}(t=0) = Dose$$

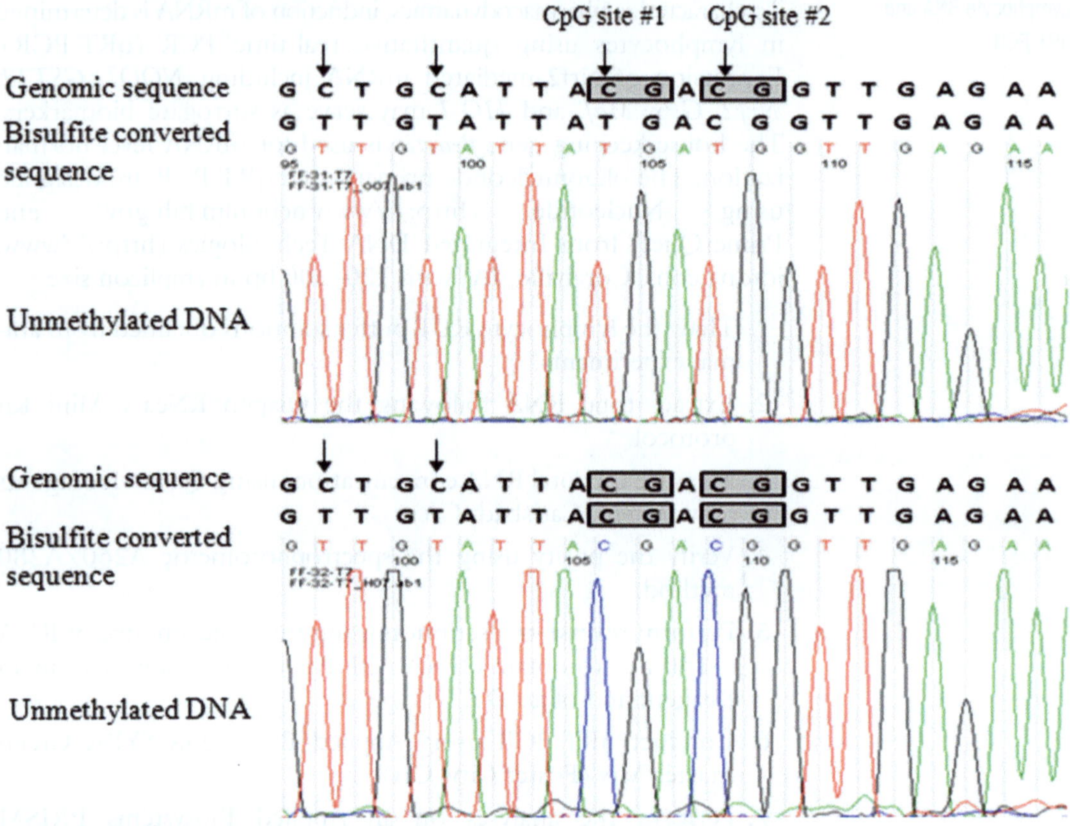

Fig. 1 Pharmacokinetic/pharmacodynamic (PK/PD) model for phase II drug metabolizing/antioxidant enzyme gene response to anticancer agent

$$\frac{\mathrm{d}A_{\mathrm{p}}(t)}{\mathrm{d}t} = -k_{pc} \cdot A_{\mathrm{p}} + k_{cp} \cdot A_{\mathrm{c}}; \quad A_{\mathrm{p}}(t=0)=0$$

Where k_{pc} and k_{cp} represent the inter-compartment rate constants between the central (c) and peripheral (p) compartments; CL, total clearance from central compartment; V_c, volume of central compartment; A_c and A_p, amount of drug in central and peripheral compartment, respectively.

2. Fit the relative mRNA expression-time profile to the indirect response model.

$$\frac{\mathrm{d}R}{\mathrm{d}t} = k_{in} \cdot E(t) - k_{out} \cdot R$$

Where,

$$E(t) = 1 + \frac{S_{\max} \cdot C_{\mathrm{c}}(t)}{SC_{50} + C_{\mathrm{c}}(t)}; \; E(0)=1$$

4 Epigenetics Approaches to Study NRF2 Regulation

DNA methylation is an essential epigenetic signal involved in development, gene regulation, imprinting, and preserving genome integrity [54]. Recently, a large amount of evidence has shown that epigenetic alterations such as DNA methylation and histone modifications consistently contribute to carcinogenesis [2, 55]. Thus, the hypermethylation of CpG islands is known to cause gene silencing of tumor suppressors and other genes with important biological functions by preventing the recruitment of transcriptional proteins from DNA, while promoters of transcriptionally active genes typically remain hypomethylated [56–58]. Furthermore, DNA methylation can interact with various methyl-CpG binding domain proteins (MBDs), such as MBD1–MBD4 and methyl CpG binding protein 2 (MeCP2), by providing a binding site [59, 60]. Thus, these binding proteins can interact with a co-repressor complex, including histone deacetylases (HDACs), resulting in transcriptional repression of genes [61, 62].

Technically, our findings have been mainly revealed by using techniques such as bisulfite genomic sequencing (BGS) and chromatin immunoprecipitation (ChIP). Bisulfite conversion and DNA sequencing are methods of choice, because together they provide detailed information on the methylation pattern of individual DNA molecules at single CpG site resolution. The BGS method is based on the deamination of cytosine residues to uracils in the presence of NaOH and sodium bisulfite [63]. Because methylcytosine is not converted under these conditions, the original methylation state of the DNA can be analyzed by sequencing of the converted DNA. After the conversion reaction, the DNA sequence under investigation is amplified by polymerase chain reaction (PCR) with primers specific for one strand of the bisulfite-converted DNA. The PCR product is cloned and individual clones are subsequently sequenced [64, 65]. On the other hand, the ChIP method relies on antibodies to identify the presence of specific histone modifications at DNA regions of interest [66]. Thus, the chromatin is extracted from cells or tissue, fragmented and incubated with antibodies against specific histone modifications. The chromatin fragments bound to the antibodies are captured using protein A/G beads, and DNA is isolated from the precipitate. This DNA is then analyzed by (quantitative) PCR to determine the abundance of a region of interest in the precipitated material [67].

Here we provide two standard protocols used in our studies to investigate the cancer chemopreventive effects of natural dietary compounds through epigenetics regulation of Nrf2.

4.1 Bisulfite Genomic Sequencing

4.1.1 Materials

Equipment

1. Bio-Rad C1000 Touch™ Thermal Cycler (Foster City, CA, USA).
2. Beckman Coulter™ Microfuge^R 18 Centrifuge (Fullerton, CA, USA).
3. Labnet International Gel XL Plus Electrophoresis System.
4. Bio-Rad Gel Doc 2000 Chemi Imaging (Foster City, CA, USA).
5. Fisher Scientific Isotemp 215 Dual-Chamber Water Bath (Pittsburgh, PA, USA).
6. New Brunswick Scientific Classic Series—C25 Incubator Shaker (Edison, NJ, USA).
7. Labnet International 211 DS Smart Check Incubator (Woodbridge, NJ, USA).
8. IEC Clinical Centrifuge with 12 × 14 mL rotor.
9. Zymo-Spin™ IC columns and collection tubes (Zymo Research).
10. BD Falcon™ 14 mL polystyrene round-bottom tube.

Reagents and Solutions

1. DNA input: Samples containing 500–600 ng of DNA (**Note 1**).
2. Commercially available bisulfite reaction kit, EZ DNA Methylation-Gold™ Kit (Zymo Research) containing: CT conversion reagent (sodium metabisulfite, ≥97 %) (**Note 2**); M-Dilution buffer (sodium hydroxid, 200 mM to 2 M); M-Dissolving buffer (dimethyl formamid, 50 %); M-Binding buffer (guanidine hydrochlorid, ≥3 M); M-Wash buffer (**Note 3**); M-Desulphonation buffer (sodium hydroxide, 200 mM to 2 M) and M-Elution buffer (*tris*-hydroxymethyl aminomethane/hydrochloric acid, ≤1 %; ethylenediaminetetraacetic acid, pH 8.0, ≤1 %).
3. TOPO TA Cloning® Kit for Sequencing (Invitrogen) containing: pCR®4-TOPO® (10 ng/μL plasmid DNA in 50 % glycerol, 50 mM Tris–HCl, pH 7.4 (at 25 °C), 1 mM EDTA, 2 mM DTT, 0.1 % Triton X-100, 100 μg/mL BSA and 30 μM phenol red); Salt Solution (1.2 M NaCl, 0.06 M $MgCl_2$); One Shot® TOP10 Chemically Competent *E. coli* and S.O.C. medium (2 % tryptone, 0.5 % yeast extract, 10 mM NaCl, 2.5 mM KCl, 10 mM $MgCl_2$, 10 mM $MgSO_4$, 20 mM glucose).
4. LB (Miller's) Broth 25 g/L, 12× (Tryptone 10.0 g/L, Yeast extract 5.0 g/L, NaCl 10.0 g/L).
5. LB plates containing 50 μg/mL ampicillin.
6. Platinum® Taq DNA Polymerase kit (Invitrogen) containing: Platinum® Taq DNA polymerase; 10× PCR buffer; 50 mM magnesium chloride and 10 mM dNTP mix.

7. BGS primers (10 μM).
8. Agarose (Low-EEO/Multi-Purpose/Molecular Biology Grade) (Fisher Scientific).
9. TrackIt™ 100-bp DNA Ladder (Invitrogen).
10. QIAquick® Gel Extraction Kit (Qiagen) containing: Buffer QG; Buffer PE; Isopropanol (100 %); QIAquick columns and Buffer EB (10 mM Tris–Cl, pH 8.5).

4.1.2 Methods

Bisulfate Reaction

1. Add 130 μL of the CT Conversion Reagent to 20 μL of your DNA sample in a PCR tube. If the volume of the DNA sample is less than 20 μL, make up the difference with water. Mix the sample by flicking the tube or pipetting the sample up and down, then centrifuge the liquid to the bottom of the tube.
2. Place the sample tube in a thermal cycler and perform the following steps: 98 °C for 10 min, 64 °C for 2.5 h and 4 °C storage up to 20 h.
3. Add 600 μL of M-Binding Buffer to a Zymo-Spin™ IC Column and place the column into a Collection Tube provided.
4. Load the sample (from **step 2**) into the Zymo-Spin™ IC Column containing the M-Binding Buffer. Close the cap and mix by inverting the column several times.
5. Centrifuge at full speed (<10,000 × *g*) for 30 s. Discard the flow-through.
6. Add 100 μL of M-Wash Buffer to the column. Centrifuge at full speed for 30 s.
7. Add 200 μL of M-Desulphonation Buffer to the column and let stand at room temperature (20–30 °C) for 15–20 min. After the incubation, centrifuge at full speed for 30 s.
8. Add 200 μL of M-Wash Buffer to the column. Centrifuge at full speed for 30 s. Add another 200 μL of M-Wash Buffer and centrifuge for an additional 30 s.
9. Place the column into a 1.5 mL microcentrifuge tube. Add 30 μL of M-Elution Buffer directly to the column matrix. Centrifuge for 30 s at full speed to elute the DNA (**Note 4**).

Bisulfite PCR Amplification

1. Bisulfite PCR primer design is critical for successful implementation of subsequent bisulfite sequencing analysis. The detailed guidelines for primer design of bisulfite treated-DNA templates are discussed in **Note 5**.
2. Add 2–3 μL of the bisulfite-converted DNA as template for the PCR reaction in a total volume of 20 μL (2 μL of PCR buffer, 1.5 μL of magnesium chloride, 0.6 μL of dNTP mix, 1 μL of BGS primers, 0.2 μL of Platinum® Taq DNA polymerase and 11.7 μL of water).

3. Perform PCR reaction with the following program: 94 °C 3 min; 94 °C 30 s, 70/55 °C 45 s, 72 °C 1 min, 15 cycles; 94 °C 30 s, 60 °C 45 s, 72 °C 1 min, 25 cycles; 72 °C 5 min (**Note 6**).
4. Verify by gel-based electrophoresis (1.5 % w/v) the PCR product using 10 μL of reaction.

PCR Purification (**Note 7**)

1. Excise the DNA fragment from the agarose gel with a clean, sharp scalpel.
2. Weigh the gel slice. Add 3 volumes Buffer QG to 1 volume gel (100 mg–100 μL).
3. Incubate at 50 °C for 10 min or until the gel slice has completely dissolved.
4. Add 1 gel volume of isopropanol to the sample and mix.
5. Apply the sample to the QIAquick column and centrifuge for 1 min. Discard flow-through. For sample volumes of >800 μL, load and spin again.
6. Add 0.5 mL Buffer QG to the QIAquick column and centrifuge for 1 min. Discard flow-through.
7. To wash, add 0.75 mL Buffer PE to QIAquick column and let the column stand 2–5 min after addition of Buffer PE. Centrifuge for 1 min and discard flow-through.
8. Centrifuge the QIAquick column once more for 1 min at 17,900 × *g* (13,000 rpm) to remove residual wash buffer.
9. Place QIAquick column into a clean 1.5 mL microcentrifuge tube.
10. To elute DNA, add 30 μL Buffer EB to the center of the QIAquick membrane, let the column stand for 1 min, and then centrifuge for 1 min.

TA Cloning of Target DNA Fragment

1. To perform the TOPO® cloning reaction, add 4.5 μL of fresh purified PCR product from PCR purification step, 1 μL of salt solution and 0.5 μL of TOPO® vector. Mix reaction gently and incubate for 10 min at room temperature (22–23 °C).
2. Add 2 μL of the TOPO® cloning reaction into 25 μL of One Shot® Chemically Competent *E. coli* and mix gently.
3. Incubate on ice for 20 min.
4. Heat-shock the cells for 30 s at 42 °C without shaking.
5. Immediately transfer the tubes to ice for 2 min.
6. Add 180 μL of room temperature S.O.C. medium and shake the tube horizontally (200 rpm) at 37 °C for 1 h.
7. Spread all the content from each transformation on a prewarmed selective LB plate and incubate overnight at 37 °C.

Miniprep and Sequencing

1. Pick ~10 single colonies from each treatment and inoculate a culture of 3 mL of LB medium containing ampicillin (100 μg/mL). Incubate for 12–16 h at 37 °C with vigorous shaking (200 rpm).
2. Harvest the bacterial cells by centrifugation at >8,000 rpm (6.800 × *g*) for 3 min at room temperature (15–25 °C) and discard the supernatant fraction.
3. Resuspend pelleted bacterial cells in 250 μL Buffer P1 and transfer to a microcentrifuge tube.
4. Add 250 μL Buffer P2 and mix thoroughly by inverting the tube 4–6 times (**Note 8**).
5. Add 350 μL Buffer N3 and mix immediately and thoroughly by inverting the tube 4–6 times.
6. Centrifuge for 10 min at 13,000 rpm (~17,900 × *g*).
7. Apply the supernatant fractions from **step 6** to the QIAprep spin column by decanting or pipetting.
8. Centrifuge for 30–60 s. Discard the flow-through.
9. Wash the QIAprep spin column by adding 0.5 mL Buffer PB and centrifuging for 30–60 s. Discard the flow-through.
10. Wash QIAprep spin column by adding 0.75 mL Buffer PE and centrifuging for 30–60 s.
11. Discard the flow-through, and centrifuge for an additional 1 min to remove residual wash buffer.
12. Place the QIAprep column in a 1.5 mL microcentrifuge tube. To elute DNA, add 30 μL Buffer EB to the center of each QIAprep spin column, let stand for 1 min, and centrifuge for 1 min.
13. Add 2 μL of eluted DNA into 8 μL of nuclease-free water and proceed with standard sequencing analysis (Genwiz, Piscataway, NJ) using T7 primer (5′-TAATACGACTCACTATAGGG-3′).

Data Analysis

1. Extract the sequencing results in FASTA format and create the alignment using regular sequence alignment software (e.g., MEGA5). An example of sequencing results of 2 single clones is shown in Fig. 2.
2. During this process, the data with incomplete bisulfite conversion or low-sequence identity can be excluded either with the software or manually.
3. Perform basic statistics of the methylation level (%) of at least 3 biological replicates, and generate the methylation pattern map.

4.2 Chromatin Immunoprecipitation Assay (CHIP)

4.2.1 Materials

Equipment

1. Bio-Rad C1000 Touch™ Thermal Cycler (Foster City, CA, USA).
2. DynaMag™-PCR Magnet (Invitrogen), or other magnet capable of holding 0.2-mL PCR tubes or strip wells.
3. Bioruptor® UCD-200 Sonicator (UCD-200, Diagenode).

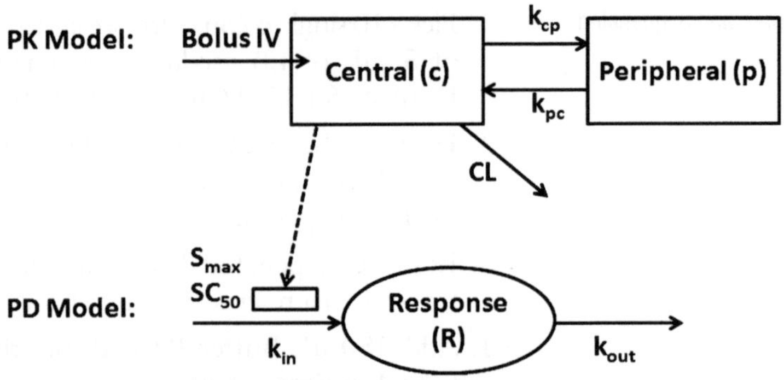

Fig. 2 Bisulfite sequencing traces for amplicons derived from an unmethylated (*top*) and methylated (*bottom*) single clone from the murine *Nrf2* promoter. After bisulfite conversion, the unmethylated cytosines are converted to thymines, leaving the methylated cytosine in the CpG site unaltered

4. Labnet International Gel XL Plus Electrophoresis System.
5. Bio-Rad Gel Doc 2000 Chemi Imaging (Foster City, CA, USA).
6. Applied Biosystems® ViiA™ 7 Real-Time PCR System (Carlsbad, CA, USA).
7. ABI PRISM™ 384-Well Clear Optical Reaction Plate (Carlsbad, CA, USA).
8. Eppendorf Centrifuge 5415 R (4 °C) (Hamburg, Germany).
9. Labnet International Spectrafuge™ Mini Centrifuge.
10. Vertical rotating mixer capable of holding 0.2-mL PCR tubes or strip wells.
11. Cell counter (hemacytometer).
12. Microcentrifuge tubes, RNase/DNase-free.
13. Fisher Touch Mixer Model 231 (Pittsburgh, PA, USA).

Reagents and Solutions

1. RPMI-1640 medium with 10 % fetal bovine serum (FBS, Gibco).
2. Dimethyl sulfoxide (DMSO) (St. Louis, MO, USA).
3. 5-Azadeoxycytidine (5-Aza) (St. Louis, MO, USA).
4. Trichostatin A (TSA) (St. Louis, MO, USA).
5. MAGnify™ Chromatin Immunoprecipitation System Kit (Invitrogen) containing: Glycine (1.25 M); Dynabeads® Protein A/G; Reverse Cross-linking Buffer; DNA Purification Magnetic Beads; DNA Purification Buffer; Proteinase K (20 mg/mL); IP Buffer 1; IP Buffer 2; DNA Wash Buffer; DNA Elution Buffer; Protease Inhibitors (200×); Mouse IgG (1 μg/μL); Rabbit IgG (1 μg/μL); Dilution Buffer and Lysis Buffer (**Note 9**).

6. Trypsin, 0.25 % (1×) with EDTA 4Na, liquid (Gibco).
7. Nuclease-free water.
8. Formaldehyde, 37 %, Molecular Biology Grade.
9. Phosphate Buffered Saline (PBS), PH 7.4, 1× liquid (Gibco).
10. SYBR® Green Real-Time PCR Master Mixes (Applied Biosystems).
11. qPCR primers for specific sequence of interest.
12. Antibodies: anti-Pol II, anti-MBD2, anti-MeCP2, anti-trimethyl-histone H3-Lys9 (H3K9me3), anti-H3Ac, and Rabbit IgG antibodies (Millipore, MA).

4.2.2 Methods

Coupling the Antibody to Dynabeads® (**Note 10**)

1. Resuspend the Dynabeads® using gentle up-and-down pipetting while taking care to avoid creating air bubbles.
2. Add 100 μL of cold Dilution Buffer to each tube (individual 0.2-mL PCR tubes).
3. Add 10 μL of fully resuspended Dynabeads® Protein A/G to each tube, and pipet up and down gently 5 times to mix.
4. Place the tubes in the DynaMag™-PCR Magnet and wait at least 30 s, or until the beads form a tight pellet.
5. With the tubes on the magnet, remove and discard the liquid, being careful not to disturb the bead pellet.
6. Remove the tube containing the pelleted magnetic beads from the magnet and add 100 μL of cold Dilution Buffer to each tube.
7. Add the antibody of interest to the appropriate experimental tubes (5 μg of anti-Pol II, 5 μg of anti-MBD2, 5 μg of anti-MeCP2, 5 μg of anti-trimethyl-histone H3-Lys9 (H3K9me3), 5 μg of anti-H3Ac, and 1 μg Rabbit IgG antibodies).
8. Cap the tubes and flick gently to resuspend the beads.
9. Rotate the tubes end-over-end at 4 °C for 1 h.

Collecting and Cross-linking Adherent Cells

1. Aspirate the media and wash cells with 10 mL of room temperature 1× PBS.
2. Aspirate the PBS and add enough trypsinizing reagent to cover the cells.
3. Incubate at 37 °C for ~3 min or until cells dislodge from the plate surface.
4. When all the cells have detached, add 10 mL of room-temperature PBS and pipet the cells gently up and down to mix.
5. Transfer the cell suspension to a centrifuge tube and spin at 200 × *g* for 5 min to pellet.
6. Discard the supernatant fraction and resuspend the pellet in room-temperature PBS. (Estimate the resuspension volume so

the cell density is more concentrated than your planned dilution.) Mix the cell solution gently.

7. Collect a small aliquot to verify that the cells are at the desired concentration. Determine cell density using a hemacytometer chamber.
8. Determine the volume of cell suspension required for the total number of immunoprecipitations (IPs) planned (number of cells per IP times the total number of IPs). Transfer this volume to a new tube.
9. If the volume is ≤500 μL, bring the final volume to 500 μL with room temperature PBS. If the volume is >500 μL, spin the cell suspension at 200 × *g* for 5 min, aspirate the supernatant fraction, and resuspend the pellet in 500 μL of PBS.
10. Add 13.5 μL of 37 % formaldehyde to the 500 μL of sample, for a final concentration of 1 %. Invert the tube to mix, and incubate for 10 min at room temperature.
11. To stop the reaction, add 57 μL of room-temperature 1.25 M glycine to the sample. Invert the tube to mix, and incubate for 5 min at room temperature.
12. In a cold centrifuge at 4 °C, spin the cross-linked cells at ~200 × *g* for 10 min. From this point on, keep all tubes on ice.
13. Remove and discard the supernatant fraction, leaving ~30 μL behind so as to not disturb the pellet.
14. Resuspend the cells in 500 μL of cold PBS, and spin at 200 × *g* for 10 min at 4 °C to pellet.
15. Aspirate the PBS and resuspend once more in 500 μL of cold PBS. Spin cells at 200 × *g* for 10 min at 4 °C to pellet.
16. Aspirate the PBS, leaving 10–20 μL behind. Make sure not to disturb the cell pellet.
17. Add 50 μL of Lysis Buffer with Protease Inhibitors per 1 million cells (e.g., add 100 μL for 2 million cells or 150 μL for 3 million cells) (**Note 11**).
18. Resuspend by mild pulses on the vortex mixer.
19. Incubate the tube on ice for at least 5 min.

Shearing the Chromatin into ~200–500 bp Fragments

1. Precool the water reservoir with ice.
2. Remove the ice and add ice-cold water to the water level mark.
3. Set the Bioruptor® UCD-200 to High Power, and sonicate the cell lysate for 16 cycles of 30 s ON, 30 s OFF. Make sure the water in the reservoir does not overheat (**Note 12**).
4. Pellet the debris by spinning at 20,000 × *g* at 4 °C for 5 min.
5. The supernatant fraction contains the chromatin. Aliquot the freshly sonicated chromatin into new, sterile tubes.

Diluting the Chromatin

1. Dilute the sheared chromatin in cold Dilution Buffer prepared with Protease Inhibitors to the final dilution volume of 100 μL per IP reaction.
2. The starting concentration of the chromatin is 1 million cells/50 μL. The ratio of chromatin to Dilution Buffer is based on the number of cells to use in each IP reaction (**Note 13**).
3. For each treatment performed, prepare an extra 100-μL dilution. Pipet up and down gently to fully mix, and save 10 μL of this dilution in a separate 0.2-μL PCR tube (input control).
4. Reverse the cross-linking of input control sample (*see* Sect. 4.2.2.7), and isolate the DNA without performing immunoprecipitation. This isolated DNA will be used as a positive control and can also be used for data normalization using qPCR, as described in Sect. 4.2.2.9.

Binding the Chromatin

1. From "Coupling the antibody to Dynabeads®" step, spin the tubes briefly to remove any liquid trapped in the caps, then place in the DynaMag™-PCR Magnet.
2. Let stand for at least 30 s, or until the beads form a tight pellet.
3. With the tubes on the magnet, remove and discard the liquid from each tube, being careful not to disturb the bead pellet.
4. Remove the tubes from the magnet and immediately add 100 μL of diluted chromatin extract (from Diluting the Chromatin step) to each tube containing the appropriate Antibody-Dynabeads® complex.
5. Cap the tubes and flick gently to resuspend the beads.
6. Rotate the tubes end-over-end at 4 °C for 2 h.

Washing the Bound Chromatin

1. Spin the tubes briefly to remove any liquid trapped in the caps, and then place the tubes in the DynaMag™-PCR Magnet.
2. Let stand for at least 30 s, or until the beads form a tight pellet.
3. With the tubes in the magnet, remove and discard the liquid from each tube, being careful not to disturb the bead pellet.
4. Remove the tubes from the magnet and add 100 μL of IP Buffer 1 to each tube. Cap the tubes and flick gently to resuspend the beads (**Note 14**).
5. Rotate the tubes end-over-end at 4 °C for 5 min.
6. Repeat **steps 1–5** two more times.
7. Spin the tubes briefly to remove any liquid trapped in the caps, and then place the tubes in the DynaMag™-PCR Magnet.
8. Let stand for at least 30 s, or until the beads form a tight pellet.
9. With the tubes in the magnet, remove and discard the liquid from each tube, being careful not to disturb the bead pellet.

10. Remove the tubes from the magnet and add 100 μL of IP Buffer 2 to each tube. Cap the tubes and flick gently to resuspend the beads (**Note 15**).
11. Rotate the tubes end-over-end at 4 °C for 5 min. (During rotation, prepare the Reverse Cross-linking Buffer with Proteinase K as described on the following page.)
12. Repeat **steps 7–11** one more time.

Reversing the Cross-linking (**Note 16**)

1. Place the tubes from Washing with IP Buffer 2, in the DynaMag™-PCR Magnet and wait at least 30 s for a pellet to form.
2. With the tubes in the magnet, remove and discard the liquid from each tube, being careful not to disturb the bead pellet.
3. Remove the tubes from the magnet and add 54 μL of Reverse Cross-linking Buffer prepared with Proteinase K to each tube (**Note 17**). Vortex lightly to fully resuspend the beads.
4. Incubate the IP sample tubes and Input Control tubes at 55 °C for 15 min in a thermal cycler.
5. Spin the tubes briefly and then proceed uninterrupted through the following steps.
6. Place the IP sample tubes in the DynaMag™-PCR Magnet and wait at least 30 s for a pellet to form.
7. Do not discard the liquid—the liquid contains the sample. With the tubes in the magnet, carefully transfer the liquid (~50 μL) to new, sterile 0.2-mL PCR tubes. Be careful not to disturb the bead pellet, and proceed immediately to the next step.
8. Spin the IP sample tubes and Input Control tubes briefly, and then incubate at 65 °C for 15 min.
9. Cool the tubes on ice for ~5 min.
10. Discard the used magnetic beads. Do not reuse.

Purifying the DNA (**Note 18**)

1. After the tubes from Reverse Cross-linking have cooled, spin them briefly to collect the contents.
2. Add 70 μL of DNA Purification Magnetic Beads prepared with DNA Purification Buffer to each tube (**Note 19**).
3. Pipet up and down gently 5 times to mix. Incubate at room temperature for 5 min.
4. Place the tubes in the DynaMag™-PCR Magnet and wait at least 1 min for a pellet to form.
5. With the tubes in the magnet, remove and discard the liquid from each tube, leaving ~5 μL at the bottom to avoid disturbing the beads.
6. Remove the tubes from the magnet and add 150 μL of DNA Wash Buffer to each tube. Pipet up and down gently 5 times to mix.

7. Repeat **steps 4–6** one time.
8. Place the tubes in the DynaMag™-PCR Magnet and wait at least 1 min for a pellet to form.
9. With the tubes in the magnet, remove and discard the liquid from each tube, leaving ~5 μL at the bottom to avoid disturbing the beads.
10. Remove the tubes from the magnet and add 150 μL of DNA Elution Buffer to each tube. Pipet up and down gently 5 times to mix.
11. Incubate at 55 °C for 20 min in a thermal cycler.
12. Spin the tubes briefly to collect the contents. Place the tubes in the DynaMag™-PCR Magnet and wait at least 1 min for a tight pellet to form.
13. Do not discard the liquid—the liquid contains the purified sample. With the tubes in the magnet, carefully transfer the liquid to new, sterile tubes. Leave ~5 μL at the bottom to avoid disturbing the beads.
14. Discard the used magnetic beads. Do not reuse.

ChIP-qPCR

1. Perform a 2-fold serial dilution of each input control sample in MAGnify™ DNA Elution Buffer (e.g., 2, 4, 8, 16 and 32).
2. Perform a qPCR reaction (in duplicate) in a total volume of 10 μL containing 4 μL of each IP DNA or diluted input control sample as template, 5 μL of SYBR® Green Real-Time PCR Master Mix and 1 μL of ChIP primers (**Notes 20** and **21**).
3. Run the qPCR reaction with the following program: hold stage (50 °C 2 min, 95 °C 10 min); PCR stage (95 °C 15 s, 60 °C 1 min, 40 times) and melt curve stage (95 °C 15 s, 60 °C 1 min and 95 °C 15 s).

Data Analysis

1. Export the qPCR data to a spreadsheet program such as Microsoft Excel. The file should not contain omitted wells and should be in a column format containing well positions, descriptors, and CT values for each selected well.
2. Average the replicate measurements for each diluted input control reaction in a new column.
3. Create a column with the log2 of each dilution factor (e.g., the 2× dilution factor is 0.05; then the log2 of 0.05 is −4.32).
4. Calculate a linear regression equation between log2 of dilution factors and CT values.
5. Calculate the log2 of each IP from CT values.
6. The enrichment as percentage of each IP on comparison with the input is calculated by: 100 × 2 (log2 IP).

5 Notes

1. The following is a general guideline for culturing of cell lines (e.g., LNCaP). Cells are plated in 10-cm plates for 24 h and then treated with 0.1 % DMSO, 5 μM curcumin, 2.5 μM of suphoraphane, or 2.5 μM 5-Aza with 1 % FBS-containing RPMI-1640 medium. The medium must be changed every 2 days. On the sixth day, for the 5-Aza and TSA combination treatment, 500 nM TSA is then added to the 5-Aza containing medium, cultured for another 24 h, and then the cells are ready to harvest for ChIP analysis. The cell culture must be undertaken in microbiological safety cabinet using aseptic technique to ensure sterility.
2. Preparation of CT conversion reagent: Add 900 μL water, 300 μL of M-Dilution Buffer, and 50 μL M-Dissolving Buffer to a tube of CT Conversion Reagent. Mix at room temperature with frequent vortexing or shaking for 10 min. For DNA volumes >20 μL, an adjustment needs to be made during the preparation of the CT Conversion Reagent. The amount of water is decreased 100 μL for each 10 μL increase in DNA sample volume. The maximum DNA sample volume to be used for each conversion reaction is 50 μL. Do not adjust the volumes of either the M-Dissolving Buffer or M-Dilution Buffer.
3. Preparation of M-Wash Buffer: Add 24 mL of 100 % ethanol to the 6 mL l M-Wash Buffer concentrate before use.
4. The DNA is ready for immediate analysis or can be stored at or below −20 °C for later use. For long-term storage, store at or below −70 °C.
5. After bisulfite treatment, the unmethylated cytosines are converted to thymine and methylated cytosines remain as cytosines. Because the methylation status of CpG dinucleotides is unknown, the bisulfite primer sequences should strictly avoid CpG dinucleotides. Therefore, primers should be generated to replace all cytosines to thymines according to the original DNA sequence. Primer designing software (e.g.: MethPrimer http://www.urogene.org/methprimer/) can also be used to avoid potential hairpin structures and possible primer dimers based on this modified sequence. The length of the primers should be around 25–30 nucleotides and the PCR product should not exceed 400 bp due to potential DNA degradation during the bisulfite modification that might influence the PCR amplification.
6. The bisulfite PCR conditions should be carefully optimized. Thus, a gradient PCR thermocycler can help to determine the appropriate annealing temperature. If no access to a gradient PCR thermocycler is available, a touchdown PCR can be applied to increase the annealing sensitivity.

7. Purification of PCR products is necessary to remove the residue of the PCR reaction and agarose that might interfere with the outcome of sequencing results. Commercially available kits such as QIAquick Gel Extraction kit (Qiagen) can be used to purify the target PCR product from multiple nonspecific PCR bands. The purified PCR products can be directly sequenced.
8. Do not allow the lysis reaction to proceed for more than 5 min.
9. Place the magnet, tubes, and buffers on ice before performing the following steps, to cool them down.
10. Never freeze the Dynabeads® or the DNA Purification Magnetic Beads, as this will damage the beads.
11. Vortex the Lysis Buffer briefly to resuspend, and then add Protease Inhibitors (200×) to achieve a final concentration of 1×. For example, to prepare 200 μL of Lysis Buffer with Protease Inhibitors, add 1 μL of 200× Protease Inhibitors to 199 μL of stock Lysis Buffer.
12. Sonication is a critical step in the MAGnify™ procedure. Testing various sonication conditions on your samples of interest is recommended and running treated chromatin lysates on a 1.5–2.0 % agarose gel with a 100-bp ladder to determine fragment length. For example, when starting with 1 million cells per 50 μL, add 1 μL of Proteinase K to 10 μL of chromatin input and incubate at 55 °C for 20 min prior to pelleting the cell debris by spinning at 20,000 × *g* at 4 °C for 5 min. Transfer the chromatin to a new tube and run ~5 μL of chromatin input per well in a agarose gel electrophoresis.
13. For example, using 100,000 cells per IP, the volume ratio of Chromatin and Dilution Buffer is of 5 μL and 95 μL, respectively.
14. Keep the magnets, tubes, and buffer cold during the procedure.
15. Keep magnet and tubes cold during the following steps. IP Buffer 2 can remain at room temperature.
16. All tubes and buffers should be at room temperature, unless otherwise indicated.
17. Prepare 54 μL of Reverse Cross-linking Buffer per IP reaction adding 53 μL of Stock Reverse Cross-linking Buffer and 1 μL of Proteinase K. To each tube containing 10 μL of Input Control, add 43 μL of Reverse Cross-linking Buffer and 1 μL of Proteinase K, for a total volume of 54 μL.
18. All beads and buffers should be at room temperature before use.
19. Briefly vortex the DNA Purification Magnetic Beads to resuspend. Prepare 70 μL of beads per sample by adding 50 μL of DNA Purification Buffer to 20 μL of resuspended DNA Purification Magnetic Beads. Scale accordingly based on your number of samples (including Input Controls). Pipet up and down gently 5 times to mix.

20. The ChIP primers should be 20–30 bases long with a Tm of 60 °C, and should be designed for an amplicon length of approximately 80–250 bp. A final concentration of 200 nM per primer is effective for most reactions. Using a primer design software such as Primer Express 3.0 at http://frodo.wi.mit.edu/ is recommended. After primer design, perform a BLAST search of NCBI databases to ensure that primers are target-specific.
21. For each ChIP primer pair, run the Input Control DNA alongside the immunoprecipitated samples to quantify the enrichment of the eluted DNA in comparison with the inputs by qPCR.

References

1. Wattenberg LW (1985) Chemoprevention of cancer. Cancer Res 45(1):1–8
2. Su ZY, Shu L, Khor TO, Lee JH, Fuentes F, Kong AN (2013) A perspective on dietary phytochemicals and cancer chemoprevention: oxidative stress, Nrf2, and epigenomics. Top Curr Chem 329:133–162. doi:10.1007/128_2012_340
3. Chen C, Pung D, Leong V, Hebbar V, Shen G, Nair S, Li W, Kong AN (2004) Induction of detoxifying enzymes by garlic organosulfur compounds through transcription factor Nrf2: effect of chemical structure and stress signals. Free Radic Biol Med 37(10):1578–1590. doi:10.1016/j.freeradbiomed.2004.07.021, pii:S0891-5849(04)00580-5
4. Yu S, Kong AN (2007) Targeting carcinogen metabolism by dietary cancer preventive compounds. Curr Cancer Drug Targets 7(5):416–424
5. He CH, Gong P, Hu B, Stewart D, Choi ME, Choi AM, Alam J (2001) Identification of activating transcription factor 4 (ATF4) as an Nrf2-interacting protein. Implication for heme oxygenase-1 gene regulation. J Biol Chem 276(24):20858–20865. doi:10.1074/jbc.M101198200M101198200
6. Jaiswal AK (2004) Nrf2 signaling in coordinated activation of antioxidant gene expression. Free Radic Biol Med 36(10):1199–1207. doi:10.1016/j.freeradbiomed, pii: 2004.02.074S0891584904001923
7. Levy S, Forman HJ (2010) C-Myc is a Nrf2-interacting protein that negatively regulates phase II genes through their electrophile responsive elements. IUBMB Life 62(3):237–246. doi:10.1002/iub.314
8. Alam J, Stewart D, Touchard C, Boinapally S, Choi AM, Cook JL (1999) Nrf2, a Cap'n'Collar transcription factor, regulates induction of the heme oxygenase-1 gene. J Biol Chem 274(37):26071–26078
9. Ishii T, Itoh K, Takahashi S, Sato H, Yanagawa T, Katoh Y, Bannai S, Yamamoto M (2000) Transcription factor Nrf2 coordinately regulates a group of oxidative stress-inducible genes in macrophages. J Biol Chem 275(21):16023–16029. doi:275/21/16023
10. Wu TY, Saw CL, Khor TO, Pung D, Boyanapalli SS, Kong AN (2012) In vivo pharmacodynamics of indole-3-carbinol in the inhibition of prostate cancer in transgenic adenocarcinoma of mouse prostate (TRAMP) mice: involvement of Nrf2 and cell cycle/apoptosis signaling pathways. Mol Carcinog 51(10):761–770. doi:10.1002/mc.20841
11. Sun Z, Wu T, Zhao F, Lau A, Birch CM, Zhang DD (2011) KPNA6 (Importin {alpha}7)-mediated nuclear import of Keap1 represses the Nrf2-dependent antioxidant response. Mol Cell Biol 31(9):1800–1811. doi:10.1128/MCB.05036-11, MCB.05036-11
12. Lee JH, Khor TO, Shu L, Su ZY, Fuentes F, Kong AN (2013) Dietary phytochemicals and cancer prevention: Nrf2 signaling, epigenetics, and cell death mechanisms in blocking cancer initiation and progression. Pharmacol Ther 137(2):153–171. doi:10.1016/j.pharmthera.2012.09.008
13. Khor TO, Huang Y, Wu TY, Shu L, Lee J, Kong AN (2011) Pharmacodynamics of curcumin as DNA hypomethylation agent in restoring the expression of Nrf2 via promoter CpGs demethylation. Biochem Pharmacol 82(9):1073–1078. doi:10.1016/j.bcp.2011.07.065
14. Xu C, Huang MT, Shen G, Yuan X, Lin W, Khor TO, Conney AH, Kong AN (2006)

Inhibition of 7,12-dimethylbenz(a)anthracene-induced skin tumorigenesis in C57BL/6 mice by sulforaphane is mediated by nuclear factor E2-related factor 2. Cancer Res 66(16):8293–8296. doi:10.1158/0008-5472.CAN-06-0300
15. Zhang C, Su ZY, Khor TO, Shu L, Kong AN (2013) Sulforaphane enhances Nrf2 expression in prostate cancer TRAMP C1 cells through epigenetic regulation. Biochem Pharmacol 85(9):1398–1404. doi: 10.1016/j.bcp.2013.02.010
16. Shen G, Xu C, Hu R, Jain MR, Nair S, Lin W, Yang CS, Chan JY, Kong AN (2005) Comparison of (−)-epigallocatechin-3-gallate elicited liver and small intestine gene expression profiles between C57BL/6J mice and C57BL/6J/Nrf2 (−/−) mice. Pharm Res 22(11):1805–1820. doi:10.1007/s11095-005-7546-8
17. Kang HJ, Hong YB, Kim HJ, Wang A, Bae I (2011) Bioactive food components prevent carcinogenic stress via Nrf2 activation in BRCA1 deficient breast epithelial cells. Toxicol Lett 209(2):154–160. doi:10.1016/j.toxlet.2011.12.002, pii: S0378-4274(11)01653-5
18. Barve A, Khor TO, Nair S, Reuhl K, Suh N, Reddy B, Newmark H, Kong AN (2009) Gamma-tocopherol-enriched mixed tocopherol diet inhibits prostate carcinogenesis in TRAMP mice. Int J Cancer 124(7):1693–1699. doi:10.1002/ijc.24106
19. Yu S, Khor TO, Cheung KL, Li W, Wu TY, Huang Y, Foster BA, Kan YW, Kong AN (2010) Nrf2 expression is regulated by epigenetic mechanisms in prostate cancer of TRAMP mice. PLoS One 5(1):e8579. doi:10.1371/journal.pone.0008579
20. Cho HY, Reddy SP, Debiase A, Yamamoto M, Kleeberger SR (2005) Gene expression profiling of NRF2-mediated protection against oxidative injury. Free Radic Biol Med 38(3):325–343. doi:10.1016/j.freeradbiomed.2004.10.013, pii: S0891-5849(04)00835-4
21. Kwak MK, Wakabayashi N, Itoh K, Motohashi H, Yamamoto M, Kensler TW (2003) Modulation of gene expression by cancer chemopreventive dithiolethiones through the Keap1-Nrf2 pathway. Identification of novel gene clusters for cell survival. J Biol Chem 278(10):8135–8145. doi:10.1074/jbc.M211898200M211898200
22. Lee JM, Calkins MJ, Chan K, Kan YW, Johnson JA (2003) Identification of the NF-E2-related factor-2-dependent genes conferring protection against oxidative stress in primary cortical astrocytes using oligonucleotide microarray analysis. J Biol Chem 278(14):12029–12038. doi:10.1074/jbc.M211558200M211558200
23. Rangasamy T, Cho CY, Thimmulappa RK, Zhen L, Srisuma SS, Kensler TW, Yamamoto M, Petrache I, Tuder RM, Biswal S (2004) Genetic ablation of Nrf2 enhances susceptibility to cigarette smoke-induced emphysema in mice. J Clin Invest 114(9):1248–1259. doi:10.1172/JCI21146
24. Thimmulappa RK, Mai KH, Srisuma S, Kensler TW, Yamamoto M, Biswal S (2002) Identification of Nrf2-regulated genes induced by the chemopreventive agent sulforaphane by oligonucleotide microarray. Cancer Res 62(18):5196–5203
25. Rushmore TH, Morton MR, Pickett CB (1991) The antioxidant responsive element. Activation by oxidative stress and identification of the DNA consensus sequence required for functional activity. J Biol Chem 266(18):11632–11639
26. Villeneuve NF, Lau A, Zhang DD (2010) Regulation of the Nrf2-Keap1 antioxidant response by the ubiquitin proteasome system: an insight into cullin-ring ubiquitin ligases. Antioxidants Redox Signal 13(11):1699–1712. doi:10.1089/ars.2010. 3211
27. Hayes JD, McMahon M, Chowdhry S, Dinkova-Kostova AT (2010) Cancer chemoprevention mechanisms mediated through the Keap1-Nrf2 pathway. Antioxidants Redox Signal 13(11):1713–1748. doi:10.1089/ars.2010.3221
28. Yu R, Mandlekar S, Lei W, Fahl WE, Tan TH, Kong AN (2000) p38 mitogen-activated protein kinase negatively regulates the induction of phase II drug-metabolizing enzymes that detoxify carcinogens. J Biol Chem 275(4):2322–2327
29. Saw CL, Cintron M, Wu TY, Guo Y, Huang Y, Jeong WS, Kong AN (2011) Pharmacodynamics of dietary phytochemical indoles I3C and DIM: Induction of Nrf2-mediated phase II drug metabolizing and antioxidant genes and synergism with isothiocyanates. Biopharm Drug Dispos 32(5):289–300. doi:10.1002/bdd.759
30. Chen C, Yu R, Owuor ED, Kong AN (2000) Activation of antioxidant-response element (ARE), mitogen-activated protein kinases (MAPKs) and caspases by major green tea polyphenol components during cell survival and death. Arch Pharm Res 23(6):605–612
31. Wu TY, Khor TO, Saw CL, Loh SC, Chen AI, Lim SS, Park JH, Cai L, Kong AN (2011) Anti-inflammatory/anti-oxidative stress activities and differential regulation of Nrf2-mediated genes by non-polar fractions of tea Chrysanthemum zawadskii and licorice Glycyrrhiza uralensis. AAPS J 13(1):1–13. doi:10.1208/s12248-010-9239-4

32. Prawan A, Keum YS, Khor TO, Yu S, Nair S, Li W, Hu L, Kong AN (2008) Structural influence of isothiocyanates on the antioxidant response element (ARE)-mediated heme oxygenase-1 (HO-1) expression. Pharm Res 25(4):836–844. doi:10.1007/s11095-007-9370-9
33. Jeong WS, Keum YS, Chen C, Jain MR, Shen G, Kim JH, Li W, Kong AN (2005) Differential expression and stability of endogenous nuclear factor E2-related factor 2 (Nrf2) by natural chemopreventive compounds in HepG2 human hepatoma cells. J Biochem Mol Biol 38(2):167–176
34. Kim BR, Hu R, Keum YS, Hebbar V, Shen G, Nair SS, Kong AN (2003) Effects of glutathione on antioxidant response element-mediated gene expression and apoptosis elicited by sulforaphane. Cancer Res 63(21):7520–7525
35. Yuan X, Xu C, Pan Z, Keum YS, Kim JH, Shen G, Yu S, Oo KT, Ma J, Kong AN (2006) Butylated hydroxyanisole regulates ARE-mediated gene expression via Nrf2 coupled with ERK and JNK signaling pathway in HepG2 cells. Mol Carcinog 45(11):841–850. doi:10.1002/mc.20234
36. Saw CL, Huang Y, Kong AN (2010) Synergistic anti-inflammatory effects of low doses of curcumin in combination with polyunsaturated fatty acids: docosahexaenoic acid or eicosapentaenoic acid. Biochem Pharmacol 79(3):421–430. doi:10.1016/j.bcp.2009.08.030
37. Chan K, Lu R, Chang JC, Kan YW (1996) NRF2, a member of the NFE2 family of transcription factors, is not essential for murine erythropoiesis, growth, and development. Proc Natl Acad Sci U S A 93(24):13943–13948
38. Yoh K, Itoh K, Enomoto A, Hirayama A, Yamaguchi N, Kobayashi M, Morito N, Koyama A, Yamamoto M, Takahashi S (2001) Nrf2-deficient female mice develop lupus-like autoimmune nephritis. Kidney Int 60(4):1343–1353. doi:10.1046/j.1523-1755.2001.00939.x, pii: kid939
39. Chanas SA, Jiang Q, McMahon M, McWalter GK, McLellan LI, Elcombe CR, Henderson CJ, Wolf CR, Moffat GJ, Itoh K, Yamamoto M, Hayes JD (2002) Loss of the Nrf2 transcription factor causes a marked reduction in constitutive and inducible expression of the glutathione S-transferase Gsta1, Gsta2, Gstm1, Gstm2, Gstm3 and Gstm4 genes in the livers of male and female mice. Biochem J 365(Pt 2):405–416. doi:10.1042/BJ20020320BJ20020320
40. Cho HY, Jedlicka AE, Reddy SP, Kensler TW, Yamamoto M, Zhang LY, Kleeberger SR (2002) Role of NRF2 in protection against hyperoxic lung injury in mice. Am J Respir Cell Mol Biol 26(2):175–182
41. Bauer AK, Cho HY, Miller-Degraff L, Walker C, Helms K, Fostel J, Yamamoto M, Kleeberger SR (2011) Targeted deletion of Nrf2 reduces urethane-induced lung tumor development in mice. PLoS One 6(10):e26590. doi:10.1371/journal.pone.0026590PONE-D-11-06632
42. Itoh K, Chiba T, Takahashi S, Ishii T, Igarashi K, Katoh Y, Oyake T, Hayashi N, Satoh K, Hatayama I, Yamamoto M, Nabeshima Y (1997) An Nrf2/small Maf heterodimer mediates the induction of phase II detoxifying enzyme genes through antioxidant response elements. Biochem Biophys Res Commun 236(2):313–322, S0006291X97969436
43. Chan K, Kan YW (1999) Nrf2 is essential for protection against acute pulmonary injury in mice. Proc Natl Acad Sci U S A 96(22):12731–12736
44. Yu X, Kensler T (2005) Nrf2 as a target for cancer chemoprevention. Mutat Res 591(1–2):93–102. doi:10.1016/j.mrfmmm.2005.04.017, pii: S0027-5107(05)00309-X
45. Goerttler K, Loehrke H, Schweizer J, Hesse B (1979) Systemic two-stage carcinogenesis in the epithelium of the forestomach of mice using 7,12-dimethylbenz(a)anthracene as initiator and the phorbol ester 12-O-tetradecanoylphorbol-13-acetate as promoter. Cancer Res 39(4):1293–1297
46. Bartsch H, Nair J (2006) Chronic inflammation and oxidative stress in the genesis and perpetuation of cancer: role of lipid peroxidation, DNA damage, and repair. Langenbecks Arch Surg 391(5):499–510. doi:10.1007/s00423-006-0073-1
47. Coussens LM, Werb Z (2002) Inflammation and cancer. Nature 420(6917):860–867. doi:10.1038/nature01322nature01322
48. Hussain SP, Harris CC (2007) Inflammation and cancer: an ancient link with novel potentials. Int J Cancer 121(11):2373–2380. doi:10.1002/ijc.23173
49. Ekbom A, Helmick C, Zack M, Adami HO (1990) Ulcerative colitis and colorectal cancer. A population-based study. N Engl J Med 323(18):1228–1233. doi:10.1056/NEJM199011013231802
50. Boismenu R, Chen Y (2000) Insights from mouse models of colitis. J Leukoc Biol 67(3):267–278
51. Khor TO, Huang M-T, Kwon KH, Chan JY, Reddy BS, Kong A-N (2006) Nrf2-deficient

mice have an increased susceptibility to dextran sulfate sodium–induced colitis. Cancer Res 66(24):11580–11584. doi:10.1158/0008-5472.can-06-3562

52. Wang H, Khor TO, Yang Q, Huang Y, T-y W, Saw CL-L, Lin W, Androulakis IP, Kong A-NT (2012) Pharmacokinetics and pharmacodynamics of phase II drug metabolizing/antioxidant enzymes gene response by anticancer agent sulforaphane in rat lymphocytes. Mol Pharm 9(10):2819–2827. doi:10.1021/mp300130k
53. Dayneka NL, Garg V, Jusko WJ (1993) Comparison of four basic models of indirect pharmacodynamic responses. J Pharmacokinet Biopharm 21(4):457–478
54. Sadikovic B, Al-Romaih K, Squire JA, Zielenska M (2008) Cause and consequences of genetic and epigenetic alterations in human cancer. Curr Genomics 9(6):394–408. doi:10.2174/138920208785699580
55. Link A, Balaguer F, Goel A (2010) Cancer chemoprevention by dietary polyphenols: promising role for epigenetics. Biochem Pharmacol 80(12):1771–1792. doi:10.1016/j.bcp.2010.06.036
56. Prendergast GC, Ziff EB (1991) Methylation-sensitive sequence-specific DNA binding by the c-Myc basic region. Science 251(4990):186–189
57. Suzuki MM, Bird A (2008) DNA methylation landscapes: provocative insights from epigenomics. Nat Rev Genet 9(6):465–476
58. Esteller M (2002) CpG island hypermethylation and tumor suppressor genes: a booming present, a brighter future. Oncogene 21(35):5427–5440
59. Hendrich B, Bird A (1998) Identification and characterization of a family of mammalian methyl-CpG binding proteins. Mol Cell Biol 18(11):6538–6547
60. Lewis JD, Meehan RR, Henzel WJ, Maurer-Fogy I, Jeppesen P, Klein F, Bird A (1992) Purification, sequence, and cellular localization of a novel chromosomal protein that binds to methylated DNA. Cell 69(6):905–914
61. Feng Q, Zhang Y (2001) The MeCP1 complex represses transcription through preferential binding, remodeling, and deacetylating methylated nucleosomes. Genes Dev 15(7):827–832
62. Nan X, Ng HH, Johnson CA, Laherty CD, Turner BM, Eisenman RN, Bird A (1998) Transcriptional repression by the methyl-CpG-binding protein MeCP2 involves a histone deacetylase complex. Nature 393(6683):386–389
63. Li LC, Dahiya R (2002) MethPrimer: designing primers for methylation PCRs. Bioinformatics 18(11):1427–1431
64. Clark SJ, Harrison J, Paul CL, Frommer M (1994) High sensitivity mapping of methylated cytosines. Nucleic Acids Res 22(15):2990–2997
65. Grunau C, Clark SJ, Rosenthal A (2001) Bisulfite genomic sequencing: systematic investigation of critical experimental parameters. Nucleic Acids Res 29(13):E65–E75
66. Solomon MJ, Larsen PL, Varshavsky A (1988) Mapping protein–DNA interactions in vivo with formaldehyde: evidence that histone H4 is retained on a highly transcribed gene. Cell 53(6):937–947, pii: S0092-8674(88)90469-2
67. Haring M, Offermann S, Danker T, Horst I, Peterhansel C, Stam M (2007) Chromatin immunoprecipitation: optimization, quantitative analysis and data normalization. Plant Methods 3:11. doi:10.1186/1746-4811-3-11, pii: 1746-4811-3-11

Chapter 4

Methods to Analyze Chemopreventive Effect of Silibinin on Prostate Cancer Biomarkers Protein Expression

Gagan Deep, Swetha Inturi, and Rajesh Agarwal

Abstract

Prostate cancer is now diagnosed mostly at an early stage, and therefore, chemopreventive strategies could be useful to prevent further progression of the disease and to reduce the morbidity and mortality due to this malignancy. Here, we have described methods (immunoblotting, immunofluorescence, and immunohistochemistry) that could be employed to screen and validate the effect of chemopreventive agents on the protein expression of various cancer-related biomarkers for proliferation, apoptosis, angiogenesis, and metastasis. As an example, we have discussed chemopreventive efficacy of silibinin against prostate cancer as well as its effect on several molecular biomarkers associated with this malignancy. Overall, the methods used to study cancer biomarker protein expression that we describe in this chapter are extremely useful in cancer chemopreventive studies.

Key words Prostate cancer, Chemoprevention, Silibinin, Immunoblotting, Immunofluorescence, Immunohistochemistry, Confocal, Biomarkers

1 Introduction

1.1 Prostate Cancer Chemoprevention

Prostate cancer (PCA) is the most common non-cutaneous malignancy and, second to lung cancer, the most common cause of cancer-associated deaths in American men [1]. According to the American Cancer Society in 2012, ~241,740 new cases were diagnosed and 28,170 deaths occurred due to this cancer in the USA [1]. Patients with localized PCA have a high 5-year survival rate and a relatively low mortality to incidence ratio compared to other cancer types [2]. However, in PCA patients with metastasis, the median survival is reduced to only 12–15 months [2–4] suggesting the importance of early diagnosis and targeting the disease progression to metastatic stage to reduce mortality. Due to existing screening measures, PCA could be diagnosed at early stages when the disease is still localized in the prostate or surrounding tissues; however, existing curative measures, including anti-androgen therapy, radiotherapy, and chemotherapy, are studded with significant side

Ann M. Bode and Zigang Dong (eds.), *Cancer Prevention: Dietary Factors and Pharmacology*, Methods in Pharmacology and Toxicology, DOI 10.1007/978-1-4614-9227-6_4, © Springer Science+Business Media New York 2014

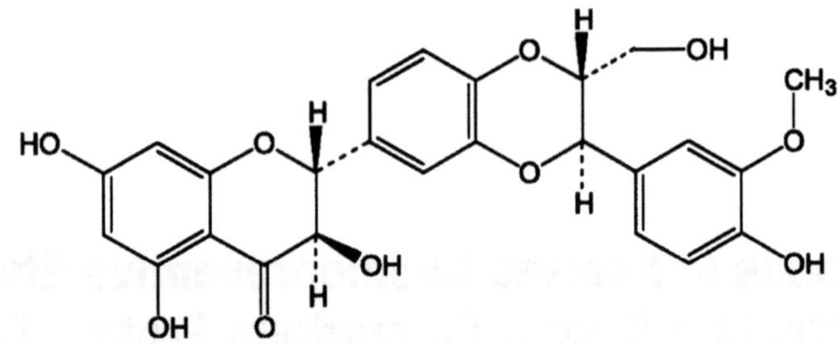

Fig. 1 Chemical structure of silibinin

effects [5–8]. Therefore, often, patients diagnosed with localized indolent disease are not treated initially, known as the "watchful waiting" regime, to avoid treatment sides effects such as hair loss, pain, urinary incontinence, permanent impotence, compromised sexual potential, nausea, vomiting, and diarrhea. We believe that chemoprevention strategies could fill this gap and prevent the disease progression without significant side effects. The administration of chemopreventive agents has been shown to prevent initiation, promotion, and progression stages of carcinogenesis in different animal models, and is suggested to effectively reduce cancer morbidity and mortality [9–13]. These agents are usually inexpensive, nontoxic to normal cells, selectively target cancer cells through pleiotropic mechanisms, and are biologically available following oral administration [9, 10, 14]. Therefore, preventing or inhibiting the growth and progression of PCA through nontoxic chemopreventive agents could be an ideal strategy considering the fact that prostate carcinogenesis involves multiple processes and usually requires more than a decade for the development of clinically significant disease. Among various groups of chemopreventive agents, extensive epidemiological and preclinical data have been generated in recent years supporting the efficacy of phytochemicals against human PCA [11, 12, 15, 16]. Here, we have briefly described the chemopreventive potential of a flavonoid, *silibinin*, against PCA.

1.2 Cancer Chemopreventive Efficacy of Silibinin

Silibinin ($C_{25}H_{22}O_{10}$, molecular weight, 482.44, Fig. 1) is isolated from the seeds of *Silybum marianum* (L.) Gaertn (Family Asteraceae), which is also known as milk thistle. Both milk thistle extract and silibinin have a long history of use in traditional medicine to treat a variety of diseases especially related to the liver [17, 18]. A large body of literature illustrates the cancer chemopreventive efficacy of silibinin in cell culture, animal models and human studies [14, 19–23]. Silibinin has been reported to be effective against multiple cancer sites including prostate, skin, lung, colon, breast, glioblastoma, ovarian, bladder, leukemia, cervical, kidney, laryngeal, osteosarcoma, oral, and gastric [14]. Several molecular mechanisms have been propounded to describe silibinin's broad spectrum of cancer chemopreventive efficacy, including the induction of CDK (cyclin dependent kinase) inhibitors, and inhibition of epidermal growth factor receptor (EGFR) and NF-κB pathways [9, 14, 24–27]. In addition, silibinin has also been reported to target tumor microenvironment components (e.g., endothelial cells, cancer-associated fibroblasts, macrophages, osteoclasts) to exert its cancer chemopreventive efficacy [16, 28–30].

An abundant amount of literature has focused on the cancer chemopreventive efficacy of silibinin against PCA [9, 14, 16, 19, 27, 28, 31]. Silibinin has been reported to target the deregulated cell cycle to inhibit PCA cell proliferation [32, 33]. Furthermore, oral administration of silibinin has also been reported to reduce the growth of human PCA PC3 and DU145 cells implanted in nude mice as xenografts [28, 34–36]. More relevant to clinical conditions, silibinin feeding was shown to significantly prevent the disease progression in the TRAMP (transgenic adenocarcinoma of the mouse prostate) mouse model [13, 31, 37]. Recently, clinical trials are being conducted to examine the chemopreventive usefulness of silibinin in PCA patients [20, 21].

1.3 Prostate Cancer Biomarkers Employed in Establishing the Chemopreventive Efficacy of Silibinin

To assess the chemopreventive efficacy of silibinin, others and we have employed several biomarkers associated with growth, progression, and metastasis of PCA cells. For example, silibinin was reported to target androgen receptor (AR) signaling and to decrease the expression of prostate specific antigen (PSA) in PCA cells [33, 38, 39]. Importantly, AR is considered a major driver as well as a relevant drug target at each stage of prostate carcinogenesis; and until recently, PSA was widely accepted as the most useful biomarker for the diagnosis and prognosis of PCA [40]. Another biomarker employed frequently to study the inhibitory effect of silibinin on the proliferation rate of PCA cells is PCNA (proliferating cell nuclear antigen) that plays a role in DNA synthesis and repair [28, 35, 37, 41, 42]. Similarly, Ki-67, cyclins, CDKs, and CDKIs have also been used to understand the growth inhibitory effects of silibinin against PCA [13, 37, 41]. To understand the effect of silibinin on apoptosis induction in PCA cells, the TUNEL (terminal deoxynucleotidyl transferase dUTP nick end labeling) assay and cleaved caspase 3 are utilized [28, 35, 41, 42]. Angiogenesis biomarkers such as CD31, VEGF (vascular endothelial growth factor), VEGF receptor (VEGFR), HIF-1α (hypoxia inducible factor alpha), and FGF (fibroblast growth factor) have been extensively used to establish angiopreventive efficacy of silibinin against PCA [13, 28, 31, 41, 42]. Further, the protein expression of IGF (insulin-like growth factors), IGF receptor, and IGF binding protein (IGFBP) have also been frequently studied as endpoint biomarkers to understand the molecular underpinnings of silibinin's chemopreventive efficacy against PCA [35, 36, 43].

The epithelial to mesenchymal transition (EMT) is now considered an integral component of metastasis [8, 15]; and metastasis could be prevented by targeting EMT in primary PCA cells. We have reported that silibinin targets EMT by enhancing the protein expression of epithelial biomarker E-cadherin and inhibiting the protein expression of several mesenchymal biomarkers (e.g., snail1, fibronectin, vimentin) [13, 19, 31]. Importantly, inhibition of EMT by silibinin translated into a significant prevention of PCA metastasis [13, 31], signifying the importance of studying biomarkers in establishing the efficacy as well as the mechanism(s) of action of silibinin against PCA.

The above-mentioned biomarkers for proliferation, apoptosis, angiogenesis, and EMT could be employed for the testing of novel chemopreventive agents both in cell culture and animal models. The techniques that are usually used to study the protein expression of these biomarkers are immunoblotting, immunofluorescence, and immunohistochemistry. The underlying principle in all three techniques is similar, and the protein of interest is probed with primary and secondary antibodies. However, the final signal is detected differently. For example, in immunoblotting, proteins are separated based upon their molecular weight and electric charge and probed for the protein of interest using a primary antibody. Subsequently, a species-specific secondary antibody, usually linked to a reporter enzyme such as horseradish peroxidase (HRP), is directed at the primary antibody. HRP-tagged to the secondary antibody catalyzes a reaction involving hydrogen peroxide (H_2O_2), luminol, and a signal enhancer. This reaction results in the emission of a blue luminescence, which is in proportion to the amount of protein in the sample. Similarly, in immunohistochemistry, following primary and secondary antibodies incubation, HRP-tagged streptavidin (directed towards the secondary antibody) is used to catalyze a reaction involving H_2O_2 and DAB (3,3'-diaminobenzidine) producing a brown color precipitate in the area of the antibody binding with the antigen and reflects the protein level in the tissue. In immunofluorescence, a secondary antibody is tagged with a fluorescent dye, which on excitation emits light of specific wavelength and is detected by a fluorescent microscope. Immune-fluorescence has an added advantage because in addition to detecting the protein of interest cellular localization of the protein as well as its co-localization with other proteins can also be studied.

2 Materials

2.1 Equipment

1. Tissue-Tearor (BioSpec Products, Markham, Ontario, Canada) for homogenizing tissues.
2. Vortex-Genie 2 (Scientific Industries Inc., Bohemia, NY).

3. Precision 280-Series Microprocessor based water bath (Thomas Scientific, Swedesboro, NJ).
4. Centrific Centrifuge Model 225 bench top centrifuge (Thermo Fisher Scientific, Pittsburg, PA).
5. Table top 5415R microcentrifuge (Eppendorf, Hamburg, Germany).
6. Smartspec 3000 spectrophotometer (Bio-Rad, Philadelphia, PA) for protein estimation.
7. PowerPac™ Basic power supply (Bio-Rad, Philadelphia, PA) and XCell SureLock™ Mini-Cell electrophoresis system (Life Technologies, Grand Island, NY) for SDS-PAGE gel electrophoresis.
8. Nikon D Eclipse C1 Plus Confocal Microscope with Nikon EZ-C1 FreeViewer software (Nikon Instruments, Melville, NY) to analyze the immunofluorescence staining.
9. Tissue Processing Center TPC 15 (Medite GmbH, Wollenweberstraße, Burgdorf, Germany).
10. Leica EG1160 Embedding Center with dispenser and hot Plate (Leica Microsystems Inc., Buffalo Grove, IL) for paraffin tissue embedding.
11. Leica RM2255 Automated Rotary Microtome (Leica Microsystems Inc., Buffalo Grove, IL) and Tissue Flotation Bath (Triangle Biomedical Sciences Inc., Durham, NC) for sectioning of the paraffin-embedded tissue specimens.
12. Decloaking Chamber (Biocare medical, Concord, CA) for antigen retrieval during immunohistochemical staining.
13. Axioskop 2 upright microscope equipped with AxiocamMrc5 color camera to examine and AxioVision Rel. 4.8.2 software (Carl Zeiss, Oberkochen, Germany) to analyze the immunohistochemical staining.

2.2 Reagents and Solutions

1. Protease inhibitor 100× stocks: 100 mM phenylmethylsulfonyl fluoride (PMSF) (Thermo Fisher Scientific, Rockford, IL) in Iso-propanol, 1 mg/mL Aprotinin (Roche Diagnostics Corporation, Indianapolis, IN).
2. Lysis buffer: 10 mM Tris pH 7.4 (Sigma), 150 mM NaCl (Sigma), 1 % Triton X-100 (Sigma), 1 mM EDTA, 1 mM EGTA, 0.2 mM sodium orthovanadate, 0.5 % IGEPAL (Sigma), with protease inhibitors.
3. Buffer A: 10 mM HEPES (pH 7.9), 10 mM KCl, 0.1 mM EDTA, 0.1 mM EGTA.
4. Buffer C: 20 mM HEPES, 0.4 M NaCl, 1 mM EDTA, 1 mM EGTA.
5. Nonidet P-40 (Sigma-Aldrich Corp., St. Louis, MO).

6. DC™ Protein Assay kit (Bio-Rad, Philadelphia, PA).
7. 2× Sample buffer: 0.125 M Tris pH 6.8 (Sigma), 4 % SDS (Roche), 20 % glycerol (Sigma), 10 % BME (Sigma), 0.4 mg/mL bromophenol blue.
8. Novex® Tris-Glycine precast 12 % gels (Life Technologies, Grand Island, NY).
9. Running buffer: 24 mM Tris–HCl pH 8.3, 192 mM glycine, 0.1 % (w/v) SDS.
10. Transfer buffer: 25 mM Tris–HCl pH 8.3, 192 mM glycine, 20 % (v/v) methanol.
11. Wash buffer: 10 mM Tris–HCl, 100 mM NaCl, pH 7.5.
12. Blocking buffer: 5 g of nonfat dry milk in 100 mL of wash buffer.
13. Amersham Hybond ECL Nitrocellulose Membrane (GE Healthcare Biosciences, Pittsburgh, PA).
14. Developer and Fixer (Kodak).
15. Autoradiography cassettes (Thermo Fisher Scientific, Pittsburg, PA).
16. Amersham Hyperfilm ECL (GE Healthcare Biosciences, Pittsburgh, PA).
17. Amersham ECL Detection Reagents RPN 2105 (GE Healthcare Biosciences, Pittsburgh, PA).
18. Stripping buffer: 100 mL 62.5 mM Tris, 10 mL 20 % SDS, 8 mL 2-mercaptoethanol.
19. PBS-B: 0.2 % Brij in 1× PBS.
20. CAS block blocking buffer (Life Technologies, Grand Island, NY) for blocking the tissue sections in immunochemistry.
21. Scott's Water: 10 g magnesium sulfate and 2 g sodium bicarbonate in 1,000 mL ddH_2O.
22. 10 mM sodium citrate solution, pH 6.
23. Super PAP Pen HT™ Slide Markers (Research Products International Corp., Mount Prospect, IL).
24. Fluoromount™ Aqueous Mounting Medium (Sigma).
25. Permaslip mounting medium (Alban Scientific Inc., St. Louis, MO) to mount cover glasses on microscope slides.
26. Tissue-Tek® Mega-Cassette® System, Sakura® Finetek (VWR, Radnor, PA).
27. Streptavidin, Horseradish peroxidase conjugate (Life Technologies, Grand Island, NY).
28. DAB Peroxidase Substrate Kit (Vector Laboratories, Inc., Burlingame, CA).

3 Methods

3.1 Whole Cell Lysate Preparation from Cell Cultures

The protocol described below is for a 100-mm cell culture plate

1. Cells are cultured and treated with drug(s) as required.
2. At the end of the treatment, place the cell culture plate on ice and collect the culture media along with floating cells ("floaters") into a labeled 15 mL tube. Centrifuge tubes at 800 × *g* for 5 min and discard the supernatant fraction.
3. Wash the plate twice with ice-cold 1× PBS and add it to the tube containing the floaters.
4. Collect the cells by centrifugation at 800 × *g* for 5 min. Discard the supernatant fraction, repeat the wash twice and place the tube with the washed cell pellet on ice.
5. Add 150 μL of the lysis buffer to the tube and vortex until the pellet is dispersed. Now, add the lysis buffer from the tube to the culture plate and let it stand on ice for 20 min (**Note 1**).
6. Tilt the plate and scrape the cells using a cell lifter to collect the cells at one edge of the plate.
7. Transfer the contents to a labeled eppendorf tube and store at −80 °C or continue with a freeze-thaw cycle.
8. Freeze the sample at −80 °C for 10 min followed by thawing the sample by placing it in a 37 °C water bath using a floater for 3 min or until the samples are completely thawed. Repeat this process two more times, vortexing the samples in between (10–15 s).
9. Centrifuge the lysate at 16,000 × *g* for 30 min at 4 °C using a microcentrifuge.
10. Carefully collect the supernatant fraction into a fresh, labeled eppendorf tube. Freeze the lysates at −80 °C until needed.

3.2 Cytosolic and Nuclear Fraction Preparation from Cell Cultures

The following reagent amounts pertain to an 80–90 % confluent 100-mm cell culture plate:

1. Place the cell culture plate on ice. Discard the culture medium and wash the cell culture plate twice using ice-cold 1× PBS.
2. Add 120–150 μL of Buffer A with 1 mM PMSF and 1 mM DTT to the culture plate and let it stand on ice for 15 min.
3. Tilt the plate and scrape the cells using a cell lifter to collect the cells at one edge of the plate and transfer to a labeled eppendorf tube.
4. Add 20 μL of 10 % Nonidet P-40 solution and gently vortex for 15 s.
5. Centrifuge the sample at 16,000 × *g* for 40 s at 4 °C using a microcentrifuge.

6. Carefully, without disturbing the pellet, collect the supernatant fraction into a fresh, labeled eppendorf tube and store at –80 °C. This is the Cytosolic Fraction.
7. Wash the pellet twice with 500 μL of Buffer A by centrifuging at 13,000 × *g* for 40 s.
8. Add 50 μL of Buffer C with 1 mM PMSF and 1 mM DTT to the pellet and resuspend by gently pipetting the solution up and down.
9. Gently rock the tube at 4 °C for 15 min using a nutator.
10. Centrifuge at 16,000 × *g* for 10 min at 4 °C.
11. Collect the supernatant fraction in to a fresh tube and store at –80 °C. This is the Nuclear Fraction.

3.3 Whole Cell Lysate Preparation from Prostate Tumor Tissue

1. Thaw frozen tissue on ice or use fresh tissue and weigh out 75–100 mg.
2. Wash the tissue in ice-cold PBS to remove any blood present.
3. Place the tissue in a petri dish and mince the tissue into very small pieces using a blade or a scalpel.
4. Transfer the minced pieces of tissue into a 2 mL tube.
5. Add 750–1,000 μL tissue lysis buffer to the tissue.
6. Disrupt the tissue using the Tissue-Tearor at 2,300 × *g* for about 90–150 s while still keeping the tube containing tissue on ice. Do not let the tissue become heated.
7. Leave the tissue on ice for 15 min with intermittent vortexing.
8. Freeze the sample at –80 °C for 10 min followed by thawing the sample by placing it in a 37 °C waterbath using a floater for 3 min or until the samples are completely thawed Repeat this process two more times, vortexing the samples in between.
9. Centrifuge the samples at 16,000 × *g* for 5 min at 4 °C using a microcentrifuge. Collect the supernatant fraction into a fresh tube.
10. Centrifuge the supernatant fraction collected in the previous step at 16,000 × *g* for 30 min at 4 °C.
11. Carefully collect the supernatant fraction into a fresh tube. Freeze the lysates at –80 °C until needed.

3.4 Cytosolic and Nuclear Fraction Preparation from Prostate Tumor Tissue

1. Thaw frozen tissue on ice or use fresh tissue and weigh out 75–100 mg.
2. Wash the tissue in ice-cold PBS to remove any blood present.
3. Place the tissue in a petri dish and mince the tissue into very small pieces using a blade or a scalpel.
4. Transfer the minced pieces of tissue into a 2 mL tube.

5. Add 800 μL of Buffer A with 1 mM PMSF and 1 mM DTT to the tissue.
6. Disrupt the tissue using the Tissue-Tearor at 2,300×*g* for about 90–150 s while still keeping the tube containing tissue on ice.
7. Leave the tissue on ice for 40 min and vortex the tube for 30 s every 10 min.
8. To the sample tube, add 50 μL of 10 % NP-40 and, every 5 min, vortex the sample tube at high speed for 45 s and repeat this five times.
9. Centrifuge the samples at 16,000×*g* for 90 s at 4 °C using a microcentrifuge.
10. Collect the supernatant fraction into a fresh tube and store at −80 °C until needed. This is the Cytosolic Fraction.
11. Take care not to disturb the pellet and gently wash it twice with 100 μL of Buffer A.
12. Add 100 μL of Buffer C with 1 mM PMSF and 1 mM DTT to the pellet and resuspend by gently pipetting the solution up and down.
13. Vortex the sample 3 times at high speed for 45 s at 5 min intervals.
14. Gently rock the tube at 4 °C for 15 min using a nutator.
15. Vortex the sample 2 times at high speed for 45 s at 5 min intervals.
16. Centrifuge at 16,000×*g* for 20 min at 4 °C.
17. Collect the supernatant fraction into a fresh tube and store at −80 °C. This is the Nuclear Fraction.

3.5 Protein Estimation

We have used the DC™ Protein Assay kit (Bio-Rad, Philadelphia, PA), a colorimetric assay for estimating protein content in whole cells and the nuclear and cytosolic fractions, which have undergone detergent solubilization. The assay is a modified version of the Lowry assay and is based on the reaction of protein with an alkaline copper tartrate solution and Folin reagent.

1. Thaw the samples to be assayed on ice.
2. Label 15 mL tubes, including a tube for blank or background measurement.
3. Add 90 μL of ddH_2O to the sample tubes and 100 μL of ddH_2O the blank tube.
4. Prepare a standard curve with a range of 0–5 mg/mL protein using the appropriate volume of BSA standard supplied with the kit.
5. Add 10 μL of the protein lysate sample to the labeled tubes.

6. Add 20 μL of reagent S to each mL of reagent A that will be needed for the assay.
7. Add 500 μL of "reagent A + S" in each tube.
8. Add 4 mL of reagent B to each tube in the dark. Vortex the tubes gently.
9. Incubate for 20 min in the dark.
10. Measure the protein content at 750 nm using a spectrophotometer.
11. Plot the sample absorbance values against the standard absorbance values to determine the sample protein concentration.

3.6 SDS-PAGE

Depending on the protein to be analyzed, 40–80 μg of protein is used

3.6.1 Sample Preparation

1. Mix each sample with an equal volume of 2× sample buffer (**Note 2**).
2. Heat samples in a boiling water bath for 5 min.
3. Centrifuge the samples at 16,000 × *g* for 5 min at room temperature.
4. Use 10 μL of the Bio-Rad Kaleidoscope molecular weight marker to load in one well of each gel.

3.6.2 Electrophoresis

Novex® Tris-Glycine precast gels, set up in XCell SureLock™ Mini Cell electrophoresis system, are used for the separation of proteins. Electrophoresis is conducted using the PowerPac™ Basic power supply.

1. Take the gel out from the pouch and rinse with deionized water.
2. Peel off the tape covering the bottom of the cassette.
3. Pull the comb out of the cassette gently to free the gel loading wells.
4. Wash the cassette wells twice with 1× running buffer.
5. Orient the gel in the Mini Cell unit so that the "notched well" side of the cassette faces the buffer core.
6. Clamp the Mini Cell unit properly to avoid any leakage of the running buffer.
7. Fill the unit with 1× running buffer making sure to take out all the bubbles from the cassette wells.
8. Load the samples into the wells using a sample-loading tip. For the best results load sample buffer in all the remaining empty wells to ensure uniform running of the samples.
9. Turn power on to a voltage of 125 V.

10. The run is complete when the bromophenol blue-colored samples reach the bottom, in about 2 h.
11. Turn the power off and take the gel out of the unit.

3.6.3 Western Blotting Transfer

1. During the gel electrophoresis, prepare and cool the transfer buffer (**Note 3**).
2. Wash the gel cassette after removing from the running buffer and carefully separate the cassette plates to reveal the gel.
3. Placing a filter paper on the gel, remove the gel from the cassette and sandwich the gel with nitrocellulose membrane and filter paper. Transfer pads are kept both below and above the sandwich of the filter paper–gel–nitrocellulose membrane–filter paper.
4. Set the gel in the transfer apparatus along with the transfer pads and fill the apparatus with cold transfer buffer.
5. Transfer proteins at 100 mA for 210 min. Then take out the membrane and place in a small box containing blocking buffer.

3.6.4 Immunoblotting

1. Block the transferred membrane for 1 h using 5 % nonfat milk.
2. Incubate the membrane with a primary antibody (targeted at the protein of interest) diluted in blocking buffer by gentle shaking for 2 h at room temperature or incubate overnight at 4 °C. This step is conducted in sealable plastic pouches.
3. Thereafter, membranes are removed and washed 3 times with wash buffer containing 0.1 % Tween-20.
4. Incubate the membrane with the secondary antibody diluted in blocking buffer by gentle shaking for 1 h.
5. Wash the membrane 3 times with wash buffer containing 0.1 % Tween-20.

3.6.5 Enhanced Chemiluminescence (ECL)

Amersham ECL Detection Reagents are used for the detection of proteins.

1. Place 1 mL each of reagents A and B included in the kit into two separate tubes.
2. In a dark room, place the membrane on a plastic wrap.
3. Mix the reagents A and B.
4. Pour the solution on to the membrane and incubate for 1–3 min.
5. Drain the liquid off of the membrane and place the membrane in a plastic pouch.
6. Place the plastic pouch in a film cassette.
7. Expose the film to the membrane for the appropriate time.

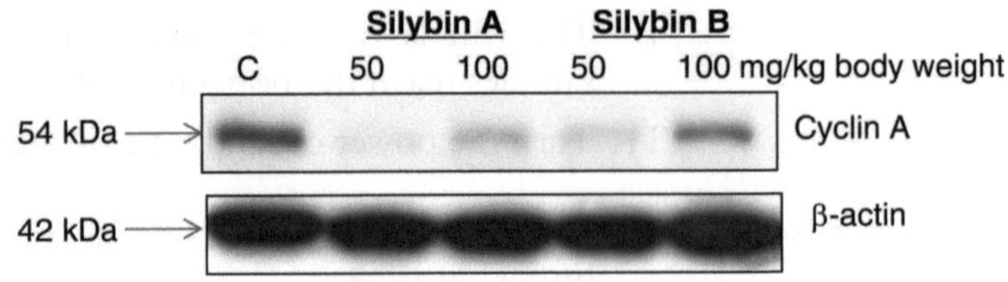

Fig. 2 Effect of silibinin isomers (silybin A and silybin B) on the cyclin A protein level in human prostate cancer cells DU145 xenograft tissues measured by western blotting. Membrane was stripped and re-probed with β-actin to confirm equal protein loading

8. Place the film in developing solution for 30 s and then wash in water for 30 s followed by incubation in fixer solution until the film doesn't appear milky and is clear.
9. Wash in tap water adequately and dry the film.

3.6.6 Stripping the Membrane and Re-probing for Another Protein

Membranes are often stripped and re-probed with other proteins. Stripping is also essential to check for protein loading, and for that, stripped membranes are re-probed to detect the relevant loading control such as β-actin or α-tubulin.

1. Membranes are washed twice in wash buffer (10 min each) at room temperature.
2. Membranes are incubated (with gentle shaking) with stripping buffer at 55 °C in a water bath in a chemical fume hood for about 20 min.
3. Thereafter, membranes are washed for about 30 min frequently changing the wash buffer. Make sure to cover the box because stripped membranes have a strong odor due to BME.
4. Membranes are blocked again and re-probed with primary and secondary antibodies for another protein as indicated above.

As an example, we have presented western blotting data for a cell cycle regulatory molecule cyclin A (Fig. 2). This blot shows the effect of two doses (50 and 100 mg/kg body weight) of silibinin isomers (silybin A and silybin B) on cyclin A expression in DU145 xenograft tissues. The membrane was stripped and re-probed with β-actin to check equal protein loading.

3.7 Immunofluorescence in Cell Cultures

1. Place sterile round cover slips in the wells of a 12-well plate.
2. Plate approximately 30,000 cells in each well of the plate and let the cells attach overnight.
3. At the end of the desired treatments, aspirate the media and rinse with PBS.
4. Aspirate the PBS and cover the cells with 4 % formaldehyde and incubate for 30 min.

5. Aspirate the fixative and rinse 3 times with PBS for 5 min each.
6. Cover the cells with ice-cold 100 % methanol and incubate for 10 min.
7. Rinse the cells with PBS for 5 min. Repeat twice.
8. Add the Cas-block blocking buffer to the cells and let stand for 1 h at room temperature.
9. Remove the blocking buffer and without rinsing add the primary antibody diluted in 0.3 % Triton-X in PBS and incubate overnight at 4 °C (**Note 4**).
10. Rinse the cells with PBS for 5 min. Repeat twice.
11. Add the Alexa fluor- or Texas Red-tagged secondary antibody and 1 μg/mL DAPI diluted in 0.3 % Triton-X in PBS and incubate in the dark for 30 min to 1 h at room temperature.
12. Rinse the cells with PBS for 5 min. Repeat twice.
13. Remove the coverslip using sharp forceps and mount on a labeled slide using 20–25 μL of mounting media.
14. Let the slides dry for 15 min in the dark.
15. Capture and analyze the cell images using for example a Nikon D Eclipse C1 Plus Confocal Microscope connected to a computer installed with Nikon EZ-C1 FreeViewer software.

3.8 Tissue Processing and Histological Staining

3.8.1 Paraffin Tissue Processing

All the tissues are placed in a cassette, locked and immediately fixed in 10 % buffered formalin overnight and then are exchanged into 70 % ethanol and stored at 4 °C until further processing. The Tissue Processing Center TPC 15 is used for tissue processing. Below are the steps of incubation for paraffin tissue processing.

Tissues used should be small in size to facilitate efficient wax infiltration.

1. 10 % formalin for 60 min at 30 °C.
2. 70 % ethanol for 45 min at 30 °C.
3. 95 % ethanol for 45 min at 30 °C.
4. 95 % ethanol for 60 min at 30 °C.
5. 100 % ethanol for 45 min at 35 °C.
6. 100 % ethanol for 60 min at 35 °C.
7. 100 % ethanol for 60 min at 35 °C.
8. Toluene for 45 min at 38 °C.
9. Toluene for 60 min at 38 °C.
10. Toluene for 75 min at 38 °C.
11. Paraffin for 60 min at 61 °C.
12. Paraffin for 75 min at 61 °C.
13. Paraffin for 90 min at 61 °C (**Note 5**).

3.8.2 Embedding Tissues in Paraffin Blocks

Paraffin tissue embedding is performed using the Leica EG1160 Embedding Center with dispenser and hot plate.

1. Turn the embedding center on at least 1 h prior to beginning the embedding process.
2. Place the processed tissue cassettes into the 65 °C paraffin bath in the embedding center.
3. Place an embedding mold on the hot plate and place the tissues at the bottom of the mold in the desired orientation using a heated forceps.
4. Add the labeled cassette top to the top of the mold and fill the mold with paraffin, taking care not to introduce any bubbles into the paraffin.
5. Gently slide the mold from the hot plate onto the cold surface of the embedder.
6. Let the mold cool down and become hardened for about 30 min.
7. Place the molds at −80 °C for about 15 min and pop the paraffin block out of the mold.
8. The tissue blocks can be stored at room temperature until further use.

3.8.3 Tissue Sectioning

The Leica RM2255 Automated Rotary Microtome and Tissue Flotation Bath are used for sectioning of the paraffin-embedded tissue samples.

1. Turn on the tissue floatation water bath and heat it to 35 °C.
2. Fit the microtome with a fresh blade and set the thickness of the sections to 5 μm.
3. Fit the block into the microtome and cut the sections (**Note 6**).
4. Float the tissue section ribbon in the water bath.
5. Mount the sections onto lysine pre-coated histological slides.
6. Dry the slides overnight at 37 °C. Store the slides in slide storage boxes at room temperature until needed.
7. The slides can be used to detect proteins through immunofluorescence or immunohistochemistry.

3.9 Immunofluorescence in Tumor Tissue

3.9.1 Deparaffinization and Rehydration

1. Incubate the formalin fixed, paraffin embedded tissue sections for 5 min in xylene. Repeat.
2. Rehydrate the tissue sections using graded ethanol concentrations of 100, 100, 95, 95, and 70 % for 5 min each.
3. Rinse the slides in PBS-B for 5 min. Repeat twice.

3.9.2 Antigen Retrieval

1. Conduct the antigen retrieval using 10 mM sodium citrate solution for 10 min in a decloaking chamber at suboptimal boiling temperature (85 °C).

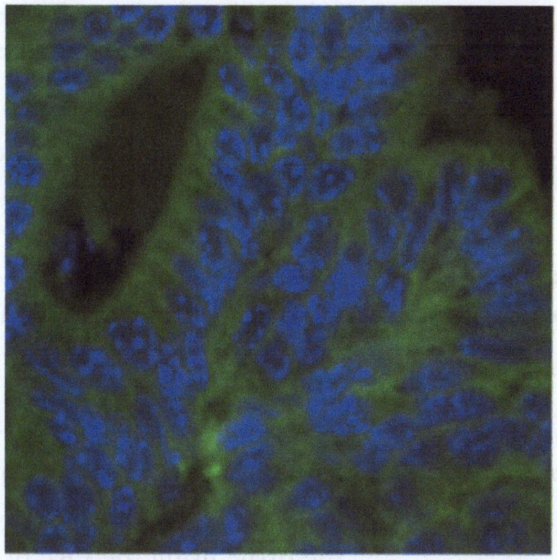

Fig. 3 Immunofluorescence method was used to analyze silibinin effect on the E-cadherin (green-Alexa fluor 488 rabbit anti-mouse IgG) expression in 12 week old TRAMP prostate tissue. DAPI was used to stain the nuclei

2. Let the slides cool slowly to room temperature for about 30 min.
3. Rinse the slides 3 times in PBS for 5 min each.

3.9.3 Immunofluorescence

1. Wipe the slides to remove excess PBS and draw circles around the tissue using the PAP pen (**Note 7**).
2. Add CAS-block blocking buffer to the slides and let stand for 1 h at room temperature.
3. Remove the blocking buffer and add the primary antibody diluted in 12 % BSA and incubate overnight in a humidified chamber at 4 °C.
4. Rinse the slides 3 times in PBS for 5 min each.
5. Incubate the slides in the dark with Alexa fluor- or Texas Red-tagged secondary antibody along with 1.0 μg/mL DAPI in 12 % BSA for 2 h at room temperature.
6. Rinse the slides 3 times in PBS for 5 min each.
7. Mount the slides using Fluoromount or any other mounting media, which doesn't scatter light and let slides dry in the dark (**Note 8**).
8. Capture and analyze the cell images using for example the Nikon D Eclipse C1 Plus Confocal Microscope connected to a computer installed with Nikon EZ-C1 FreeViewer software.

As an example, we have presented an immunofluorescence image for E-cadherin in PCA tissue from TRAMP mice treated with silibinin (Fig. 3). In this staining, sections were stained with the primary antibody against E-cadherin followed by incubation with Alexa fluor 488-tagged secondary antibody and DAPI as described above.

3.10 Immunohistochemistry

3.10.1 Deparaffinization and Rehydration: See Sect. 3.9.1 (Note 9)

3.10.2 Antigen Retrieval

1. Conduct the antigen retrieval using 10 mM sodium citrate solution for 10 min in a decloaking chamber at suboptimal boiling temperature (85 °C).
2. Let the slides cool slowly to room temperature.
3. Rinse the slides 3 times in PBS-B for 5 min each.

3.10.3 Immunohistochemical Staining

1. Incubate the slides in 3 % H_2O_2 in methanol for 10 min.
2. Rinse the slides 3 times in PBS-B for 5 min each.
3. Wipe the slides to remove excess PBS and draw circles around the tissue using the PAP pen.
4. Add CAS-block blocking buffer to the slides and let stand for 1 h at room temperature. Blocking is needed to reduce the background.
5. Remove the blocking buffer and incubate the tissue sections with the primary antibody diluted in PBS overnight at 4 °C.
6. Rinse the slides 3 times in PBS-B for 5 min each.
7. Incubate the tissue sections with a biotin-conjugated species-specific secondary antibody for 45 min at room temperature.
8. Incubate the slides with Streptavidin-HRP conjugate for 45 min at room temperature.
9. Rinse the slides 3 times in PBS-B for 5 min each.
10. Immediately before use, prepare the DAB substrate solution by adding 2 drops of Buffer Stock Solution, 4 drops of DAB Stock Solution and 2 drops of the Hydrogen Peroxide Solution to 5.0 mL of distilled water, and mixing well after adding of each of the solutions. Cover each tissue section with DAB and incubate in the dark until brown color appears (2–10 min).
11. Rinse the slides 3 times in deionized water for 2 min each.

3.10.4 Counterstaining

1. Dip the slides in 1:10 diluted Harris Hematoxylin solution in water for 2 min.
2. Rinse the slides 2 times in tap water for 1 min each with intermittent dips.
3. Dip the slides in Scott's water for 2 min.
4. Rinse the slides 2 times in tap water for 1 min each with intermittent dips.

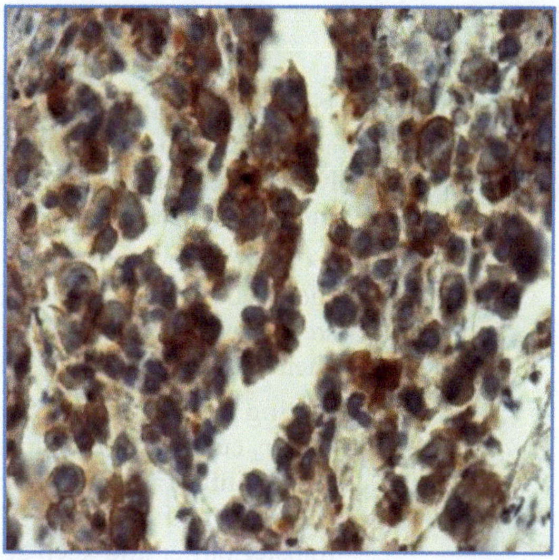

Fig. 4 Immunohistochemical analyses of Integrin β1 (*brown* staining) in PC3 xenograft tissues, which were counterstained with hematoxylin (*blue* staining) to stain nuclei

3.10.5 Dehydration and Mounting

1. Dip the slides in increasing concentrations of ethanol (70, 95, 95, 100, and 100 %) for 2 min each.
2. Place the slides 3 times in xylene for 5 min each and continue with mounting.
3. Drain the xylene from the slide and add three drops of Permaslip mounting medium and cover with a cover slip. Avoid getting bubbles.
4. Tilt the slide on edge onto a paper towel to let the excess xylene or mounting medium drain.
5. Let the slides air-dry at room temperature overnight.

3.10.6 Microscopic Observation and Analysis

Microscopic immunohistochemical and histopathological analyses can be performed using the Carl Zeiss Axioskop 2 upright microscope (Carl Zeiss, Inc., Germany) equipped with Carl Zeiss AxioCam MrC5 color camera and the images can be analyzed using Axiovision Rel 4.5 software.

As an example, we have presented the immunohistochemical data for integrin β1 (brown staining) (Fig. 4). The expression of integrin β1 was analyzed in human prostate cancer PC3 xenograft tissues following the detailed methods above. For more examples of western blotting, immunofluorescence, and immunohistochemistry, please see following Refs. [13, 16, 19, 31].

4 Notes

1. Protease inhibitors (PMSF and Aprotinin) and DTT should be added fresh to the lysis buffers before each use. The amount of lysis buffer added depends upon the cell type as well as the number of cells/confluency in the plate.
2. 2× Sample buffer can be stored at room temperature, but should be stored at −20 °C once BME is added. BME in this step, as well as in any other step, should be added only inside a chemical fume hood.
3. During the gel electrophoresis, prepare and cool the transfer buffer, cut one nitrocellulose membrane and two filter papers per gel into transfer pad size, and then immerse them in transfer buffer and keep at 4 °C. Similarly, immerse transfer pads in transfer buffer and keep at 4 °C.
4. For immunofluorescence detection, if detection of protein co-localization is required, make sure to use the primary antibodies of different host sources, and secondary antibodies of different fluorescence emissions.
5. After the tissue processing, do not let the tissues stand in paraffin for a long time, and proceed to tissue embedding as soon as possible.
6. Blocks to be sectioned should be kept at −20 °C for approximately 10 min and taken out one at a time to obtain smoother tissue section ribbons.
7. Before using the PAP pen, make sure to clean out the PBS around the tissue section and make sure not to touch the sections with the PAP pen because its hydrophobic nature will inhibit the antibody from interacting with the tissue.
8. For mounting immunofluorescence slides, use Fluoromount or any other mounting media which preserves fluorescence and doesn't scatter light.
9. As much as possible, immunohistochemical steps should be performed inside a chemical fume hood.

5 Conclusions

PCA is the main cause of mortality and morbidity in men; therefore, additional and alternative measures are urgently needed to control this malignancy. In this regard, chemopreventive approaches could be useful in preventing the growth and progression of PCA. Now an abundant amount of literature suggests a broad spectrum of efficacy of silibinin against PCA. Protein estimation methods described in this chapter have been extensively used to establish the effect of silibinin on various proliferation, apoptosis, angiogenesis, and metastasis biomarkers in PCA cells, both in vitro and in vivo. In future studies, these methods could be employed to further study the effect of silibinin, as well as of other agents, on the protein expression/localization of additional biomarkers in PCA cells such as those involved in cancer cell metabolism and tumor microenvironment.

References

1. Siegel R, Naishadham D, Jemal A (2012) Cancer statistics, 2012. Cancer J Clin 62(1):10–29. doi:10.3322/caac.20138
2. Kingsley LA, Fournier PG, Chirgwin JM, Guise TA (2007) Molecular biology of bone metastasis. Mol Cancer Ther 6(10):2609–2617
3. Tantivejkul K, Kalikin LM, Pienta KJ (2004) Dynamic process of prostate cancer metastasis to bone. J Cell Biochem 91(4):706–717
4. Hadaschik BA, Gleave ME (2007) Therapeutic options for hormone-refractory prostate cancer in 2007. Urol Oncol 25(5):413–419
5. Koivisto P, Kolmer M, Visakorpi T, Kallioniemi OP (1998) Androgen receptor gene and hormonal therapy failure of prostate cancer. Am J Pathol 152(1):1–9
6. Feldman BJ, Feldman D (2001) The development of androgen-independent prostate cancer. Nat Rev Cancer 1(1):34–45
7. Harzstark AL, Ryan CJ (2008) Novel therapeutic strategies in development for prostate cancer. Expert Opin Investig Drugs 17(1):13–22
8. Petrylak DP (2005) The current role of chemotherapy in metastatic hormone-refractory prostate cancer. Urology 65(Suppl 5):3–7, Discussion 7–8
9. Deep G, Agarwal R (2007) Chemopreventive efficacy of silymarin in skin and prostate cancer. Integr Cancer Ther 6(2):130–145. doi:10.1177/1534735407301441
10. Wattenberg LW (1997) An overview of chemoprevention: current status and future prospects. Proc Soc Exp Biol Med 216(2):133–141
11. Agarwal R (2000) Cell signaling and regulators of cell cycle as molecular targets for prostate cancer prevention by dietary agents. Biochem Pharmacol 60(8):1051–1059
12. Surh YJ (2003) Cancer chemoprevention with dietary phytochemicals. Nat Rev Cancer 3(10):768–780
13. Raina K, Rajamanickam S, Singh RP, Deep G, Chittezhath M, Agarwal R (2008) Stage-specific inhibitory effects and associated mechanisms of silibinin on tumor progression and metastasis in transgenic adenocarcinoma of the mouse prostate model. Cancer Res 68(16):6822–6830. doi:10.1158/0008-5472.CAN-08-1332
14. Deep G, Agarwal R (2010) Antimetastatic efficacy of silibinin: molecular mechanisms and therapeutic potential against cancer. Cancer Metastasis Rev 29(3):447–463. doi:10.1007/s10555-010-9237-0
15. Singh RP, Agarwal R (2006) Mechanisms of action of novel agents for prostate cancer chemoprevention. Endocr Relat Cancer 13(3):751–778
16. Kavitha CV, Deep G, Gangar SC, Jain AK, Agarwal C, Agarwal R (2012) Silibinin inhibits prostate cancer cells- and RANKL-induced osteoclastogenesis by targeting NFATc1, NF-kappaB, and AP-1 Activation in RAW264.7 cells. Mol Carcinog. doi:10.1002/mc.21959
17. Agarwal R, Agarwal C, Ichikawa H, Singh RP, Aggarwal BB (2006) Anticancer potential of silymarin: from bench to bed side. Anticancer Res 26(6B):4457–4498
18. Pradhan SC, Girish C (2006) Hepatoprotective herbal drug, silymarin from experimental pharmacology to clinical medicine. Indian J Med Res 124(5):491–504
19. Deep G, Gangar SC, Agarwal C, Agarwal R (2011) Role of E-cadherin in antimigratory and antiinvasive efficacy of silibinin in prostate cancer cells. Cancer Prev Res (Phila) 4(8):1222–1232. doi:1940-6207.CAPR-10-0370.10.1158/1940-6207.CAPR-10-0370
20. Flaig TW, Glode M, Gustafson D, van Bokhoven A, Tao Y, Wilson S, Su LJ, Li Y, Harrison G, Agarwal R, Crawford ED, Lucia MS, Pollak M (2010) A study of high-dose oral silybin-phytosome followed by prostatectomy in patients with localized prostate cancer. J Prostate 70(8):848–855. doi:10.1002/pros.21118
21. Flaig TW, Gustafson DL, Su LJ, Zirrolli JA, Crighton F, Harrison GS, Pierson AS, Agarwal R, Glode LM (2007) A phase I and pharmaco-

kinetic study of silybin-phytosome in prostate cancer patients. Investig New Drugs 25(2): 139–146

22. Hoh C, Boocock D, Marczylo T, Singh R, Berry DP, Dennison AR, Hemingway D, Miller A, West K, Euden S, Garcea G, Farmer PB, Steward WP, Gescher AJ (2006) Pilot study of oral silibinin, a putative chemopreventive agent, in colorectal cancer patients: silibinin levels in plasma, colorectum, and liver and their pharmacodynamic consequences. Clin Cancer Res 12(9):2944–2950
23. Singh RP, Deep G, Chittezhath M, Kaur M, Dwyer-Nield LD, Malkinson AM, Agarwal R (2006) Effect of silibinin on the growth and progression of primary lung tumors in mice. J Natl Canc Inst 98(12):846–855
24. Roy S, Gu M, Ramasamy K, Singh RP, Agarwal C, Siriwardana S, Sclafani RA, Agarwal R (2009) p21/Cip1 and p27/Kip1 are essential molecular targets of inositol hexaphosphate for its antitumor efficacy against prostate cancer. Cancer Res 69(3):1166–1173. doi:10.1158/0008-5472.CAN-08-3115
25. Tyagi A, Sharma Y, Agarwal C, Agarwal R (2008) Silibinin impairs constitutively active TGFalpha-EGFR autocrine loop in advanced human prostate carcinoma cells. Pharm Res, 25:2143–2150
26. Zi X, Grasso AW, Kung HJ, Agarwal R (1998) A flavonoid antioxidant, silymarin, inhibits activation of erbB1 signaling and induces cyclin-dependent kinase inhibitors, G1 arrest, and anticarcinogenic effects in human prostate carcinoma DU145 cells. Cancer Res 58(9): 1920–1929
27. Singh RP, Agarwal R (2006) Prostate cancer chemoprevention by silibinin: bench to bedside. Mol Carcinog 45(6):436–442
28. Deep G, Gangar SC, Rajamanickam S, Raina K, Gu M, Agarwal C, Oberlies NH, Agarwal R (2012) Angiopreventive efficacy of pure flavonolignans from milk thistle extract against prostate cancer: targeting VEGF-VEGFR signaling. PloS One 7(4):e34630. doi:10.1371/journal.pone.0034630
29. Singh RP, Dhanalakshmi S, Agarwal C, Agarwal R (2005) Silibinin strongly inhibits growth and survival of human endothelial cells via cell cycle arrest and downregulation of survivin, Akt and NF-kappaB: implications for angioprevention and antiangiogenic therapy. Oncogene 24(7):1188–1202
30. Deep G, Agarwal R (2013) Targeting tumor microenvironment with silibinin: promise and potential for a translational cancer chemopreventive strategy. Curr Cancer Drug Target 13:486–499
31. Singh RP, Raina K, Sharma G, Agarwal R (2008) Silibinin inhibits established prostate tumor growth, progression, invasion, and metastasis and suppresses tumor angiogenesis and epithelial-mesenchymal transition in transgenic adenocarcinoma of the mouse prostate model mice. Clin Cancer Res 14(23):7773–7780. doi:10.1158/1078-0432.CCR-08-1309
32. Deep G, Singh RP, Agarwal C, Kroll DJ, Agarwal R (2006) Silymarin and silibinin cause G1 and G2-M cell cycle arrest via distinct circuitries in human prostate cancer PC3 cells: a comparison of flavanone silibinin with flavanolignan mixture silymarin. Oncogene 25(7):1053–1069
33. Zi X, Agarwal R (1999) Silibinin decreases prostate-specific antigen with cell growth inhibition via G1 arrest, leading to differentiation of prostate carcinoma cells: implications for prostate cancer intervention. Proc Natl Acad Sci U S A 96(13):7490–7495
34. Singh RP, Raina K, Deep G, Chan D, Agarwal R (2009) Silibinin suppresses growth of human prostate carcinoma PC-3 orthotopic xenograft via activation of extracellular signal-regulated kinase 1/2 and inhibition of signal transducers and activators of transcription signaling. Clin Cancer Res 15(2):613–621. doi:10.1158/1078-0432.CCR-08-1846
35. Singh RP, Deep G, Blouin MJ, Pollak MN, Agarwal R (2007) Silibinin suppresses in vivo growth of human prostate carcinoma PC-3 tumor xenograft. Carcinogenesis 28(12): 2567–2574. doi:10.1093/carcin/bgm218
36. Singh RP, Dhanalakshmi S, Tyagi AK, Chan DC, Agarwal C, Agarwal R (2002) Dietary feeding of silibinin inhibits advance human prostate carcinoma growth in athymic nude mice and increases plasma insulin-like growth factor-binding protein-3 levels. Cancer Res 62(11):3063–3069
37. Raina K, Blouin MJ, Singh RP, Majeed N, Deep G, Varghese L, Glode LM, Greenberg NM, Hwang D, Cohen P, Pollak MN, Agarwal R (2007) Dietary feeding of silibinin inhibits prostate tumor growth and progression in transgenic adenocarcinoma of the mouse prostate model. Cancer Res 67(22): 11083–11091
38. Zhu W, Zhang JS, Young CY (2001) Silymarin inhibits function of the androgen receptor by reducing nuclear localization of the receptor in the human prostate cancer cell line LNCaP. Carcinogenesis 22(9):1399–1403

39. Thelen P, Wuttke W, Jarry H, Grzmil M, Ringert RH (2004) Inhibition of telomerase activity and secretion of prostate specific antigen by silibinin in prostate cancer cells. J Urol 171(5):1934–1938
40. Hansen J, Rink M, Graefen M, Shariat S, Chun FK (2013) Assays for prostate cancer : changing the screening paradigm? Mol Diagn Ther 17(1):1–8. doi:10.1007/s40291-013-0014-y
41. Singh RP, Sharma G, Dhanalakshmi S, Agarwal C, Agarwal R (2003) Suppression of advanced human prostate tumor growth in athymic mice by silibinin feeding is associated with reduced cell proliferation, increased apoptosis, and inhibition of angiogenesis. Cancer Epidemiol Biomarkers Prev 12(9): 933–939
42. Deep G, Raina K, Singh RP, Oberlies NH, Kroll DJ, Agarwal R (2008) Isosilibinin inhibits advanced human prostate cancer growth in athymic nude mice: comparison with silymarin and silibinin. Int J Cancer 123(12):2750–2758. doi:10.1002/ijc.23879
43. Zi X, Zhang J, Agarwal R, Pollak M (2000) Silibinin up-regulates insulin-like growth factor-binding protein 3 expression and inhibits proliferation of androgen-independent prostate cancer cells. Cancer Res 60(20):5617–5620

Chapter 5

An Approach to the Evaluation of Berries for Cancer Prevention with Emphasis on Esophageal Cancer

Gary D. Stoner, Li-Shu Wang, Laura A. Kresty, Dan Peiffer, Chieh-Ti Kuo, Yi-Wen Huang, Dian Wang, Ben Ransom, Steven Carmella, and Stephen S. Hecht

Abstract

Our laboratory has been developing a food-based approach to cancer prevention using freeze-dried berries, mainly black raspberries, for more than two decades. Berries contain many known agents with chemopreventive potential including certain vitamins, minerals, simple and complex polyphenols, phytosterols, and various fiber constituents. Because berries are approximately 80–90 % water, the freeze-drying process concentrates these bioactive constituents approximately tenfold. This chapter describes methods we use to harvest the berries, grind them into a powder, and determine the nutrient, chemical, and microbial content of the powder before use in both preclinical and clinical studies. We have found that berry powder, when added at 5.0–10 % of the diet, protects against chemically induced cancer in the rodent esophagus and colon, and other laboratories have demonstrated protective effects in the rodent oral cavity, mammary gland, and skin. Bio-fractionation studies indicate that the anthocyanins in black raspberries are important for their chemopreventive effects. The berries function to reduce cell proliferation, inflammation, and angiogenesis and to stimulate apoptosis and differentiation, and they influence the expression levels of multiple genes and signaling pathways associated with these cellular functions. Black raspberry and strawberry powders are well tolerated by humans for at least 6–9 months when consumed orally at doses as high as 60 g/day. As an example of their effects in humans, we describe here the ability of black raspberries and strawberries (STRW) to modulate the development of premalignant lesions (Barrett's esophagus and esophageal dysplasia) in the esophagus. We hope that the information and methods in this review will be helpful to others who are considering the use of food-based approaches to cancer prevention.

Key words Berries, Cancer prevention, Esophagus, Colon, Anthocyanins, Animal, Human

1 Introduction

Berries are among the most widely consumed fruits in the human diet. They are richly abundant in antioxidant flavonoids and phenolic acids, as well as antioxidant vitamins, tannins, lignans, stilbenes, and carotenoids [1]. The most important berries in commercial production include members of the genus *Rubus* (blackberry, red

Ann M. Bode and Zigang Dong (eds.), *Cancer Prevention: Dietary Factors and Pharmacology*, Methods in Pharmacology and Toxicology, DOI 10.1007/978-1-4614-9227-6_5, © Springer Science+Business Media New York 2014

raspberry, cloudberry, black raspberry), *Vaccinium* (blueberry, lingonberry, bilberry, cranberry), *Fragaria* (strawberry), and *Sambucus* (elderberry, red elderberry). Recently, factors influencing the chemical composition of berries, and their use for nutritional and medicinal purposes have been described [1]. Experimental studies with berries have increased dramatically in the past 10–15 years and have shown that berries exhibit protective effects against multiple human diseases including cardiovascular disease, diabetes, neurological diseases and cancer. This increase in research activity has led to a significant increase in the demand for berries worldwide. For example, in the year 2000, strawberry production in the UK was 16,000 tons, whereas in 2009, it rose to 55,000 tons [2]. Similarly, worldwide blueberry production has increased dramatically with about 50,000 acres planted in 1995 to 190,000 acres in 2010 [3]. These increases in production reflect, at least in part, the benefits of berry research to the berry industry. Unfortunately, however, the increase in demand for berries has often been accompanied by significant increases in cost which reduces their utility for disease prevention, particularly in developing countries.

Our laboratories have been evaluating a "food-based" approach to cancer prevention using black raspberries (BRBs; *Rubus occidentalis*) since 1993. BRBs were chosen for study because they have amongst the highest levels of ellagitannins and anthocyanins [4] and exhibit higher antioxidant activity [5] when compared to most other berry types. BRBs contain multiple compounds with chemopreventive potential including simple polyphenols such as chlorogenic, ferulic and coumaric acids, quercetin and kaempferol, complex polyphenols such as anthocyanins and ellagitannins, vitamins A, C, E and folic acid, minerals such as calcium and zinc, carotenoids, and phytohormones such as β-sitosterol [6]. Moreover, BRBs likely contain additional compounds with chemopreventive potential that have not, as yet, been identified. Because BRBs are about 80–90 % water, the process of freeze-drying the berries and removing the water results in about an eight- to ninefold concentration of these putative chemopreventive agents. The freeze-drying process is conducted under anoxic conditions so that relatively little degradation of berry constituents can occur. Typically, for experimental studies, the dried berries are ground into a fine powder and the powder added to synthetic diets for animal studies or to water or other vehicles for use by humans.

The approach that we have used for evaluating the chemopreventive effects of black raspberry powder in different formulations has been discussed in detail in a recent Commentary [6] and is shown in Fig. 1. In the present chapter, we reiterate this approach and specifically describe methods used to evaluate berries for chemopreventive efficacy in both rodent and human esophagus. The reader is referred to other papers [7–10] that describe

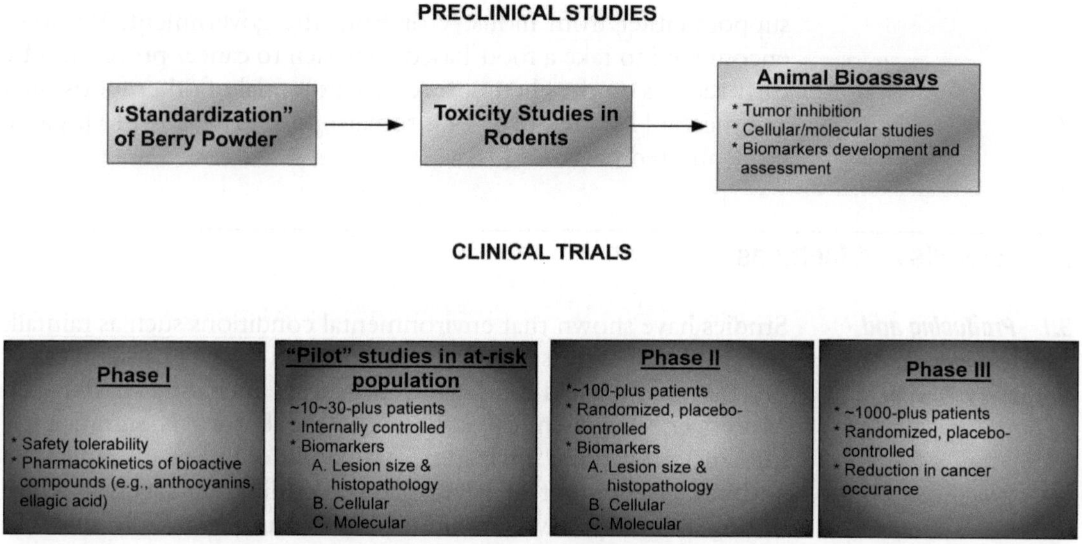

Fig. 1 Stepwise approach to evaluate berries for cancer prevention

methods used for evaluation of berries in other organ sites such as colon and oral cavity. Our hope is that this information will be useful for other laboratories interested in evaluating specific foodstuffs for cancer prevention.

2 Approach Used to Evaluate the Chemopreventive Activity of BRBs (Fig. 1)

1. Develop "standardized" BRB powder using nutrient, non-nutrient, microbial, and chemical analyses.
2. Evaluate potential toxicity in rodents.
3. Determine anti-tumorigenic effects in rodents and the mechanism(s) of these effects.
4. Conduct phase I clinical trials of toxicity and pharmacokinetics in humans.
5. Conduct "pilot" trials in 20–30 high-risk individuals to examine effects on precancerous lesions and relevant biomarkers.
6. Conduct randomized, placebo-controlled phase II biomarker trials typically involving 100–200 high-risk individuals.
7. Conduct phase III trials typically involving more than a thousand individuals to determine cancer prevention efficacy.

This approach is not unlike that proposed by Kelloff et al. [11] for the preclinical and clinical evaluation of individual natural compounds and synthetic drugs for chemopreventive efficacy. The most difficult step in this approach is conducting large, phase III trials because of the difficulty in obtaining financial support either from industry or from the government. We were encouraged to take a food-based approach to cancer prevention by early reports on the chemopreventive potential of other foods such as broccoli [12], tea [13, 14], tomato juice [15], soy [16], garlic [17], and red beetroot [18].

3 Materials and Methods

3.1 Producing and Standardizing Black Raspberry Powder

Studies have shown that environmental conditions such as rainfall, soil conditions, stress and microbial load can have a profound effect on the yearly yield of berries per acre, including BRBs [4]. Moreover, the chemical content of the berries is significantly influenced by these environmental conditions. For example, the anthocyanin content of BRBs grown on different farms in Ohio during a single year was found to vary as much as two- to fourfold [4]. Similarly, the ellagic acid content of BRBs was found to vary as much as 35–40 % from year to year [19]. To minimize this variability, we have obtained all BRBs from a single farm in Ohio, or more recently, from a farm in Oregon that maintains similar USDA standards for berry production, harvest, and storage. The steps used for preparing black raspberry powder from these berries are shown in Fig. 2. Each year, BRBs of the Jewel (Ohio) or Bristol

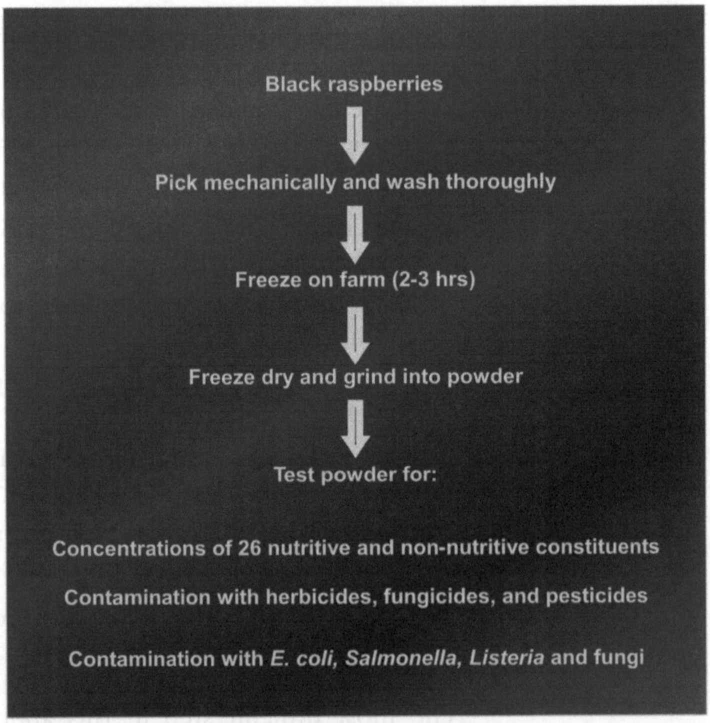

Fig. 2 Method for preparing and testing berry powder

(Oregon) varieties are grown in the same soil, picked mechanically when ripe, washed immediately with water and frozen at −20 °C on the farm within 2–3 h of picking. The berries are then shipped frozen to either Van Drunen Farms in Momence, IL (Ohio berries) or Oregon Freeze Dry (Albany, OR) where they are freeze-dried under Good Manufacturing Practice (GMP) conditions. After freeze-drying, whole BRBs are ground into a fine powder and used as such in experimental studies. Alternatively, the seeds can be removed by forcing the dried berries through a sieve, and the dried pulp ground into a powder. The seeds can also be ground into a fine powder; however, we have not evaluated the chemopreventive potential of BRB seeds, which contain significant quantities of ellagitannins. Berry powder prepared from pulp only is preferred for human studies because some subjects in clinical trials have developed mild gastrointestinal disturbances from consuming berry seeds. In our laboratory, powders prepared from either whole berries (pulp + seed) or berry pulp only, have been about equal in their ability to reduce chemically induced tumors in the rat esophagus (data not published). Typically, the berry powder is shipped frozen from the freeze-drying facilities to our laboratories where it is stored at −20 °C until used for experiments. For standardization purposes, each yearly batch of berry powder is analyzed by Covance Laboratories (Madison, WI) for its content of 20+ nutrient and non-nutrient components, including agents with chemopreventive potential [6]. During the past several years, quantitative analysis of the four anthocyanins in BRB powder has been performed in the Stephen Hecht laboratory at the University of Minnesota Cancer Center (Minneapolis, MN). Recently, we have observed that the levels of the four anthocyanins in BRB powder remain within 20–25 % of the initial analysis for at least 10 years when the powder is stored in sealed plastic bags at −20 °C (data not published).

Recent events have emphasized the importance of evaluating the safety of food products for human consumption. Therefore, we recommend that each batch (100–500 lbs) of freeze-dried BRB powder, and powder from other berry types, be analyzed for contamination with microbes (e.g., *Listeria*, *Escherichia coli*, *Salmonella*, *Shigella*, and fungi), and potentially harmful chemicals (pesticides, herbicides, and fungicides) (Fig. 2). These analyses are routinely performed by commercial firms that require only about 100–200 g of powder to test for microbial and chemical contamination, as well as nutrient and non-nutrient content. In addition, to prevent degradation of nutrients and non-nutritive constituents, as well as the growth of microbes (especially fungi), berry powders should be stored frozen at −20 °C or colder in sealed bags before and during use in animal studies and in human clinical trials.

Table 1 illustrates some of the potential chemopreventive agent content of powders that were prepared from BRBs obtained from an Ohio farm in 1997, 2001 and 2006 [20] and from an

Table 1
Some potential chemopreventive agents in powder made from black raspberries harvested in 1997, 2001, 2006, and 2010

	Crop year[a]			
Component	**1997**	**2001**	**2006**	**2010**
Minerals				
Calcium	215.00	175.00	188.00	234.00
Selenium[a]	<5.00	<5.00	<5.00	<5.00
Zinc	2.69	2.34	2.16	2.00
Vitamins				
α-Carotene	<0.02	<0.02	<0.03	<0.02
β-Carotene	<0.02	0.06	<0.07	<0.02
α-Tocopherol	n.d.	n.d.	10.40	n.d.
γ-Tocopherol	n.d.	n.d.	11.20	n.d.
Folate	0.06	0.08	0.14	0.12
Sterols				
β-Sitosterol	80.10	88.80	110.00	84.20
Campesterol	3.40	5.90	5.50	4.60
Simple phenols				
Ellagic acid	166.30	185.00	225.00	320.00
Ferulic acid	17.60	<5.00	47.10	90.80
ρ-Coumaric acid	9.23	6.82	6.92	n.d.
Chlorogenic acid	n.d.	n.d.	0.14	0.11
Quercetin	n.d.	43.60	36.50	143.00
Anthocyanins				
Cyanidin-3-*O*-glucoside	n.d.	250.00	278.50	277.80
Cyanidin-3-*O*-sambubioside	n.d.	220.00	56.00	76.49
Cyanidin-3-*O*-rutinoside	n.d.	2,002.00	1,790.00	1,981.43
Cyanidin-3-*O*-xylosylrutinoside	n.d.	510.00	853.50	373.21

Abbreviation: *n.d.* not determined
[a]All measures in the crop-year columns are mg/100 g dry weight, except for that of selenium, which is μg/100 g dry weight. Berries in crop years 1997, 2001, and 2006 were obtained from a farm in Ohio. Those from the year 2010 were obtained from a farm in Oregon

Oregon farm in 2010. The content of these components in the Ohio berries appears to be similar to that of the Oregon berries; however, further studies are needed to provide an adequate comparison of the chemical composition of Ohio and Oregon berries. Note that BRBs contain relatively high levels of the four anthocyanins, calcium, ß-sitosterol, ellagic acid and quercetin. The amounts of calcium, zinc, ß-sitosterol, α-carotene, ellagic acid, ρ-coumaric acid, cyanidin-3-*O*-glucoside, and cyanidin-3-*O*-rutinoside in the yearly powders varied from 10 to 40 %, whereas the amounts of other constituents (ß-carotene, folate, ferulic acid, quercetin, cyanidin-3-*O*-sambubioside and cyanidin-3-*O*-xylosylrutinoside) varied from 60 to 90 %. The relatively high variability in levels of ß-carotene and folate is likely due to problems in accurately measuring the low levels of these agents in the powder. Selenium is present in microgram quantities in BRBs, so values for selenium are reported as <5 μg/100 g dry weight. Because only a small percentage of the overall number of compounds in BRBs is analyzed, BRBs likely contain potential chemopreventive agents in addition to those listed in Table 1.

Importantly, in spite of the variability in content of the above-mentioned constituents in BRB powder on a year-to-year basis, all yearly batches of powder tested so far have exhibited similar inhibitory effects on the development of chemically induced tumors in the rat esophagus when the powder is added at 5 % of the diet. These results suggest that the effectiveness of BRBs is not compromised by significant variations in some of their bioactive constituents. This may be due to the fact that the fiber component of black raspberries is almost as effective in preventing tumor development in the rat esophagus as whole BRB powder and its content is routinely about 45 % of the dry weight of the powder.

3.2 Testing for Toxicity in Rodents

Chemopreventive agents may be administered to humans for periods of months to years. Therefore, they should elicit chemopreventive effects at concentrations that cause little or no toxicity. To evaluate the potential toxicity of BRB powder, the powder was mixed into a synthetic AIN-76A diet at a concentration of 2.5, 5.0, or 10 % using a Hobart mixer. To maintain an isocaloric diet, the starch in the AIN-76A diets containing BRB powder was reduced by 2.5, 5.0, or 10 %. BRB powder was mixed into the diet for at least 20 min to ensure even mixing of the powder throughout the diet. Even mixing was confirmed by routine sampling of the mixed diet and analyzing the samples for content of the four anthocyanins in BRBs. Five to six week-old male Fischer 344 rats were fed either control AIN-76A diet or control diet containing 2.5, 5.0, or 10 % BRB powder for a period of 36 weeks. Control and berry diet groups each contained a minimum of ten rats. The diet was placed in feeding jars and changed once per week. The anthocyanins in BRBs remain stable in the diet for a period of at least 1 week. Weight data on each rat and food consumption data was obtained weekly. At 36 weeks, the rats were euthanized by inhalation of CO_2 and about 1 mL of blood is collected from the heart. The following organs were harvested and placed in 10 % buffered formalin for subsequent histopathologic evaluation: nasal cavity, oral cavity, esophagus, lung, stomach, small intestine, colon, liver, pancreas, thymus, heart, brain, kidney, spleen, urinary bladder and testis. After fixation in buffered formalin for at least 24 h, the formalin was replaced by phosphate buffered saline (PBS) and the tissues refrigerated until prepared for evaluation by routine histopathology. All tissues from each of the ten rats per group were examined by a board-certified pathologist for evidence of toxicity.

Table 2
BRB diets to prevent the development of carcinogen-induced and spontaneously occurring tumors in animal models

Species	Site	Carcinogen	Berries	% Tumor reduction	References
Hamster	Cheek pouch	DMBA	5, 10 % in diet	8–56	[21]
Rat	Colon	AOM	2.5, 5, 10 % in diet	42–71	[7]
Rat	Esophagus	NMBA	5, 10 % in diet	43–68	[20]
Rat	Mammary gland	Estrogen	1, 2.5 % in diet	43–51	[22]
Min mouse	Intestine	Spontaneous	10 % in diet	57	[23]
Muc2+ mouse	Intestine, colon	Spontaneous	10 % in diet	50–55	[23]
SKH-1 mouse	Skin	UVB	500 mg extract	77	[24]

DMBA 7,12-dimethylbenz[a]anthracene, *AOM* azoxymethane, *NMBA* N-nitrosomethylbenzylamine

Body weight and food consumption data did not vary significantly between control- and BRB-fed rats during the 36-week study. Histopathologic evaluation revealed no obvious toxic effects in any of the organs examined from rats treated with either control or BRB diets. Similarly, no significant differences were observed in white blood cell counts or in hematocrits between rats on control versus BRB diets. Interestingly, about a 10 % reduction in blood cholesterol in rats treated with the berry diets was observed compared to the control diet at 36 weeks [7, 20].

Note that rat diets containing as high as 10 % BRB powder would be equivalent to approximately 1.8 oz of BRB powder in the daily human diet, as calculated on a body surface area basis [6]. Because 1 oz of berry powder is equivalent in content to about 10 oz of fresh berries, 1.8 oz of powder averages to about 1.1 lb of fresh whole BRBs per day. The observation that little or no toxicity was observed in rats treated for 36 weeks with BRBs at 10 % of the diet suggested that high doses of berries might also be well tolerated in humans.

3.3 Evaluating Anticarcinogenic Effects in Animals and Mechanisms of Action

Table 2 summarizes the results of numerous studies to evaluate the ability of BRB diets to prevent the development of carcinogen-induced and spontaneously occurring tumors in animal models. AIN-76A diets containing either 1.0, 2.5, 5.0, or 10 % BRB powder have been shown to reduce carcinogen-induced tumors in the Syrian hamster cheek pouch [21], in the F344 rat colon and esophagus [7, 20] and in the ACI rat mammary gland [22]. A 10 % BRB diet inhibited the development of spontaneous intestinal tumors in $Apc^{+/-}$ Min mice and both intestinal and colon tumors in $Muc2^{-/-}$ mice [23]. Finally, an anthocyanin-rich extract of BRBs was shown to inhibit UVB-induced skin tumors in SKH-1 mice [24].

The most reliable measure of tumor inhibition in these model systems is tumor multiplicity and depending upon the temporal sequence of administration of the carcinogen and the berry diet, the extent of reduction in tumor multiplicity ranges from about 30 to 70 %. BRB diets do not inhibit 100 % of tumorigenesis, suggesting that the inhibitory components in BRBs and/or their metabolites are not fully absorbed, which is most certainly the case for the anthocyanins and ellagitannins [25]. Typically, the uptake of BRB anthocyanins and ellagitannins into the blood of rodents and humans is less than 1 % of the administered dose [25, 26]. In addition, BRB compounds may not sufficiently affect all of the critical signaling pathways of carcinogenesis.

3.3.1 Rat Esophagus Model of Squamous Cell Carcinoma

Most studies in our laboratory have evaluated the anticarcinogenic effects of BRB powder in a rat model of esophageal squamous cell carcinoma [27]. Because the objective of this chapter is to present methods used to evaluate BRB effects in preclinical animal models (Fig. 1), we describe in detail the development and use of the rat esophageal model for berry studies. In this model system, esophageal tumors are produced by repeated subcutaneous (s.c.) injection of a carcinogen, *N*-nitrosomethylbenzylamine (NMBA), into the interscapular region of male Fischer 344 (F-344) rats and tumors on the surface of the esophagus are counted after 25–35 weeks. The time required for tumor development varies with the dose of carcinogen and the time-frame in which the carcinogen is administered. Most tumors are papillomas because the emerging papillomas restrict transit of food through the esophagus leading to severe weight loss of the animals before many carcinomas can develop. With the exception of the nasal cavity, we have not observed tumor development at any organ site other than the esophagus in this animal model. Nasal cavity tumors are rare.

Two protocols have been used to evaluate the potential inhibitory effects of BRBs on the development of NMBA-induced esophageal tumors (Fig. 3). In the "complete carcinogenesis protocol" (Fig. 3A), 10 control rats, 5–7 weeks-old, are injected with the solvent for NMBA (DMSO/water; 80:20; vehicle control); another 10 rats are fed the highest dietary dose of BRBs (berry control); 30 rats are treated with NMBA only (carcinogen control); and 30 rats per group are treated with NMBA + BRBs (2.5, 5.0, or 10 %). Rats are fed BRB diets for 2 weeks before initial treatment with NMBA, during the NMBA treatments, and until the end of the bioassay. Beginning at week 3, the animals are injected s.c. with NMBA (0.35–0.5 mg/kg body weight) once per week for 15 weeks. All rats are sacrificed at 25–30 weeks. Esophageal papillomas do not develop spontaneously and have not been observed in any vehicle control or berry control rats to date. NMBA control rats usually have develop between 7 and 10 papillomas per esophagus, and the BRB diets typically reduce the average number of

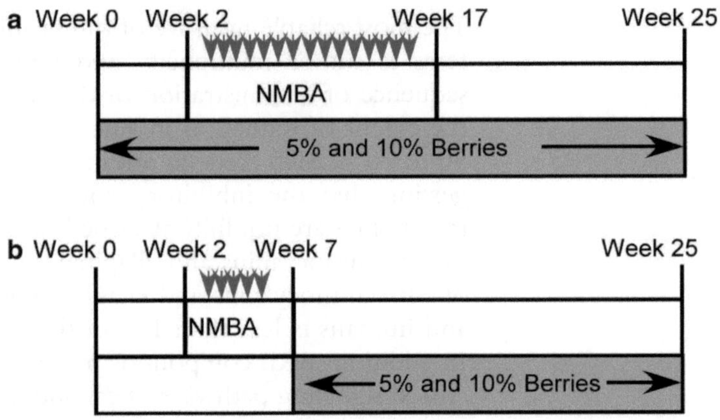

Fig. 3 Two protocols for evaluation of the potential inhibitory effects of BRBs on the development of NMBA-induced esophageal tumors

esophageal papillomas by about 30–80 % relative to the number in NMBA controls. The inhibitory effects of the 5.0 and 10 % BRB diets on tumor multiplicity are usually significant ($p < 0.05$) whereas the effects of the 2.5 % BRB diet are usually not significant ($p > 0.05$). Because NMBA is a strong carcinogen, BRBs rarely produce a significant reduction in tumor incidence when compared to the incidence in NMBA control rats. Tumor size data in rats treated with NMBA only, versus NMBA+BRBs is often too variable to demonstrate a significant inhibitory effect of the berries on tumor size. The complete carcinogenesis protocol permits an evaluation of both the anti-initiation and anti-promotion/progression effects of the berries. In recent studies, additional rats have been added to the bioassay to permit the sampling of esophageal tissues at intermediate time points (i.e., 10 and 20 weeks). This allows for examination of the effects of BRBs on morphometric, histopathologic and molecular biomarkers during tumor development. In addition, blood samples can be taken at all-time points to determine the effects of BRBs on levels of inflammatory cytokines/chemokines in the blood.

The post-initiation protocol (Fig. 3b) has been used the most frequently for chemoprevention studies in the rat model of esophageal carcinogenesis because it more closely mimics the means by which humans are treated with chemoprevention agents, including berries. In certain regions of China where the occurrence of esophageal squamous cell carcinoma is high, residents are routinely screened by upper endoscopy for the presence of esophageal dysplasia and cancer. If they have cancer or severe esophageal dysplasia, they are candidates for surgery, radiotherapy, and chemotherapy. However, esophageal lesions found to be either moderately or mildly dysplastic are not treated and individuals with these lesions are candidates for chemoprevention. In the post-initiation

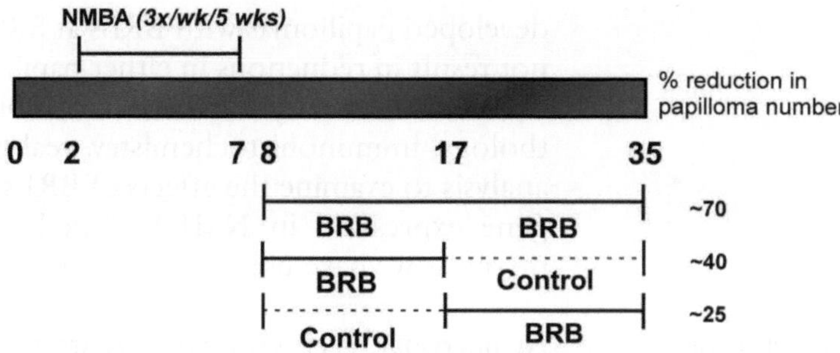

Fig. 4 Inhibition of esophageal tumor number by 5 % BRB diet in the post-initiation bioassay

protocol, beginning 1–2 weeks after they enter the animal facility, F344 male rats (5–7 weeks old) are given s.c. injections of NMBA (0.25–0.35 mg/kg B.W.) three times per week for 5 weeks. One week after cessation of NMBA treatment, the esophagus contains a mixture of normal, hyperplastic, and dysplastic (mild to moderate) epithelium resembling the histopathology of esophagi in high-risk Chinese. At that point, the rats are fed 2.5, 5.0, or 10 % BRB diets until they are sacrificed at the end of the bioassay (30–35 weeks). The control groups are the same as for the complete carcinogenesis protocol and the number of rats per group is also the same. The bioassay period is longer than in the complete carcinogenesis protocol because tumors take longer to develop. The average number of tumors per esophagus in NMBA control rats at the end of the post-initiation bioassay (2–5) is usually lower than in the complete protocol (7–10). As for the complete protocol, additional rats can be added at the beginning of the bioassay to permit intermittent sampling (e.g., at 10, 15, and 25 weeks) of esophageal tissues for histopathological and molecular studies during tumor development.

Figure 4 illustrates some results obtained by varying the time of administration of a 5 % BRB diet to rats during the post-initiation bioassay (data not published). As indicated, when the rats were initiated on the berry diet within 1 week after NMBA treatment and until the end of the bioassay, the berries reduced the number of esophageal tumors by about 60 % ($p<0.01$). However, when the berries were fed to the rats at 1 week after NMBA treatment and then removed from the diet at 15 weeks, the reduction in tumor number was only about 35 % ($p<0.05$). Finally, when the berries were withheld from the diet until 15 weeks into the bioassay the reduction in tumor number was less than 20 % ($p>0.05$). These results suggest that the most effective chemoprevention occurs when berries are fed continuously to animals that possess premalignant lesions, and that early lesions respond more effectively to BRB treatment than more advanced lesions. These results are consistent with our observation that treatment of already developed papillomas with BRBs at 5.0, 10, or 20 % of the diet did not result in reductions in either papilloma number or size [28].

Our laboratory has used a combination of routine histopathology, immunohistochemistry, real-time PCR and western blot analysis to examine the effects of BRBs on lesion development and gene expression in NMBA-treated rat esophagus. The specific methods we have used are as follows:

Histological Grading of Pre-neoplastic Lesions

At necropsy, each esophagus is stretched onto an index card and fixed in 10 % buffered formalin for no longer than 24 h. After fixation, the formalin is replaced with PBS and the tissues are kept at 4 °C in a refrigerator. Each esophagus is cut into thirds and paraffin embedded on edge. Serial 4-μm sections are cut and mounted on Superfrost Plus slides (Fisher Scientific, Pittsburgh, PA). A hematoxylin and eosin (H & E) stained slide of each esophagus is prepared and the entire esophagus of each animal scanned at 100× magnification. Each viewing field is categorized into one of five histological categories: normal epithelium, epithelial hyperplasia, low-grade dysplasia, high-grade dysplasia, and squamous cell papilloma. The classification scheme used is a modification of criteria developed by Pozharisski et al. [29], with consideration toward the gross and microscopic descriptions of hyperplasia and dysplasia given in Cotran et al. [30].

Quantitative Immunohistochemistry

The entire esophagus from five rats per group and ten tumors from the same five rats per group are stained for the antigens (e.g., biomarkers) of interest. Depending upon the biomarker, either paraffin-embedded or frozen tissues are cut at 4-μm and placed on positively charged slides. Slides with specimens are then placed in a 60 °C oven for 15 min, cooled, de-paraffinized, and rehydrated through graded ethanol solutions to water. Tissues are antigen retrieved by microwaving in sodium citrate for 5–12 min depending on the biomarker. All slides are treated for 5–10 min with a 3 % H_2O_2 solution in water to block endogenous peroxidase. The slides are then placed on a Dako Autostainer for automated staining. Primary antibodies, antibody dilutions, and incubation times and temperatures are optimized for each biomarker as previously reported [20]. The slides are then stained with their respective secondary antibody, followed by incubation with 3,3-diaminobenzidine to permit signal visualization and counterstained with hematoxylin, dehydrated through a graded series of ethanol, and coverslipped. Appropriate positive and negative controls are included in each staining run.

Slides stained for specific antigens are viewed at 200× magnification with a bright-field microscope mounted with a high-resolution spot camera. The camera is interfaced with a computer containing a Matrox frame grabber board and image analysis software (e.g., Simple PCI Imaging Systems by Compix Inc.,

Cranberry Township, PA). The basal cell layer of each esophagus is scanned, and a minimum of ten fields (1,500–2,000 cells) are quantified for each antigen under study. Papillomas are similarly quantified, but at a magnification of 100× to allow for greater visualization in a single field.

Real-Time PCR

Total cellular RNA is isolated from frozen esophageal tissues using TRIzol Reagent (Life Technologies, Gaithersburg, MD) according to the manufacturer's instructions [31]. After extraction, all RNA samples are analyzed for integrity of 18S and 28S rRNA by ethidium bromide staining of 1 μg of RNA resolved by electrophoresis on 1.2 % agarose formaldehyde gels. One-step real-time reverse-transcription PCR is performed in an appropriate sequence detection system using the QuantiTect SYBR green RT-PCR kit as described previously [32]. Briefly, the reaction of a 50 μL volume of total cellular RNA, QuantiTect RT Mix, QuantiTect SYBR green RT-PCR Master Mix, and forward and reverse primers are reverse-transcribed, and PCR is performed after the reverse transcription reaction. The expression of the genes being measured is normalized against the expression of the housekeeping gene hypoxanthineguanine-phosphoribosyltransferase (HPRT). Primers for the genes under study are designed according to published sequences with Primer Express Software v2.0 (Applied Biosystems, Foster City, CA). Each individual RNA sample for each gene is assayed in triplicate. Two controls are run with every reaction: one contains RNA and QuantiTect RT Mix to detect genomic DNA and the other contains the reaction reagents without RNA to confirm that the reagents do not display a signal. Data are collected using SDS Sequence Detector Software (PE, Applied Biosystems).

Western Blot Analysis

Proteins are extracted from frozen rat esophageal epithelium. Protein concentrations are determined using the Bio-Rad assay (Bio-Rad, Hercules, CA) according to the manufacturer's recommendations. Fifty micrograms of protein with NuPAGE LDS Sample Buffer and NuPAGE sample reducing agent are heated at 100 °C for 1 min. After cooling at room temperature for 5 min, proteins are fractionated by 7 % NuPAGE Novex Tris-acetate gel electrophoresis. Proteins are then transferred to an Invitrolon polyvinylidene difluoride membrane. The membrane is blocked with blocking buffer (e.g., concentrated saline and Hammarsten casein solution) at 4 °C overnight. The blot is then probed with appropriate antibodies against the antigen(s) (i.e., biomarker) under study at room temperature for 1 h. After extensive washing to eliminate nonspecific binding, the membrane is incubated for 1 h at room temperature with a goat anti-rabbit secondary antibody labeled with alkaline phosphatase. Western blots are visualized using a Western Breeze chromogenic immunodetection kit. h-Actin (1:1,000; Sigma) is detected in the same sample to ensure equal protein loading.

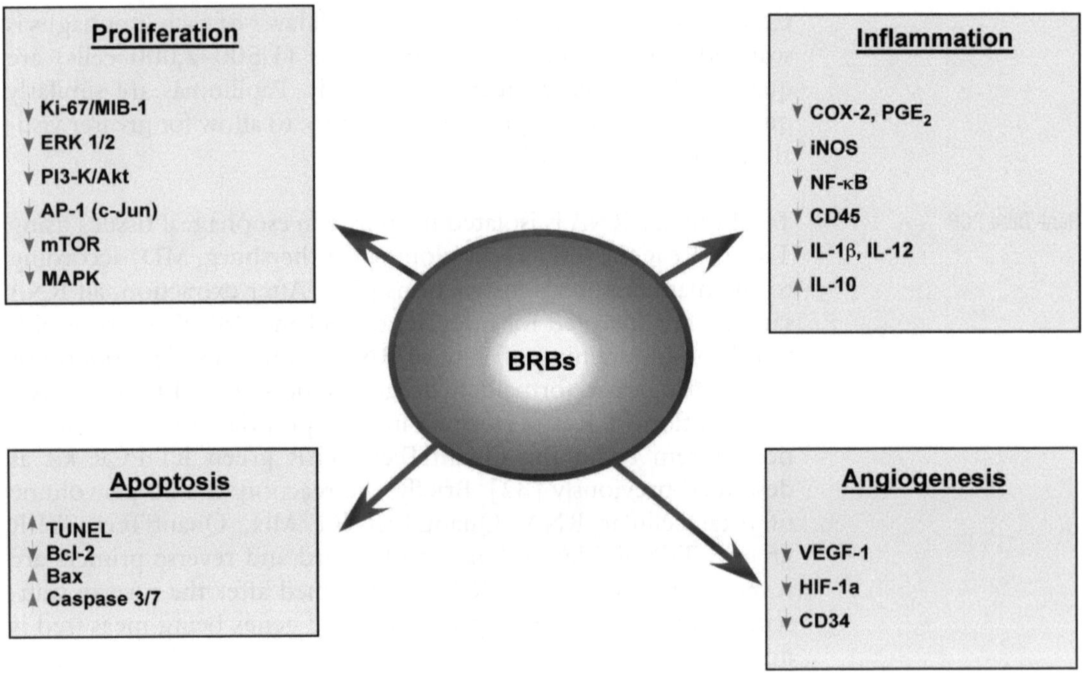

CD45-leukocyte common antigen, CDF34 - Microvessel marker

Fig. 5 Effects of BRBs on cellular events and associated genes in NMBA-treated rat esophagus

Statistical Analysis

Body weight, food consumption, tumor multiplicity (i.e., mean number of tumors/esophagus), and tumor volume data are collected for all rats fed control or experimental diets. These data and mRNA expression data are analyzed and compared using ANOVA followed by Dunnet's or Newman–Keul's multiple comparison test to identify individual differences among groups when ANOVA result is significant. Tumor incidence (i.e., percentage of animals in each group with tumors) data is analyzed using the Chi-Square test. All statistical analysis is conducted using GraphPad Prism 4.0. Differences are considered statistically significant at $p < 0.05$ and all p values are two-sided.

Some Results of Mechanistic Studies in the Rat Esophagus Model

Studies using the rat esophagus model have revealed that BRBs modulate cellular events in esophageal carcinogenesis including proliferation, apoptosis, inflammation, and angiogenesis (Fig. 5). Using the above-described methods, we have identified multiple NMBA-deregulated genes associated with cellular events that are protectively modulated by berries [31, 33, 34] (Fig. 5). These include major transcription activators such as nuclear factor kappa B (NF-κB) and activator protein-1 (AP-1), genes involved in multiple cell signaling pathways such as phosphatidylinositol 3-kinase (PI3-K)/protein kinase B (PKB/Akt), extracellular signal-regulated kinases (ERKs), p38, c-Jun N-terminal kinases (JNKs), and mammalian target of rapamycin (mTOR), apoptosis-related factors such as Bcl-2, Bax, and caspase 3/7, inflammation-related enzymes (e.g., cyclooxygenase-2, inducible nitric oxide synthase) and cytokines (e.g., interleukin [IL]-1β, IL-12, IL-10), and growth factors related to angiogenesis such as vascular endothelial growth factor (VEGF)-1 and hypoxia-inducible factor (HIF)-1α. Other genes protectively modulated by berries have been identified using DNA microarray. An early study using DNA microarray identified 462 of 2,261 NMBA-deregulated genes in the initiation stage of rat esophageal carcinogenesis that were restored to near normal levels of expression by BRBs [35]. These restored genes were associated with multiple cellular functions including carcinogen metabolism, suggesting that the active components of BRBs elicit a genome-wide effect in influencing genes involved in the early events of esophageal tumorigenesis. A more recent study using DNA microarray identified numerous genes in the late stages of rat esophageal tumorigenesis that were protectively modulated by BRBs [10]. In both pre-neoplastic tissues and in papillomas, BRBs modulated the mRNA expression of genes associated with carbohydrate and lipid metabolism, cell proliferation, apoptosis, and inflammation as well as both cyclooxygenase and lipoxygenase pathways of arachidonic acid metabolism. Matrix metalloproteinases involved in tissue invasion and metastasis were also modulated by BRBs. Therefore, as for the initiation events in carcinogenesis, BRBs elicit a genome-wide effect in modulating the expression of genes involved in the late stages of esophageal carcinogenesis.

3.4 Biofractionation of BRBs to Identify the Bioactive Constituents

In any food-based approach to cancer prevention, identifying the bioactive constituents in the foodstuff and determining their importance in the overall chemopreventive effects of the food is desirable. In attempts to accomplish this with BRBs, Dr. Stephen Hecht and his colleagues Steven Carmella and Ben Ransom (University of Minnesota) developed a procedure to isolate several extract fractions from BRB powder that could be evaluated and compared for efficacy in the rat esophagus model (Fig. 6). The methods for isolation of these extracts have been described in detail [34] and will be discussed briefly here. With appropriate modifications, these methods could be used for other foodstuffs.

3.4.1 Hexane Extract

Black raspberry powder (500 g) is placed in a 2,500 mL beaker with 1,500 mL hexane, and the mixture is stirred with an explosion proof mechanical stirrer and sonicated for 30 min at room temperature. The supernatant fraction is vacuum-filtered through a Buchner funnel. This procedure is repeated twice using fresh hexane, for a total extraction volume of 4,500 mL. After the final extraction, the residue is dried briefly on the funnel with a stream

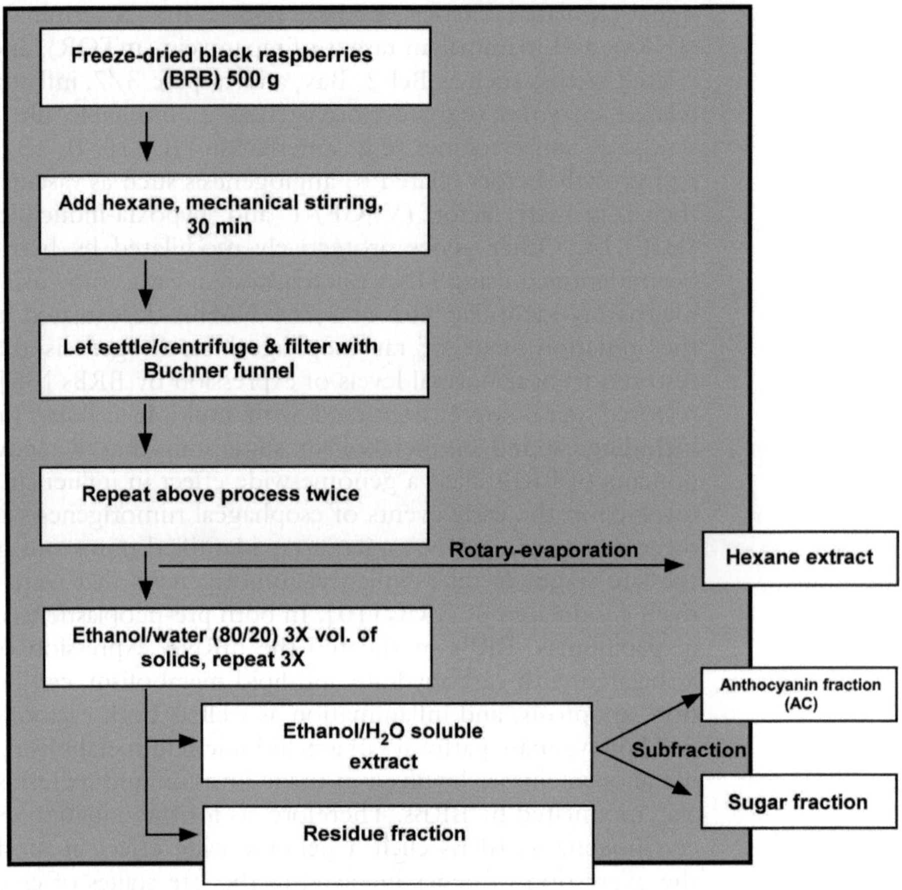

Fig. 6 Scheme for extraction of freeze-dried BRBs

of N_2. The combined hexane extracts are concentrated to dryness by rotary evaporation at reduced pressure. The final extract is stored at −20 °C.

3.4.2 Ethanol–H_2O (80:20): Soluble Extract

The residue from the hexane extract is placed in a 2,500 mL beaker with 1,500 mL of ethanol–H_2O (80:20), and the mixture is stirred and sonicated for 30 min at room temperature as described above. The resulting mixture is filtered as above, and the procedure is repeated three times with fresh 1,500 mL batches of ethanol–H_2O (80:20). The solvents are removed to the extent possible by rotary evaporation at reduced pressure. This process yields a syrup and the remaining solvent is removed by freeze-drying, as described below.

3.4.3 Ethanol–H_2O: Insoluble (Residue) Fraction

The berry mass obtained above after removal of the ethanol–H_2O (80:20) solvent is allowed to dry for several minutes under vacuum, placed in a vacuum desiccator for 4 days, and then stored at 4 °C. This fraction represents the solids in BRB and is termed the "residue" fraction.

3.4.4 Anthocyanin Fraction and Sugar Fraction

A polystyrene-based resin, SP-700 (Mitsubishi Chemical Co.; 1.5 L, 825 g) is activated by overnight treatment with 1.2 L of 96 % ethanol, followed by rinsing with 1.2 L of doubly distilled H_2O. The resin is stirred in the H_2O for 10 min and then filtered. The filtered resin is mixed with 1.5 L of doubly distilled H_2O and introduced into a 7.5 cm (diameter) × 50 cm glass column containing a glass frit. The height of the resin in the column is about 36 cm. The packed column is washed thoroughly with 4 L of H_2O to remove any ethanol. The washed resin is poured back into a 3-L beaker, and about 150 g of the ethanol–H_2O (80:20) extract (as a concentrated syrup equivalent to about 93 g of the dried extract, or 11 % of the resin weight) is then added. The mixture is stirred for 10 min to allow the anthocyanins to adsorb onto the resin and then placed back into the column. The column is eluted with about 2 L of H_2O at a rate of about 20 mL/min. This eluant contains the "sugar fraction." Then, 3 L of 95 % ethanol are added to the column in steps. The first 800 mL, containing H_2O that was already on the column, is collected separately and combined with the sugar fraction. The next 2 L of the now deeply colored ethanol eluant is collected and it contains the anthocyanin fraction. The anthocyanin fraction is concentrated to a tar-like consistency using a centrifugal vacuum concentrator (e.g., SpeedVac, Thermo Savant) using a preparative rotor. The sugar fraction is concentrated by rotary evaporation under reduced pressure.

3.4.5 Freeze-Drying of the Ethanol–H_2O (80:20)-Soluble Extract and Sugar Fractions

During conventional freeze-drying, the sugar fraction remains as a syrup and the 80:20 extract expands to a semisolid tar. The initial water content of each of these fractions is determined by freeze-drying or rotary-evaporating a small aliquot to dryness. The fractions are then adjusted to approximately 75–80 % H_2O content. A metal colander with numerous 4-mm circular openings in the bottom is placed over a stainless-steel beaker, which is approximately two thirds full with 4 L of liquid N_2. Seven hundred milliliters of the sugar or the ethanol–H_2O (80:20) fraction is poured into the colander over a 2-min period. The majority of the extract forms 5-mm frozen spheres at the bottom of the beaker. The liquid N_2 and the spheres are poured through a wire mesh strainer. The spheres in the strainer are immediately placed in a precooled (−80 °C) 10 × 6 × 1.2-in. metal tray. The tray is placed on a prechilled (−25 °C) shelf in a freeze drier and vacuum is applied. The sample remains under these conditions for 4 days. The freezing shelf temperature is then allowed to equilibrate, and the sample remains under these conditions for 3 days. The result is a dry foam for the ethanol–H_2O (80:20) extract and the sugar fraction. These fractions are then stored at −20 °C.

Anthocyanin levels in BRBs, the ethanol–H_2O (80:20) extract, and the anthocyanin fraction are determined by high-performance liquid chromatography before incorporation into the diet [36]. The molar percentages of the three major anthocyanins in BRB are cyanidin-3-O-glucoside (12 %), cyanidin-3-O-(2G-xylosylrutinoside) (34 %), and cyanidin-3-O-rutinoside (53 %). These molar percentages are very similar for the ethanol–water-soluble extract and the anthocyanin fraction.

3.4.6 Testing the BRBs and Their Component Extracts/Fractions for Anticarcinogenic Activity in the Rat Esophagus Model

The extract fractions isolated above are tested for their relative ability to inhibit the development of NMBA-induced esophageal tumors in F344 rats using the post-initiation protocol [34]. Two weeks after arrival in the animal facility, rats are randomly assigned into eight groups and placed on control AIN-76A diet or AIN-76A diet containing BRB powder or its fractions for the entire 30-week bioassay. The amount of each fraction added to the diet is based on the weight percentage contribution of each fraction to BRB. For the fractions containing anthocyanins (i.e., anthocyanin extract and ethanol–H_2O (80:20) extract) the amount of each fraction is increased to compensate for losses of anthocyanins during isolation of the fraction (as determined by high-performance liquid chromatography analysis of the anthocyanins), so that the amount of anthocyanins in each of these fractions, when added to the diet, is approximately 3.8 μmol/g diet, the same as that in the 5 % BRB powder diet. The groups are as follows: group 1, vehicle control group; group 2, NMBA control group; group 3, 5 % BRB powder and NMBA; group 4, the anthocyanin extract and NMBA; group 5, the ethanol–H_2O (80:20) extract and NMBA; group 6, the residue fraction (containing only 0.02 μmol anthocyanins/g diet) and NMBA; group 7, the hexane extract and NMBA; and group 8, the sugar fraction and NMBA (groups 7 and 8 contain only trace quantities of anthocyanins). After 2 weeks on the diet, rats in group 1 are injected s.c. with 0.2 mL of a solution containing 20 % DMSO in water once per week for 15 weeks (vehicle control). Rats in groups 2–8 are injected s.c. with NMBA (0.3 mg/kg body weight) in 0.2 mL vehicle once per week for 15 weeks. At 30 weeks, the animals are sacrificed by CO_2 asphyxiation. The esophagus of each animal is opened longitudinally, and the surface tumors are mapped, counted, and sized. Lesions > 0.5 mm in a single dimension (length, width, and height) are considered to be tumors. Tumor volume is calculated using the formula for a prolate spheroid: length × width × height × $\pi/6$, and expressed in mm^3, which can also be considered as an estimate of tumor size. About one half of each esophagus and each individual tumor is fixed in 10 % neutral buffered formalin for subsequent histopathologic evaluation, and the remaining esophagus and tumors are snap-frozen in liquid nitrogen for western blot analysis.

The effects of the diets on the number and volume of NMBA-induced esophageal papillomas at 30 weeks are shown in Fig. 7a, b, respectively. As indicated, diets containing either 5 % whole BRB powder, the anthocyanin extract, or the ethanol–H_2O-soluble extract (each containing ~3.8 μmol anthocyanins/g diet) were

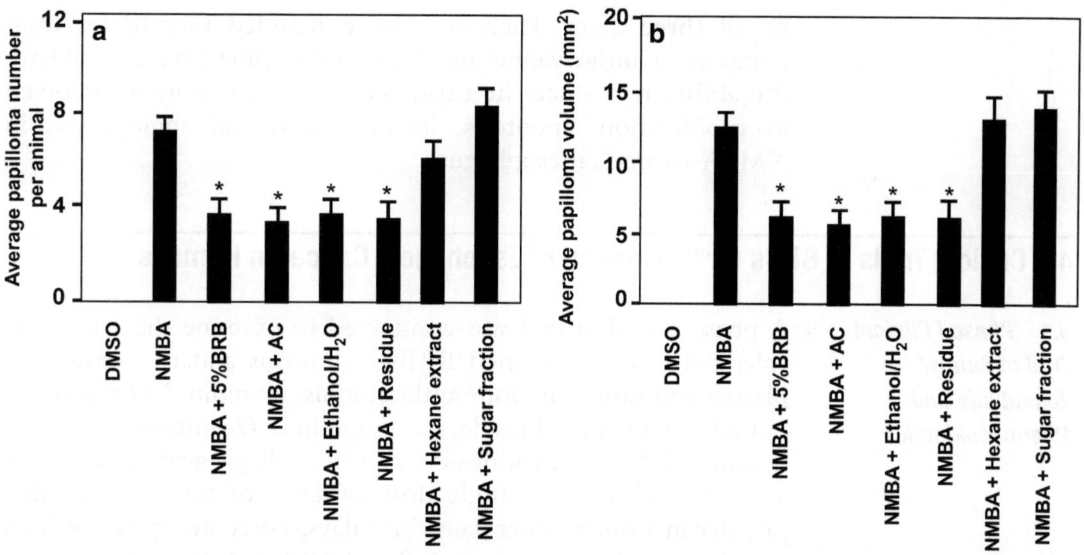

Fig. 7 Effect of diets containing BRB or BRB residues/fractions on papilloma development in NMBA-treated rat esophagus. Rats treated with NMBA + 5 % BRB, NMBA + anthocyanin (AC) fraction, NMBA + ethanol–H_2O-soluble extract (Ethanol–H_2O), and NMBA + residue fraction (Residue) had fewer papillomas (**a**) and smaller papilloma volume (**b**) than rats treated with NMBA only. Columns, mean ($n = 15$); bars, S.D. *, significantly lower ($p < 0.05$) than rats treated with NMBA only

about equally effective in reducing both the number and volume of NMBA-induced papillomas. These results provided the first in vivo evidence of the importance of the anthocyanins in the chemopreventive effects of whole BRBs. Importantly, the diet containing the residue fraction was nearly as effective as the three anthocyanin-containing diets in reducing both the number and volume of NMBA-induced papillomas. This fraction might be expected to contain multiple fiber constituents including pectin, lignans, cellulose, hemicellulose, as well as protein and ellagitannins. The ellagitannins do not appear to be responsible for the inhibitory effects of the residue fraction because the residue fraction of blueberries was also shown to inhibit esophageal tumorigenesis in rats and blueberries have only trace amounts of ellagitannins [37]. As expected, the hexane extract (mainly nonpolar compounds) and the sugar fraction (mainly glucose and fructose) were ineffective in reducing the number and volume of esophageal papillomas in NMBA-treated rats.

Mechanistic studies revealed that diets containing either 5 % BRBs or the anthocyanin or residue fractions all reduced Ki-67 cell proliferation rates in preneoplastic esophagus and in papillomas from NBMA-treated rats [34]. Similarly, all three diets stimulated apoptosis in the papillomas as measured by TUNEL assay. In addition, the upregulation of COX-2, CD45, NF-κB p50, CD34, VEGF, and HIF-1α in NMBA-treated rat esophagus was reduced by all three diets. Therefore, we concluded that BRBs, their component anthocyanins and their residue (fiber) fraction all have the ability to reduce the expression levels of proteins involved in proliferation, apoptosis, inflammation, and angiogenesis in NMBA-treated rat esophagus.

4 Clinical Trials of BRBs for Prevention of Esophageal Cancer in Humans

4.1 Phase I Clinical Trial of Safety/Tolerability and Pharmacokinetics

A phase I clinical trial was conducted to examine the safety and tolerability of freeze-dried BRBs in humans and to measure, in plasma and urine, the four anthocyanins: cyanidin-3-*O*-glucoside, cyanidin-3-*O*-sambubioside, cyanidin-3-*O*-rutinoside, and cyanidin-3-*O*-xylosylrutinoside, as well as ellagic acid [25]. Eleven subjects consumed a single dose of 45 g of freeze-dried BRB powder in a slurry water daily for 7 days. Forty-five grams of BRB powder would contain about 2.0 g of BRB anthocyanins and 0.2 g of ellagic acid. Moreover, this dose in humans is comparable to the daily consumption of a 5 % BRB diet in rats that exhibit consistently reduced NMBA-induced esophageal tumorigenesis. Blood samples were collected pre-dose on days 1 and 7 and at 10 time points post-dose. Urine was collected for 12 h pre-dose on days 1 and 7 and at three 4-h intervals post-dose.

Overall, the BRB powder was well tolerated. All 11 subjects completed the study and compliance was 100 %. Four subjects reported a total of three adverse events: (1) constipation, mild to moderate and possibly or probably related to the consumption of the BRB powder; (2) dark stools, mild and related to the consumption of the BRB powder; and (3) hematoma at the venipuncture site related to collection of blood samples. Maximum concentrations of the four anthocyanins and ellagic acid in plasma occurred at 1–2 h, and maximum quantities in urine appeared from 0 to 4 h. Overall, less than 1 % of these compounds were absorbed and excreted in urine. None of the pharmacokinetic parameters changed significantly between days 1 and 7. We concluded from this study that 45 g of freeze-dried BRB daily is well tolerated and it results in quantifiable anthocyanins and ellagic acid in plasma and urine.

4.2 "Pilot" Trial of BRBs for Chemopreventive Efficacy in Patients with Barrett's Esophagus

We have conducted a 6-month chemoprevention pilot trial administering 32 or 45 g (female and male, respectively) of freeze-dried BRB powder per day to 20 patients with Barrett's esophagus [37]. Barrett's esophagus (BE) [2] is a premalignant lesion in which the normal stratified squamous epithelium changes to a metaplastic columnar-lined epithelium, and its importance lies in the fact that it confers a 30–40-fold increased risk for the development of esophageal adenocarcinoma. Esophageal adenocarcinoma (EAC), an extremely deadly malignancy, is linked with gastroesophageal reflux disease and its incidence has increased dramatically in the past 20 years [37]. Inclusion criteria for the trial included 18 years of age or older, complete medical history, a physical examination, completion of a food-frequency questionnaire, positive endoscopy for BE (columnar lined esophagus, with specialized intestinal metaplasia/goblet cells) extending ≥1 cm above the gastroesophageal junction on the prescreening biopsy and on two previous biopsies, no history of invasive cancer within the past 5 years, normal organ function, normal serum chemistries, and signed informed consent. Exclusion criteria included any severe chronic or life-threatening diseases (pulmonary or cardiac disease, malignancy within 5 years, or severe rheumatologic or neurological disease), inability to return for follow-up visits, abnormal wound healing, esophageal varices or a history of varices or variceal bleeding, BE with high-grade dysplasia, coagulopathy that precedes taking esophageal biopsies safely, and excessive use of multivitamins or micronutrient supplements daily.

Eligible subjects were instructed to mix the BRB powder (32 g for females and 45 g for males) with 170 mL of water and orally consume the berries each morning at a designated time of their choosing for 26 weeks. This gram quantity is equivalent to consuming approximately 1.5 cups (females) and 2.0 cups of fresh berries for females and males, respectively. Biopsies of BE were taken before and after berry treatment. Each subject collected urine for a 3-h period of time in the morning, at study baseline (pre-berry treatment), at week 12 and at the final time point of 26 weeks. The urine was stored at −80 °C without preservatives.

Urine samples were analyzed, in triplicate, for 8-hydroxy-2′-deoxyguanosine (8-OHdG) and 8-epiprostaglandin F2α (8-Iso-PGF2) using immunoaffinity chromatography–monoclonal antibody-based enzyme-linked immunosorbent assays (ELISAs) as described [38, 39]. In addition, urinary creatinine levels were determined using the Cayman Chemical creatinine assay (Cayman Chemical, Ann Arbor, MI) according to the manufacturer's instructions. Levels of urinary 8-OHdG and 8-Iso-PGF2 were divided by levels of urinary creatinine to control for potential differences in urine volume between patients.

Immunohistochemical detection methods described above were used to measure additional outcomes in the study, including blood cholesterol levels and carotenoid profiles as well as tissue expression of Ki-67, GSTπ, CDX2, and NF-κB. Tissue markers were chosen with preference toward inflammatory signaling pathways, those altered early in the transition from normal squamous epithelium to Barrett's metaplasia, and to reflect changes in cellular proliferation, detoxification, differentiation, and transcriptional signaling. An original research paper reporting complete study results is under review.

BRBs impact markers of oxidative stress in BE patients, particularly lipid peroxidation as indicated by a significant reduction in urinary levels of 8-Iso-PGF2 following berry consumption for 6 months. Mean concentrations of 8-Iso-PGF2 at baseline, week 12 and week 26 of the study were 1.56E-10, 1.26E-10, and 1.15E-10 mg/mL of urine. In addition, 8-OHdG was reduced in approximately 50 % of the patients. However, overall, a greater variability in levels of 8-OHdG was observed and mean levels were not significantly reduced over the 26 week study duration. In conclusion, interim results are the first to show that daily consumption of BRBs significantly reduced 8-Iso-PGF2, a prostaglandin-like marker produced by cyclooxygenase-independent enzymes, and is considered to be a reliable marker of lipid peroxidation and a general indicator of oxidative stress. Elevated DNA damage in BE epithelium has been reported and is linked to increased risk for progression to dysplasia and EAC. Thus, natural agents like BRBs that reduce oxidative stress and increase detoxification may in turn reduce DNA damage and modulate cancer risk, without imparting negative side effects.

4.3 Phase II Trial of Strawberries (STRW) for Chemopreventive Efficacy in Chinese Patients with Esophageal Dysplasia

A randomized (noncomparative) phase II trial in China was conducted to investigate the effects of two doses of freeze-dried strawberries (STRW) in patients with esophageal dysplasia [40]. Esophageal dysplasia is a histologic precursor of esophageal squamous cell carcinoma (ESCC), a disease that represents almost 90 % of esophageal cancer worldwide. About 50 % of this disease occurs in China and certain provinces of China have a particularly high incidence and the reasons for this occurrence have been discussed in several reviews [27, 41, 42]. Survival from ESCC is not measurably better than from EAC, with a 5-year survival of about 7 %. We used STRW in this study because the Chinese government was reluctant to permit the import of black raspberries into China. Very few black raspberries are grown there and the most abundant berry crop in China is STRW. Fortunately, we had published that STRW are protective against NMBA-induced tumors in the rat esophagus model of ESCC [40] and, therefore, had a preclinical database in support of the trial.

Eligible patients for the trial were identified in Henan and Shandong Provinces by gastroenterologists from Beijing who conduct routine endoscopies in these provinces. To be eligible for the trial, individuals were required to meet all of the following inclusion criteria: (1) they must be over the age of 40 and give informed consent; (2) they must be diagnosed with mild or moderate esophageal dysplasia as severely dysplastic lesions are removed surgically; (3) they should be able to consume the strawberry slurry in a span of 5 min; (4) they have no prior history of intolerance or allergy to strawberry or strawberry-containing products. Individuals were excluded from the trial if they met one of the following criteria: (1) severe esophageal dysplasia; (2) a current malignancy identified histologically; (3) unable to give informed consent; (4)

undergoing radiotherapy or chemotherapy; (5) taking nonsteroidal anti-inflammatory drugs including aspirin and could not abstain from it due to a medical condition; or (6) pregnant or lactating.

Seventy-five patients were randomly assigned to receive freeze-dried STRW powder at either 30 g/day (37 patients) or 60 g/day (38 patients) for 6 months. The powder was mixed with water and consumed slowly. The patients drank one-half of their daily dose in the morning and the other half in the evening. Biopsies of dysplastic lesions were taken before and after STRW treatment. In order to observe these lesions, 20–30 mL of 1.2 % Lugol's iodine solution was sprayed onto the mucosal surface from the gastroesophageal junction to the upper pharyngoesophageal sphincter. The dysplastic lesions appear unstained relative to the surrounding normal mucosa, and biopsies were taken from unstained (whitish) areas according to the following size in diameter: 5–19 mm, one biopsy sample; 20–39 mm, two biopsy samples; and 40 mm or more, three biopsy samples. One biopsy sample was fixed in 10 % neutral buffered formalin overnight, transferred to PBS, embedded in paraffin, and sectioned in 4-μm thickness for subsequent histologic evaluation. The other biopsy samples were immediately immersed in liquid nitrogen and then transferred to a −80 °C freezer for subsequent molecular analysis.

The effects of STRW treatment on cell proliferation in the dysplastic tissues was determined by immunohistochemical staining for the Ki-67 protein in accordance with the procedures described above. Briefly, sections were de-paraffinized and blocked for non-specific binding and incubated for 1 h with a primary antibody to detect Ki-67. This was followed by a 20 min incubation with a secondary antibody (biotinylated immunoglobulin) and streptavidin–horseradish peroxidase label. The sections were then developed with diaminobenzidine chromogen, counterstained with hematoxylin, dehydrated, and mounted. Stained slides were viewed and photographed under a Nikon microscope using a high-resolution spot camera, which was interfaced with a computer loaded with image analysis software (NIS Element Research Image Analysis, version 3.1).

Western blot analysis was used to evaluate the effects of STRW on the expression levels of COX-2, iNOS, NF-κB-p65, and pS6 proteins in esophageal dysplasia specimens before and after STRW treatment. One of the downstream targets of mTOR is p70S6 kinase, whose substrate is pS6, a component of the S40 ribosome subunit [43]. Measurement of pS6 by western blot is used to assess the activity of mTOR [44]. The methods used for western blot analysis were essentially as described above.

Results of this study indicated that STRW were exceptionally well tolerated at both dose levels. Only 1 participant who consumed 30 g/day of STRW powder had diarrhea for only 1 day. Compliance was excellent with 94.7 % and 97.4 % for 60 g/day

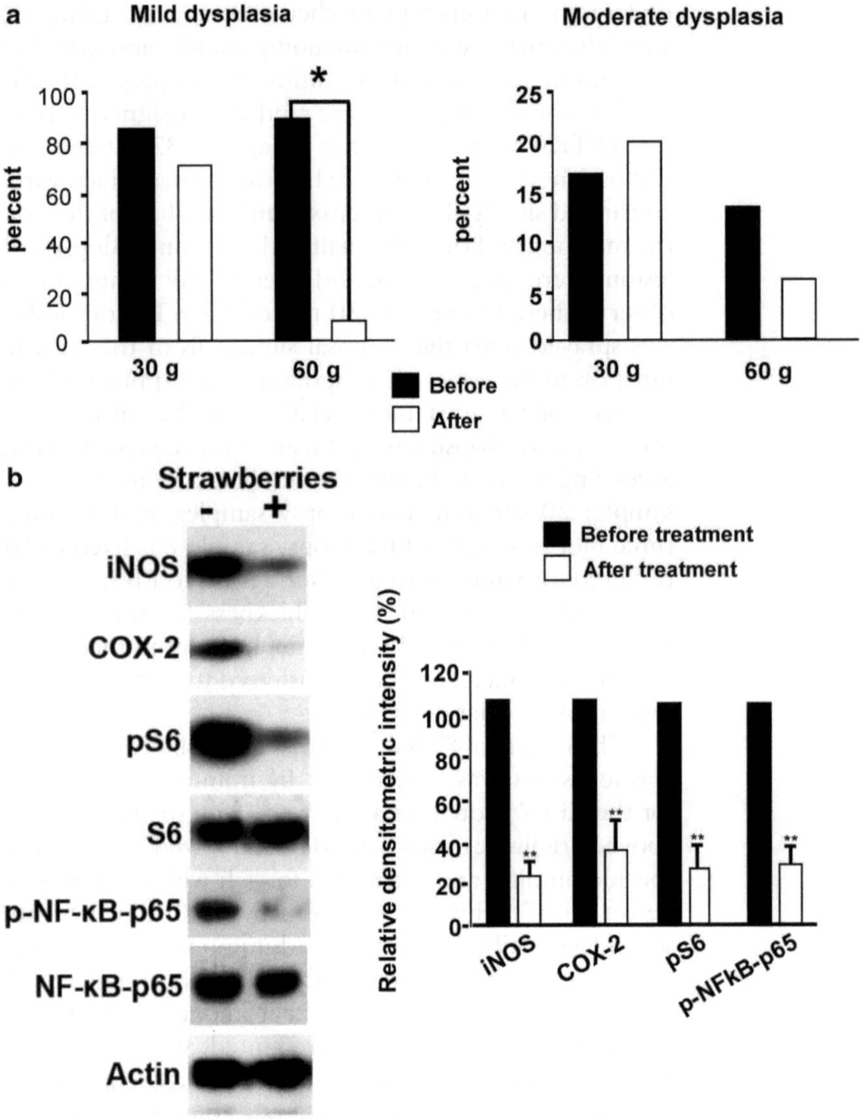

Fig. 8 Berries reduce esophageal dysplasia in China and protectively modulate biomarkers of cellular proliferation and inflammation

and 30 g/day of STRW, respectively. The lower daily dose (30 g/day) of STRW had no significant effect on the regression of either mild or moderately dysplastic lesions in the esophagi of berry-treated patients (Fig. 8a). However, in patients treated with 60 g/day of STRW for 6 months, 31 were diagnosed with mild dysplasia (86.1 %) and five patients with moderate dysplasia (13.9 %). After 6 months of treatment, no change was observed in 4 patients with mild dysplasia but a decrease was observed in 26 patients ($p < 0.0001$) with mild dysplasia. An increase in histologic grade was observed in 1 patient. In patients with moderate dysplasia, no change was observed in 2 patients and a decrease in histologic grade was observed in 3 patients. Overall, 29 of 36 patients (80.6 %) treated with the high dose of STRW powder experienced a decrease in histologic grade of the premalignant lesions during the study ($p < 0.0001$).

Western blot analysis indicated that 6 months of a total of 30 g/day of STRW treatment nonsignificantly decreased the expression of iNOS by 35.7 %, COX-2 by 25.5 %, pNFκB-p65 by 28.8 %, and pS6 by 8.2 % (Fig. 8b). In contrast, 6 months of a total of 60 g/day of STRW treatment significantly reduced protein expression levels of iNOS by 79.5 %, COX-2 by 62.9 %, pNFκB-p65 by 62.6 %, and pS6 by 73.2 % in human esophageal mucosa. All reductions were significant at $p < 0.001$. These data are consistent with the finding that the Ki-67 labeling index was reduced significantly only in esophageal tissues from participants treated with 60 g/day of STRW.

This study showed for the first time that the consumption of freeze-dried STRW at 60 g/day for 6 months significantly decreased the histologic grade of precancerous esophageal lesions. This reduction was associated, at least in part, by down-regulation of genes involved in cell proliferation, inflammation, and gene transcription. Based on the promising results in this study, we propose to test STRW alone and in combination with other preventative agents in randomized placebo-controlled trials in the future.

References

1. deBoer JD (ed) (2005) Berries and their role in human health. A survey of research into the health benefits of berries. DeBoer Consulting, Victoria, Canada
2. Beech MG, Simpson DW (1989) Strawberry production in the United Kingdom. Paper presented at the ISHS Acta Horticulture 265: international strawberry symposium
3. Brazelton C (2011) World blueberry acreage and production. 2008 World blueberry acreage and production report 1–51
4. Tulio AZ, Reese RN, Wyzgoski FJ, Rinaldi PL, Fu R, Scheerens JC, Miller AR (2008) Cyanidin 3-rutinoside and cyanidin 3-xylosylrutinoside as primary phenolic antioxidants in black raspberry. J Agric Food Chem 56(6):1880–1888. doi:10.1021/jf072313k
5. Moyer RA, Hummer KE, Finn CE, Frei B, Wrolstad RE (2001) Anthocyanins, phenolics, and antioxidant capacity in diverse small fruits: Vaccinium, Rubus, and Ribes. J Agric Food Chem 50(3):519–525. doi:10.1021/jf011062r
6. Stoner GD (2009) Foodstuffs for preventing cancer: the preclinical and clinical development of berries. Cancer Prev Res 2(3):187–194. doi:10.1158/1940-6207.capr-08-0226
7. Harris GK, Gupta A, Nines RG, Kresty LA, Habib SG, Frankel WL, LaPerle K, Gallaher DD, Schwartz SJ, Stoner GD (2001) Effects of lyophilized black raspberries on azoxymethane-induced colon cancer and 8-hydroxy-2′-deoxyguanosine levels in the Fischer 344 rat. Nutr Cancer 40(2):125–133. doi:10.1207/s15327914nc402_8
8. Mallery SR, Zwick JC, Pei P, Tong M, Larsen PE, Shumway BS, Lu B, Fields HW, Mumper RJ, Stoner GD (2008) Topical application of a bioadhesive black raspberry gel modulates gene expression and reduces cyclooxygenase 2 protein in human premalignant oral lesions. Cancer Res 68(12):4945–4957. doi:10.1158/0008-5472.can-08-0568
9. Shumway BS, Kresty LA, Larsen PE, Zwick JC, Lu B, Fields HW, Mumper RJ, Stoner GD, Mallery SR (2008) Effects of a topically applied bioadhesive berry gel on loss of heterozygosity indices in premalignant oral lesions. Clin Cancer Res 14(8):2421–2430. doi:10.1158/1078-0432.ccr-07-4096

10. Wang LS, Dombkowski AA, Seguin C, Rocha C, Cukovic D, Mukundan A, Henry C, Stoner GD (2011) Mechanistic basis for the chemopreventive effects of black raspberries at a late stage of rat esophageal carcinogenesis. Mol Carcinog 50(4):291–300. doi:10.1002/mc.20634
11. Kelloff GJ, Boone CW, Malone WF, Steele VE (1992) Chemoprevention clinical trials. Mutat Res 267(2):291–295, doi:http://dx.doi.org/10.1016/0027-5107(92)90073-B
12. Fahey JW, Zhang Y, Talalay P (1997) Broccoli sprouts: an exceptionally rich source of inducers of enzymes that protect against chemical carcinogens. Proc Natl Acad Sci U S A 94(19):10367–10372
13. Khan WA, Wang ZY, Athar M, Bickers DR, Mukhtar H (1988) Inhibition of the skin tumorigenicity of (+/−) beta, 8 alpha-dihydroxy-9 alpha, 10 alpha-epoxy-7,8,9,10-tetrahydrobenzo[a]pyrene by tannic acid, green tea polyphenols and quercetin in Sencar mice. Cancer Lett 42(1–2):7–12
14. Wang Z, Huang M, Ferraro T, Wong C-Q, Lou Y-R, Reuhl K, Iatropoulos M, Yang CS, Conney AH (1992) Inhibitory effect of green tea in the drinking water on tumorigenesis by ultraviolet light and 12-O-tetradecanoylphorbol-13-acetate in the skin of SKH-1 mice. Cancer Res 52(5):1162–1170
15. Okajima E, Tsutsumi M, Ozono S, Akai H, Denda A, Nishino H, Oshima S, Sakamoto H, Konishi Y (1998) Inhibitory effect of tomato juice on rat urinary bladder carcinogenesis after N-butyl-n-(4-hydroxybutyl)nitrosamine initiation. Jpn J Cancer Res 89(1):22–26
16. Gotoh T, Yamada K, Yin H, Ito A, Kataoka T, Dohi K (1998) Chemoprevention of N-nitroso-N-methylurea-induced rat mammary carcinogenesis by soy foods or biochanin A. Jpn J Cancer Res 89(2):137–142
17. Ip C, Lisk DJ, Stoewsand GS (1992) Mammary cancer prevention by regular garlic and selenium-enriched garlic. Nutr Cancer 17(3):279–286. doi:10.1080/01635589209514197
18. Kapadia GJ, Tokuda H, Konoshima T, Nishino H (1996) Chemoprevention of lung and skin cancer by Beta vulgaris (beet) root extract. Cancer Lett 100(1–2):211–214
19. Wilkinson JT, Morse MA, Kresty LA, Stoner GD (1995) Effect of alkyl chain length on inhibition of N-nitrosomethylbenzylamine-induced esophageal tumorigenesis and DNA methylation by isothiocyanates. Carcinogenesis 16(5):1011–1015. doi:10.1093/carcin/16.5.1011
20. Kresty LA, Morse MA, Morgan C, Carlton PS, Lu J, Gupta A, Blackwood M, Stoner GD (2001) Chemoprevention of esophageal tumorigenesis by dietary administration of lyophilized black raspberries. Cancer Res 61(16):6112–6119
21. Casto BC, Kresty LA, Kraly CL, Pearl DK, Knobloch TJ, Schut HA, Stoner GD, Mallery SR, Weghorst CM (2002) Chemoprevention of oral cancer by black raspberries. Anticancer Res 22(6C):4005–4015
22. Aiyer HS, Srinivasan C, Gupta RC (2008) Dietary berries and ellagic acid diminish estrogen-mediated mammary tumorigenesis in ACI rats. Nutr Cancer 60(2):227–234. doi:10.1080/01635580701624712
23. Bi X, Fang W, Wang L-S, Stoner GD, Yang W (2010) Black raspberries inhibit intestinal tumorigenesis in Apc1638+/− and Muc2−/− mouse models of colorectal cancer. Cancer Prev Res 3(11):1443–1450. doi:10.1158/1940-6207.capr-10-0124
24. Duncan FJ, Martin JR, Wulff BC, Stoner GD, Tober KL, Oberyszyn TM, Kusewitt DF, Van Buskirk AM (2009) Topical treatment with black raspberry extract reduces cutaneous UVB-induced carcinogenesis and inflammation. Cancer Prev Res 2(7):665–672. doi:10.1158/1940-6207.capr-08-0193
25. Stoner GD, Sardo C, Apseloff G, Mullet D, Wargo W, Pound V, Singh A, Sanders J, Aziz R, Casto B, Sun X (2005) Pharmacokinetics of anthocyanins and ellagic acid in healthy volunteers fed freeze-dried black raspberries daily for 7 days. J Clin Pharmacol 45(10):1153–1164. doi:10.1177/0091270005279636
26. He J, Magnuson BA, Lala G, Tian Q, Schwartz SJ, Giusti MM (2006) Intact anthocyanins and metabolites in rat urine and plasma after 3 months of anthocyanin supplementation. Nutr Cancer 54(1):3–12. doi:10.1207/s15327914nc5401_2
27. Stoner GD, Chen T, Kresty LA, Aziz RM, Reinemann T, Nines RG (2006) Protection against esophageal cancer in rodents with lyophilized berries: potential mechanisms. Nutr Cancer 54(1):33–46. doi:10.1207/s15327914nc5401_5
28. Stoner GD, Aziz RM (2007) Prevention and therapy of squamous cell carcinoma of the rodent esophagus using freeze-dried black raspberries. Acta Pharmacol Sin 28(9):1422–1428
29. Pozharisski KM (1973) Tumors of the oesophagus. In: V. S. Turusov (ed), Pathology of Tumors in Laboratory Animals, 1-Tumors of the Rat, IARC Sci. Publ., Part 1, Lyon, France: IARC, pp 87–100
30. Contran RS, Kumar V, Robbins SL (1994) Neoplasia Ed. 5 Schoen F. J. eds. Robbins Pathologic Basis of Disease, W. B. Saunders Company Philadelphia, pp 245–248

31. Chen T, Hwang H, Rose ME, Nines RG, Stoner GD (2006) Chemopreventive properties of black raspberries in N-nitrosomethylbenzylamine-induced rat esophageal tumorigenesis: down-regulation of cyclooxygenase-2, inducible nitric oxide synthase, and c-Jun. Cancer Res 66(5):2853–2859. doi:10.1158/0008-5472.can-05-3279
32. Chen LC, Chen BK, Chang JM, Chang WC (2004) Essential role of c-Jun induction and coactivator p300 in epidermal growth factor-induced gene expression of cyclooxygenase-2 in human epidermoid carcinoma A431 cells. Biochim Biophys Acta 1683(1–3):38–48, doi:http://dx.doi.org/10.1016/j.bbalip.2004.04.003
33. Chen T, Rose ME, Hwang H, Nines RG, Stoner GD (2006) Black raspberries inhibit N-nitrosomethylbenzylamine (NMBA)-induced angiogenesis in rat esophagus parallel to the suppression of COX-2 and iNOS. Carcinogenesis 27(11):2301–2307. doi:10.1093/carcin/bgl109
34. Wang LS, Hecht SS, Carmella SG, Yu N, Larue B, Henry C, McIntyre C, Rocha C, Lechner JF, Stoner GD (2009) Anthocyanins in black raspberries prevent esophageal tumors in rats. Cancer Prev Res 2(1):84–93. doi:10.1158/1940-6207.capr-08-0155
35. Stoner GD, Dombkowski AA, Reen RK, Cukovic D, Salagrama S, Wang LS, Lechner JF (2008) Carcinogen-altered genes in rat esophagus positively modulated to normal levels of expression by both black raspberries and phenylethyl isothiocyanate. Cancer Res 68(15):6460–6467. doi:10.1158/0008-5472.can-08-0146
36. Hecht SS, Huang C, Stoner GD, Li J, Kenney PM, Sturla SJ, Carmella SG (2006) Identification of cyanidin glycosides as constituents of freeze-dried black raspberries which inhibit anti-benzo[a]pyrene-7,8-diol-9,10-epoxide induced NFκB and AP-1 activity. Carcinogenesis 27(8):1617–1626. doi:10.1093/carcin/bgi366
37. Kresty LA, Frankel WL, Hammond CD, Baird ME, Mele JM, Stoner GD, Fromkes JJ (2006) Transitioning from preclinical to clinical chemopreventive assessments of lyophilized black raspberries: interim results show berries modulate markers of oxidative stress in Barrett's esophagus patients. Nutr Cancer 54(1):148–156. doi:10.1207/s15327914nc5401_15
38. Wang Z, Ciabattoni G, Créminon C, Lawson J, Fitzgerald GA, Patrono C, Maclouf J (1995) Immunological characterization of urinary 8-epi-prostaglandin F2 alpha excretion in man. J Pharmacol Exp Ther 275(1):94–100
39. Yin B, Whyatt RM, Perera FP, Randall MC, Cooper TB, Santella RM (1995) Determination of 8-hydroxydeoxyguanosine by an immunoaffinity chromatography-monoclonal antibody-based ELISA. Free Rad Biol Med 18(6):1023–1032, doi:http://dx.doi.org/10.1016/0891-5849(95)00003-G
40. Chen T, Yan F, Qian J, Guo M, Zhang H, Tang X, Chen F, Stoner GD, Wang X (2012) Randomized phase II trial of lyophilized strawberries in patients with dysplastic precancerous lesions of the esophagus. Cancer Prev Res 5(1):41–50. doi:10.1158/1940-6207.capr-11-0469
41. Stoner GD, Gupta A (2001) Etiology and chemoprevention of esophageal squamous cell carcinoma. Carcinogenesis 22(11):1737–1746. doi:10.1093/carcin/22.11.1737
42. Stoner GD, Wang LS, Chen T (2007) Chemoprevention of esophageal squamous cell carcinoma. Toxicol Appl Pharmacol 224(3):337–349, doi:http://dx.doi.org/10.1016/j.taap.2007.01.030
43. Iwenofu OH, Lackman RD, Staddon AP, Goodwin DG, Haupt HM, Brooks JS (2008) Phospho-S6 ribosomal protein: a potential new predictive sarcoma marker for targeted mTOR therapy. Mod Pathol 21(3):231–237
44. Sun Q, Chen X, Ma J, Peng H, Wang F, Zha X, Wang Y, Jing Y, Yang H, Chen R, Chang L, Zhang Y, Goto J, Onda H, Chen T, Wang MR, Lu Y, You H, Kwiatkowski D, Zhang H (2011) Mammalian target of rapamycin up-regulation of pyruvate kinase isoenzyme type M2 is critical for aerobic glycolysis and tumor growth. Proc Natl Acad Sci U S A 108(10):4129–4134. doi:10.1073/pnas.1014769108

Chapter 6

The Use of Mouse Models for Lung Cancer Chemoprevention Studies

Yian Wang, Michael S. You, Lucina C. Rouggly, and Ming You

Abstract

Mouse lung tumor models are widely used in lung cancer chemopreventive studies. Lung cancer is a heterogeneous disease histologically classified as small-cell lung carcinoma (SCLC) and non-small-cell lung carcinoma (NSCLC), which is usually divided into adenocarcinoma, squamous cell carcinoma (SCC), and large cell carcinoma. In order to illustrate the power of the mouse model in preclinical lung cancer investigations, comprehensive instructions for the selection of mice, genotyping, and induction of lung tumors (e.g., adenoma/adenocarcinoma, lung SCC, and SCLC) in mice are provided. We have described in detail the histological features of these tumors and the application of these features in lung cancer chemoprevention studies. We have also provided detailed information on how to semiquantitatively phenotype lung tumor development. The basic protocol described here could easily be applied to other approaches to lung cancer prevention such as chemoprevention or immunoprevention.

Key words Lung cancer, Chemoprevention, Animal models, Adenocarcinoma, Squamous cell carcinoma, Small-cell lung cancer

1 Introduction

Lung cancer is a major health concern. In the USA, 228,190 new cases and 159,480 deaths are estimated to occur in 2013 for both men and women in the USA [1]. Although the estimated number of new cases is second to prostate cancer for men and breast cancer for women, the projected number of lung cancer deaths is still higher than other common cancers, including cancers of the prostate, breast, colorectum, and pancreas [1]. Although overall cancer death rates have declined by 20 % from their peak in 1991 (215.1 per 100,000 population) to 2009 (173.1 per 100,000 population), lung cancer death rates remain the highest [1]. Epidemiological and laboratory animal studies have demonstrated that smoking is closely linked to increased lung cancer risk [2, 3]. Tobacco exposure has been implicated in 90 % of lung cancers, and

Ann M. Bode and Zigang Dong (eds.), *Cancer Prevention: Dietary Factors and Pharmacology*, Methods in Pharmacology and Toxicology, DOI 10.1007/978-1-4614-9227-6_6, © Springer Science+Business Media New York 2014

smokers have a 20-fold greater risk of developing lung cancer compared with those who have never smoked [4]. Lung cancer is positively correlated with the number of years a person has smoked [2, 5]. The percentage of smokers in America peaked at almost 50 % in the late 1960s and currently is at 26 % [6]. Many people are unable or unwilling to stop smoking even though nearly 50 % of people who had ever smoked are now former smokers.

Lung cancer is a heterogeneous disease and is histologically classified as either small-cell lung carcinoma (SCLC) or non-SCLC (NSCLC) [7]. NSCLC is usually further divided into three main histologic types: adenocarcinoma, squamous cell carcinoma (SCC), and large cell carcinoma. Lung adenocarcinoma is currently the most frequently observed histological type in Western countries. A common practice is to use the size of the primary tumor, the invasion of locoregional nodes, and the presence of distant metastases as factors to define the stage of the disease to guide cancer treatment, management, and prediction of outcome [8]. The survival rate among those with stage I disease is approximately 60–70 %, and the survival rate decreases to 40 % in patients with stages II to IIIa disease [8–10]. The current challenge is managing this deadly disease through a change in social behavior (such as cessation of tobacco use), cancer chemoprevention and immunoprevention, the development of advanced technology for early diagnosis, and identification factors that would predict tumor relapse [11].

Lung cancer is believed to arise from a multistep process with each step associated with genetic and epigenetic alterations and correlated with tumor aggressiveness. As shown in Table 1, the accumulation of genetic mutations over time is involved and results in a multistage process affecting oncogenes, tumor suppressor genes, and other related genes. For example, up to 90 % of SCLCs exhibit characteristic molecular abnormalities especially on *Rb* and *p53* tumor suppressor genes. Recent studies also found that LKB1 (liver kinase B1) modulates lung cancer differentiation and metastasis. Mutations and LOH (loss of heterozygosity) were found in about 23 % of lung adenocarcinomas. DMBT1 (deleted in malignant brain tumor 1) was altered in nearly half of the NSCLCs and in all of the SCLCs.

In recent years, our understanding of the driving forces at the molecular level in NSCLC formation and maintenance has improved dramatically. This knowledge provides new opportunities in targeted approaches against activated kinases [12]. The phosphatidylinositol 3-kinase (PI3-K) pathway plays an important role in cancer cell initiation, growth, proliferation, and survival. PI3-Ks are a conserved family of lipid kinases that phosphorylate the 3′-OH group of phosphoinositides. The resulting phosphatidylinositol (3,4,5) tris-phosphate (PIP3) is an active intracellular messenger that can in turn activate AKT and pyruvate dehydrogenase kinase (PDK). AKT promotes cellular survival through the

Table 1
Major genetic changes in lung cancers

Gene	Changes	NSCLC	SCLC
MYC	Amplifications	5–20 %	20–35 %
RAS	Mutations	15–20 %	<1 %
EGFR	Mutations	20 %	–
INK4a	Loss of heterozygosity	70 %	50 %
$p16^{ink4a}$	Mutations	20–50 %	<5 %
$p14^{arf}$	Mutations	20 %	65 %
TP53	Mutations Loss of heterozygosity	50 % 60 %	75 % 75–100 %
RB	Mutations Loss of heterozygosity	15–30 % 30 %	90 % 70 %
FHIT	Mutations	40 %	80 %
TGS101	Mutations	–	90 %
DMBT1	Mutations	40–50 %	100 %
LKB1	Mutations Loss of heterozygosity	23 %	– –
Loss of heterozygosity in various regions	3p 4p 4q 8p	70–80 % 10–20 % 30 % 80–100 %	90–100 % 50 % 80 % 80–90 %

phosphorylation of the pro-apoptotic protein Bad and phosphorylation of the transcription factor FKHLR1. AKT can also activate the NF-κB pathway, which has been shown preclinically to be a legitimate preventive target for lung cancer. Amplification of PI3-KCA appears to be quite common (>50 %) in lung SCC [13]. Mutations in PTEN (phosphatase and tensin homolog deleted from chromosome 10) have also been observed in over 10 % of lung SCCs [13]. Because either increased activity of PI3-K or decreased activity of PTEN are likely to yield similar activation of cancer cell growth, these observations emphasize the importance of this pathway, particularly in lung SCC [13]. The importance of this pathway has been confirmed by genomic data on literally hundreds of SCC samples [13, 14]. This should, in itself, encourage the testing of this class of agents (inhibitors of PI3-K) in NSCLC in preclinical models (lung adenocarcinoma and lung SCC). Both early interventions as well as later interventions similar to human trials attempting to reverse bronchial dysplasia appear warranted.

The mitogen-activated protein kinase (MAPK) signaling cascade is activated by growth factors, hormones, and chemokines that signal through their cognate tyrosine kinase receptors. These phosphorylated sites then allow docking of GRB 2 (growth factor receptor bound protein 2) and the guanine nucleotide exchange factor SOS (son-of-sevenless). The latter factor helps activate the various RAS proteins and further signaling through RAF, extracellular signal-regulated kinases (ERKs), and ERK kinase (MEK). Thus, inhibition of these downstream kinases, MEK or ERK, would be expected to modulate signaling either through the growth factor receptors or through an activated Ras. Interestingly, an activation of the MAPK pathway is highly significant with regard to activation of both lung adenocarcinomas (EGFR mutations and *KRAS* mutations) and lung SCC. In the case of lung SCC, the activation of this pathway appears to not be caused primarily by mutation, but rather by increased expression, often associated with amplification of the relevant genes [13, 14]. Thus, an examination of the use of MEK inhibitors in a prevention setting appears to be particularly promising. A MEK inhibitor (such as AZD6244) inhibits tumor cell growth in vitro and in xenograft models, including human hepatocellular carcinoma [16], thyroid cancer [17], melanoma [18], schwannoma [19], and primary NSCLC (Wang Y. et al. unpublished data). More recently, a report by Hainsworth et al. [15] has shown promising efficacy and safety of a MEK inhibitor in NSCLC patients in an open-label randomized phase II study. An oral MEK inhibitor (AZD6244) has exhibited clinical activity as second- or third-line therapy for patients with advanced NSCLC [15].

We, as well as others, have reported the use of mouse models of lung cancer in many chemopreventive studies. Lung adenocarcinoma models are perhaps the most frequently used mouse models. Several chemopreventive agents, including myo-inositol [20], budesonide [21, 22], and tea polyphenols [23–25], have been found to be highly effective in preventing lung tumor development. Our group was the first to use the NTCU-induced mouse lung SCC model in chemoprevention studies. In addition to other groups, we have identified several agents, including Antitumor mixture B (a Chinese herb mixture) [26], Pioglitazone [27], and pomegranate fruit extract [28], that are highly effective in preventing lung SCC development. Recently, we have been the first to apply a genetically engineered mouse model of small-cell lung cancer (Trp53F2-10/F2-10;Rb1F19/F19) to cancer chemoprevention studies. Using this model, we found that bexarotene is highly effective in preventing lung SCLC development in mice [29].

In this chapter, to illustrate the usefulness of mouse models of lung cancer in chemoprevention, we provide comprehensive instructions on how to conduct animal studies to determine the efficacy of a given test agent against lung tumorigenesis. Although additional animal models of lung cancer have been described by others, we focus on those that are routinely used in our group, including mouse models of lung adenocarcinoma, SCC, and SCLC.

2 Materials

2.1 Carcinogens and Other Reagents

Benzo(a)pyrene [B(a)P] (Cat. No. B1760), Tricaprylin (C8:0) (Cat. No. T-9126) and acetone are purchased from Sigma-Aldrich (St. Louis, MO). 4-(methylnitrosamino)-1-(3-pyridyl)-1-butanone (NNK) is purchased from EaglePicher Pharmaceuticals (Inkster, MI). N-nitroso-tris-chloroethylurea (NTCU) and vinyl carbamate (VC) are purchased from the Toronto Research Chemicals, Inc. (Toronto, Canada). Adeno-Cre virus (Ad5-CMV-Cre virus) is purchased from the University of Iowa Gene Transfer Vector Core (Iowa City, IA). Ketamine (NDC 0856-2013-01, Ketaset III, Ketamine HCl INJ USP) and xylazine are obtained from the Washington University School of Medicine Veterinarian Pharmacy. Saline is a 0.9 % NaCl solution. Phosphate-buffered saline (PBS) contains 137 mM NaCl, 2.7 mM KCl, 10 mM Na_2HPO_4, and 1.8 mM KH_2PO_4; pH is 7.4. Both PBS and saline can be sterilized by autoclaving for 20 min at 15 psi (1.05 kg/cm^2) on a liquid cycle or by filter sterilization, and it can be stored at room temperature or in the refrigerator (4 °C). Both can be purchased commercially.

2.2 Selection of Mice (Table 2)

A/J mice are purchased from Jackson Laboratories (Bar harbor, ME). NIH Swiss mice are obtained from the Charles River Laboratories (Wilmington, MA). *Trp53*$^{F2\text{-}10/F2\text{-}10}$;*Rb1*$^{F19/F19}$ mice were originally created in Dr. Anton Berns' laboratory (Division of Molecular Genetics, Netherlands Cancer Institute, Amsterdam, The Netherlands) [30]. The UL53–3 mice were originally developed by Lavigueur et al. [31]. Before the use of any mice in such studies, one should apply for institute approval. All mice should be treated humanely and housed in plastic cages (4–5 per cage) with

Table 2
Detailed information regarding mice used in lung cancer models

	NIH Swiss	A/J	ULp53	RFPF
Vendor	NCI Frederick	Jackson Lab	Not commercially available	Not commercially available
Mouse strain	Cr:NIH(S)	A/J	A/J and Swiss	B6(A/J × RFPF)
Strain code	01S50	000646		
Breed	Outbred	Inbred		
Appearance	Albino	Albino	Albino	Albino

hardwood bedding and dust covers of high-efficiency particulate aerosol filters in a room that is environmentally controlled at 24 ± 1 °C with a 12-h light/12-h dark cycle.

2.3 Genotyping of Transgenic Mice

2.3.1 Preparation of Tail DNA for Genotyping

The tail is clipped at ~10 mm length when the mice are at ~3 weeks of age. The tails can be stored at −80 °C or incubated in lysis buffer in a shaking-incubator at 37 °C overnight. The lysis buffer is formulated with 0.4 mg/ml Pronase, 10 % (w/v) sodium dodecyl sulfate (SDS), 10 mM Tris, 400 mM NaCl, and 2 mM ethylenediaminetetraacetic acid (EDTA)]. The lysate (300 μl) is then mixed with saturated NaCl (80 μl) and ice-cold alcohol (950 μl) to precipitate the genomic DNA. Then, the DNA is washed with 75 % ethanol twice, air-dried, and dissolved in TE buffer [Tris–HCl 1 mM (pH 7.5), EDTA 0.2 mM].

2.3.2 Genotyping for ULp53 Mice (Fig. 1)

The UL53–3 mice were originally developed through the microinjection of FVB/J mouse oocytes with a BALB/c mouse genomic clone of the *p53* gene containing a point mutation at codon 135 (Ala → Val) in exon 5 of the *p53* gene. The *p53* transgene used in the generation of the UL53–3 mice was the same as that used in a previous study [31]. The mutation, a C → T transition, created a restriction fragment length polymorphism (RFLP) with a new *Hph*I restriction enzyme cleavage site (recognition site: GGTGA). Specifically, polymerase chain reaction (PCR) primers are designed from the regions of mouse p53 exon 5 that contained the Ala-Val135 mutation (Table 3). PCR conditions are detailed in Table 4.

Table 3
Primers used for genotyping

Mouse	Gene	Primer	Sequence	RFLP	Allele: Wild type	Allele: Floxed	Allele: Mutant
RFPF	*p53*	p53-10F	5′-AAGGGGTATGA GGGACAAGG-3′	NA	460 bp	584 bp	NA
		p53-10R	5′-GAAGACAGAAAA GGGGAGGG-3′				
	pRb	Rb19E	5′-CTCAAGAGCTCAGACTC ATGG-3′	NA	200 bp	283 bp	NA
		Rb18	5′-GGCGTGTGCCATCAAT-3′				
ULp53	*p53*	ULp53-F	5′-TACTCTCCTCCCCTCAA TAAG-3′	*Hph*I	190 bp	NA	150 bp
		ULp53-R	5′-CTCGGGTGGCTCATAA GGTACCAC-3′				

NA not applicable, *RFLP* restriction fragment length polymorphism

Table 4
PCR conditions for genotyping

Gene	1 Cycle		36 Cycles						1 Cycle		Hold
ULp53	95 °C	2 min	94 °C	30 s	57 °C	30 s	72 °C	40 s	72 °C	2 min	4 °C
RFPF	95 °C	10 min	94 °C	30 s	58 °C	30 s	72 °C	50 s	72 °C	7 min	4 °C

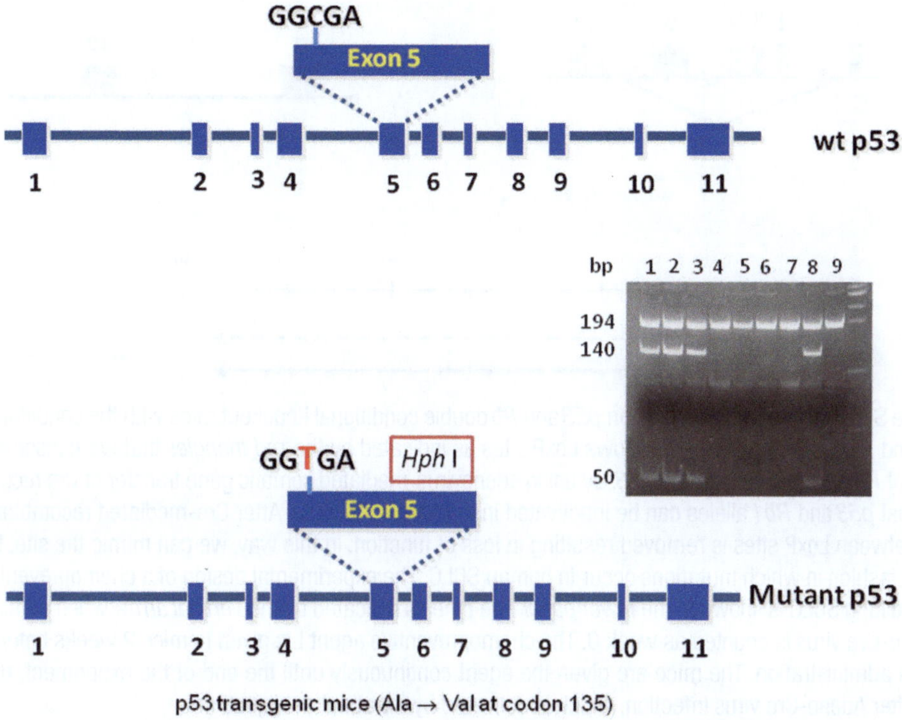

Fig. 1 The *p53* gene contains 11 exons. The mutations are usually located on exon 5 to exon 8 in human cancers. The p53 transgenic mouse model was developed with a p53 germ-line mutation at codon 135 in exon 5. At this spot, a thymine replaced cytosine, which caused an amino acid change from alanine to valine, with the sequence changing from GGCGA to GGTGA, which created a restriction enzyme cutting site. The PCR product is a 190-bp fragment with primers ULp53-F and UL-p53-R (Table 3). After digestion with restriction enzyme *Hph I*, the wild type p53 fragment is undigested, and only one 190-bp PCR fragment is seen. The transgenic allele will be cut at the GGTGA site and the 190-bp fragment will become 2 fragments (140-bp and 50-bp)

After amplification, the fragment is incubated with the restriction endonuclease *Hph*I which cleaves once within the amplified mutant transgene and does not cleave within the wild type allele. The cleaved fragments are then subjected to electrophoresis on an 8 % polyacrylamide gel along with a DNA size marker and visualized by UV light after staining with ethidium bromide (Fig. 1; [23]). A single 190-bp band is amplified for wild type p53 (Fig. 1, *lanes 4, 5, 6, 7*, and *9*) whereas three bands (190-bp, 150-bp, and 40-bp)

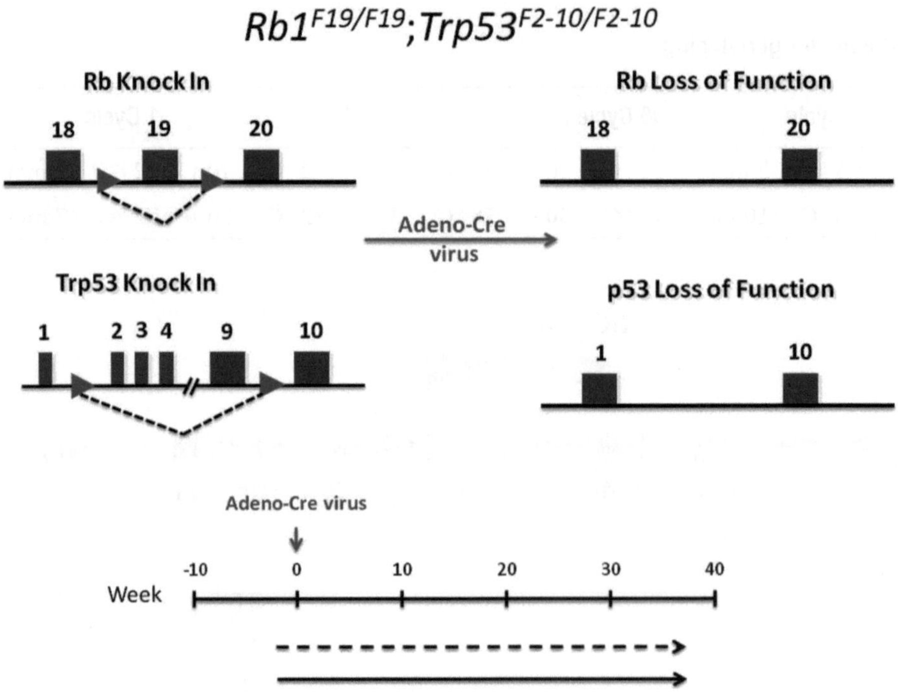

Fig. 2 The SCLC mouse model is built on *p53* and *Rb* double conditional knockout mice with the conditional alleles of *Rb1* and *Trp53*. The *upper panel* shows LoxP sites as indicated by the *red triangles* that were inserted around exon 19 of *Rb1* and exons 2–9 of *Trp53*. By using adenovirus-mediated somatic gene transfer of Cre recombinase, conditional *p53* and *Rb1* alleles can be inactivated in the lung epithelium. After Cre-mediated recombination, the region between LoxP sites is removed resulting in loss of function. In this way, we can mimic the site, time, and sporadic fashion in which mutations occur in human SCLC. The experimental design of a chemopreventive study on mouse lung SCLC is shown in the *lower panel*. The time as indicated by the *vertical arrow* when administrating the Adeno-Cre virus is counted as week 0. The chemopreventive agent t is given to mice 2 weeks before Adeno-Cre virus administration. The mice are given the agent continuously until the end of the experiment, usually 36 weeks after Adeno-Cre virus infection, which is delivered by intratracheal injection

are obtained in heterozygous *p53* transgenic mice (Fig. 1, *lanes 1, 2, 3*, and *8*). Additionally, a 2 % agarose gel is also suitable to use. With agarose gel electrophoresis, you will clearly see one fragment of 190-bp for wild type p53 and two fragments of 190-bp and 150-bp for heterozygous *p53* transgenic mice (not shown).

Genotyping for $Rb1^{F19/F19}$; $Trp53^{F2-10/F2-10}$ Mice

The $Rb1^{F19/F19}$;$Trp53^{F2-10/F2-10}$ mice (short for RFPF; Fig. 2) carrying conditional alleles for Rb1 (floxed at exon 19) and p53 (floxed at exons 2–10) can be obtained from Dr. Anton Berns' laboratory (Division of Molecular Genetics, Netherlands Cancer Institute, Amsterdam, The Netherlands) [30]. Genotyping is performed on DNA from each mouse to detect the presence of the transgenes by PCR. The PCR products are subjected to electrophoresis on a 2 % agarose gel along with a DNA size marker and visualized by ultraviolet (UV) light after staining with ethidium bromide. For the *p53*-flox allele, PCR is conducted under the conditions detailed in Table 4, with primers p53-10F and *p53*-10R to amplify a 460-bp product for the wild type allele and a 584-bp product for the *p53*-floxed allele. DNA with both wild type *p53* ($p53^{wt/wt}$) display only a single 460-bp fragment and DNA with wild type *p53* and Floxed ($p53^{Flox/wt}$) alleles will show both 460-bp and 584-bp fragments, whereas DNA with both Floxed ($p53^{Flox/Flox}$) alleles will only exhibit a single 584-bp fragment.

For *Rb*-flox, PCR is conducted with primers Rb19E and Rb18 to amplify a 200-bp product for the wild type allele and a 283-bp product for the *Rb*-floxed allele. DNA with both wild type *Rb* alleles ($Rb^{wt/wt}$) display only a single 200-bp fragment and DNA with a wild type *Rb* allele and Floxed ($Rb^{Flox/wt}$) allele show both 200-bp and 283-bp fragments, whereas DNA with both Floxed ($Rb^{Flox/Flox}$) alleles show a single 283-bp fragment (Table 3). Only $Trp53^{F2\text{-}10/F2\text{-}10}$;$Rb1^{F19/F19}$ mice should be used in the induction of SCLC.

3 Methods

3.1 General Protocols and Tumor Phenotyping Methods for Animal Studies

Three general protocols are commonly used in chemoprevention studies: (1) complete chemoprevention protocol, (2) post-initiation chemoprevention protocol, and (3) progression chemoprevention protocol [32]. In the complete chemoprevention protocol, the testing agent(s) is administrated before carcinogen initiation (i.e., about 2 weeks) and continued until the end of the experiment (20–24 weeks). In the post-initiation chemoprevention protocol, the testing agent(s) is given after carcinogen initiation (i.e., about 2 weeks after) and continues until the end of the experiment (20–24 weeks). In the tumor progression protocol, the testing agent(s) is given when benign lesions develop and continues until malignant tumors appear after carcinogen initiation.

Three tumor phenotyping methods are commonly used to assess lung tumor development in mice: (1) lung tumor incidence, (2) lung tumor multiplicity, and (3) lung tumor load. Incidence is defined as the percentage of mice that have lung tumors in a given population [% = (number of mice with lung tumors/number of total mice) × 100 %]. Multiplicity is defined as the average number of lung tumors per lung. Tumor load is the average sum of the lung tumor volume. Small animal imaging, such as micro-computerized tomography (micro-CT), magnetic resonance imaging (MRI), and positron-emission tomography (PET), can also be used to monitor lung tumor development. Advantages include readings with limited bias and the ability to monitor tumor development in live animals. Limitations include the expensive cost of equipment and the challenge that arises if a large number of mice [hundred(s)] need to be imaged in a short time period (e.g., between 3 and 5 days).

3.2 Mouse Models of Lung Adenoma and Adenocarcinoma

3.2.1 A/J Mouse Lung Adenoma Model Induced by Tobacco Specific Carcinogens such as B(a)P and NNK

B(a)P (benzo(a)pyrene) and NNK (nicotine-derived nitrosamine ketone) are tobacco specific carcinogens [33]. Many agents have been tested with positive effects using lung tumor models in A/J mice initiated with tobacco-derived carcinogens. Although the protocols vary somewhat, they are generally categorized as a complete protocol, post-initiation protocol, or progression protocol. Here, we describe a protocol generally used in our laboratories. At 6 ± 1 weeks of age, mice receive intraperitoneal (i.p.) injections of B(a)P at 100 mg/kg body weight in 0.2 ml tricaprylin (Table 5), either a single dose or two doses in 2 consecutive weeks. When NNK is the chosen initiator, mice at age of 6 ± 1 weeks receive a single intraperitoneal (i.p.) injection of NNK at 100 mg/kg body weight in 0.2 ml PBS (Table 5). In some studies, NNK has also been used concurrently with B(a)P. A mixture of B(a)P (2 μmol) and NNK (2 μmol) in 0.1 ml cottonseed oil is given to mice by oral gavage twice a week for 4 consecutive weeks [34]. The bioassay usually lasts 18–30 weeks (the time that the first dose of carcinogen was delivered is counted as week zero), but will specifically depend on the study design, including the carcinogen used, the number of doses used, and the number of carcinogens used. At the end of the final treatment, the mice are euthanized by CO_2 asphyxiation.

To maintain the integrity of the DNA and RNA in fresh tumors, the tumors along with their corresponding normal lung tissues are collected and snap frozen in liquid nitrogen as quickly as possible. In general, one to five fresh tumors and a small portion of normal lung are collected immediately upon termination and snap frozen. The rest of the lungs should be fixed in Tellyesniczky's solution [90 % ethanol (70 % v/v), 5 % glacial acetic acid, 5 % formalin (10 % v/v buffered formalin)] overnight and then kept in 70 % ethanol for evaluation prior to paraffin embedding. Alternatively, 10 % neutral-buffered formalin can be used for fixation. The fixed lungs should be evaluated by at least two investigators independently under a dissecting microscope to obtain the fixed surface tumor count. Individual tumor size is measured for volume calculation based on the following formula: ($mm^3 = V = 4/3\,\pi r^3$). The total tumor count should be obtained by adding the fixed and frozen tumor count.

A Student *t-test* is usually performed to test for significant differences in the number (multiplicity) and size (tumor load) of lung tumors per mouse between treatment and control mice. Fisher's exact test is usually used to determine the difference in the incidence. The significance of percentage changes are calculated using *Z*-statistics for proportions [35].

Histopathologically, these tumors are mostly adenomas and the tumor cells are orderly in arrangement. The cells are generally of consistent shape and size (round to polygonal). The nuclei are usually round to slightly ovoid and of consistent size. The cells and nuclei tend to line up nicely (thus giving the orderly arrangement).

Table 5
Summary of protocols for lung cancer induction

Tumor inducer			Delivery route	Dose	Term	References
Benzo(*a*)pyrene	BaP	Sigma-Aldrich (Cat. No. B1760)	Intraperitoneal (i.p.) injection	100 mg/kg B.W. in 0.2 ml of Tricaprylin (C8:0)[a]	~20 weeks	[39]
4-(methylnitrosamino)-1-(3-pyridyl)-1-butanone	NNK	Chemsyn Science Laboratories (Lenexa, KS, USA)	Intraperitoneal (i.p.) injection	100 mg/kg B.W. in 0.2 ml of PBS	18–30 weeks	[22, 35, 39]
N-nitroso-tris-chloroethylurea	NTCU	Toronto Research Chemicals, Inc. (Toronto, Canada)	Skin painting (0.04 M in 100 ml acetone) twice a week	0.04 M in 100 ml acetone twice a week	30–36 weeks	[36]
Vinyl carbamate	VC	Toronto Research Chemicals, Inc. (Toronto, Canada) V375000	Intraperitoneal (i.p.) injection	0.32 mg (in 0.2 cc saline)/female AJ mouse	~20 weeks	[40]
Ad5-CMV-Cre virus	Adeno-Cre virus	University of Iowa Gene Transfer Vector Core	Intratracheal administration	5×10^{10} particles of virus	36 weeks	[29]

[a]Tricaprylin (C8:0) is used as solvent for BaP can be purchased from Sigma-Aldrich (Cat. No. T-9126)

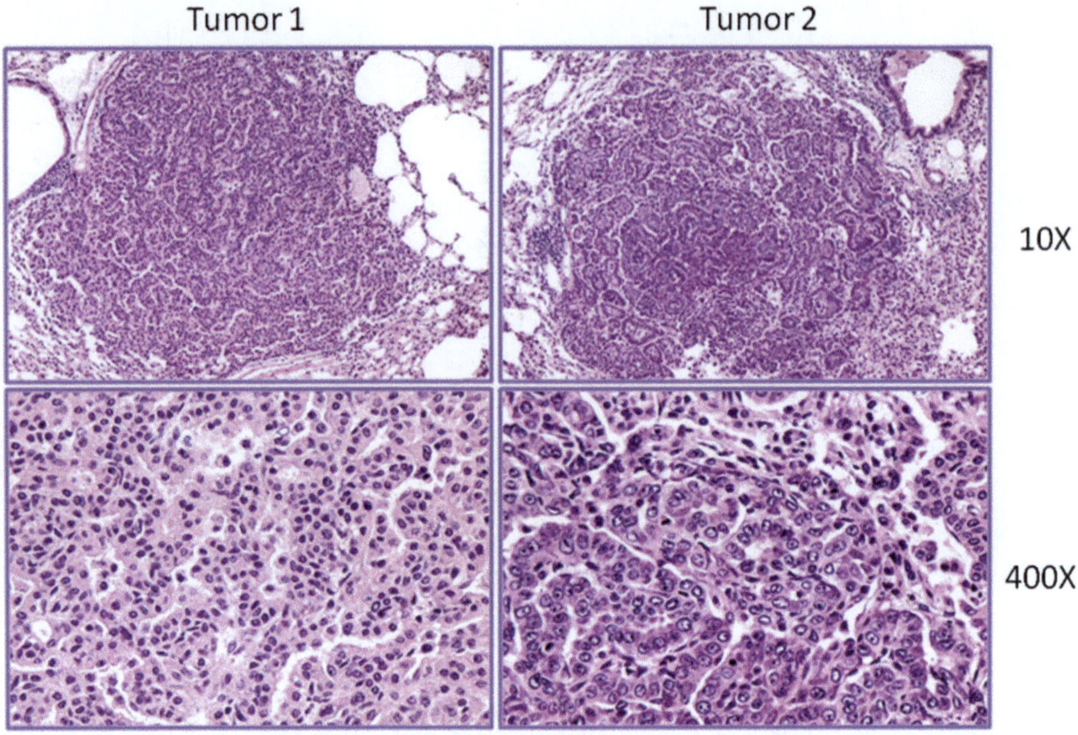

Fig. 3 p53$^{wt/Ala135Val}$ mice are given two doses of vinyl carbamate (VC) at 7 ± 1 weeks of age by i.p. injection once a week for 2 consecutive weeks (0.32 mg for females in 0.2 cc sterile saline without adjustment of pH). Twenty weeks after the initial dose of VC, mice are euthanized by CO_2 asphyxiation (Wang Y. et a. 2010; PMID: 21045137). Tumor 1, adenoma; Tumor 2, adenocarcinoma

Nuclei piled on top of one another (layering) are unusual. Prominent nucleoli are infrequently observed and the nuclei are also typically hyperchromatic or possibly contain coarse chromatin (Fig. 3; Tumor #1).

3.2.2 The A/J-p53 Transgenic Mouse and Wild Type Littermate Lung Adenocarcinoma Model Induced by VC

Lung adenocarcinoma can be readily induced by an intraperitoneal (i.p.) injection of VC in *p53*$^{wt/Ala135Val}$ as well as their wild type littermates (*p53*$^{wt/wt}$). Right before use, VC is dissolved in sterile saline (0.9 % NaCl). An intraperitoneal (i.p.) injection of VC at 0.32 mg/mouse in 0.2 ml saline is given to 6 ± 1 week old female mice either as a single dose or as two doses in 2 consecutive weeks. With two doses of VC, mice will develop multiple small adenomas in their lung 8 weeks after the first dose of VC with about 8 tumors per lung. All mice develop lung tumors at 20 weeks after the first VC injection. These tumors are diagnosed as adenocarcinomas (Fig. 3; Tumor #2). Key features suggesting carcinoma include cellular pleomorphism, anisocytosis, anisokaryosis, and other features of atypia such as prominent nucleoli. Mixing of patterns and layering of nuclei are other features that may push toward diagnosis of carcinoma. However, bronchial invasion is observed in VC-induced lung tumors in $p53^{wt/Ala135Val}$ mice. On average, ~40 lung tumors per $p53^{wt/wt}$ mouse and 50 lung tumors per $p53^{wt/Ala135Val}$ mouse are observed. The tumor load is ~25 mm^3 in $p53^{wt/wt}$ and 70 mm^3 in $p53^{wt/Ala135Val}$ mouse [27]. Recently, we found that one dose of VC is much more manageable in the evaluation of both tumor multiplicity and tumor load. Generally, <20 lung tumors per $p53^{wt/wt}$ mouse and <30 lung tumors per $p53^{wt/Ala135Val}$ mouse are observed (Wang Y. et al. unpublished data) and the average tumor load is <6 mm^3 per $p53^{wt/wt}$ mouse and <18 mm^3 per $p53^{wt/Ala135Val}$ mouse (unpublished data).

3.3 Lung SCC Mouse Model

Lung SCC can be induced in mice with NTCU skin painting as previously described [36]. NTCU is a chemical carcinogen (chlorinated nitrosotrialkylureas) and is one of only two chemical carcinogens [N-nitroso-methyl-bis-chloroethylurea (NMBCU) or NTCU] that can induce mouse SCCs [36, 37]. NMBCU is an explosive hazard. Therefore, NTCU is the only usable carcinogen for inducing SCCs. In addition, the NTCU-mouse lung SCC model is relevant to human lung SCCs in regard to the specific organ site, lesions of similar pathology, and the lack of Ras activation in both species [36].

Although lung SCCs can be induced in many strains of mice [36], NIH Swiss mice are preferred for this model. We have noticed that among ~20 strains of mice, including 129/svJ, AKR/J, BALB/cJ, C57BL/6J, FVB/J, SWR/J, A/J, and NIH Swiss ([36]; Wang Y et al. unpublished observation), the NIH Swiss mice show less skin irritations caused by NTCU and also readily develop SCC. To induce lung SCC, 8-week-old Swiss mice begin receiving NTCU treatment through repeated skin painting. The dorsal skin of each mouse is shaved 24–48 h prior to the first dose of NTCU. For the application of NTCU, 100-μl drops of 0.04 M NTCU is applied to the shaved skin with a micro-pipette (Gilson 200 μl is preferred). This process is repeated twice a week with a 3.5-day interval for the duration of the study, which is usually 32–36 weeks. Lungs are fixed in Tellyesniczky's solution [ethanol (70 % v/v), 90 %; acetic acid, glacial, 5 %; and 10 % v/v buffered formalin, 5 %]. Unlike lung adenocarcinoma, SCC does not form visible solid nodules on the surface of the lung (Fig. 4). Histopathological evaluation of the lung tumors can be carried out following the criteria previously described [36]. Approximately 100 serial tissue sections (4-μm each) are made from formalin fixed lung, and one in every 20 sections (approximately 100 μm apart) is stained with hematoxylin and eosin (H&E) and examined histologically under a light microscope. The lesions, including invasive SCC, carcinoma in situ (CIS), and the bronchial hyperplasia/metaplasia, are scored from the H&E-stained sections of each lung.

In contrast to lung adenoma and adenocarcinoma (Fig. 3), SCC lesions are distributed diffusely throughout the lungs (Fig. 4a–c,

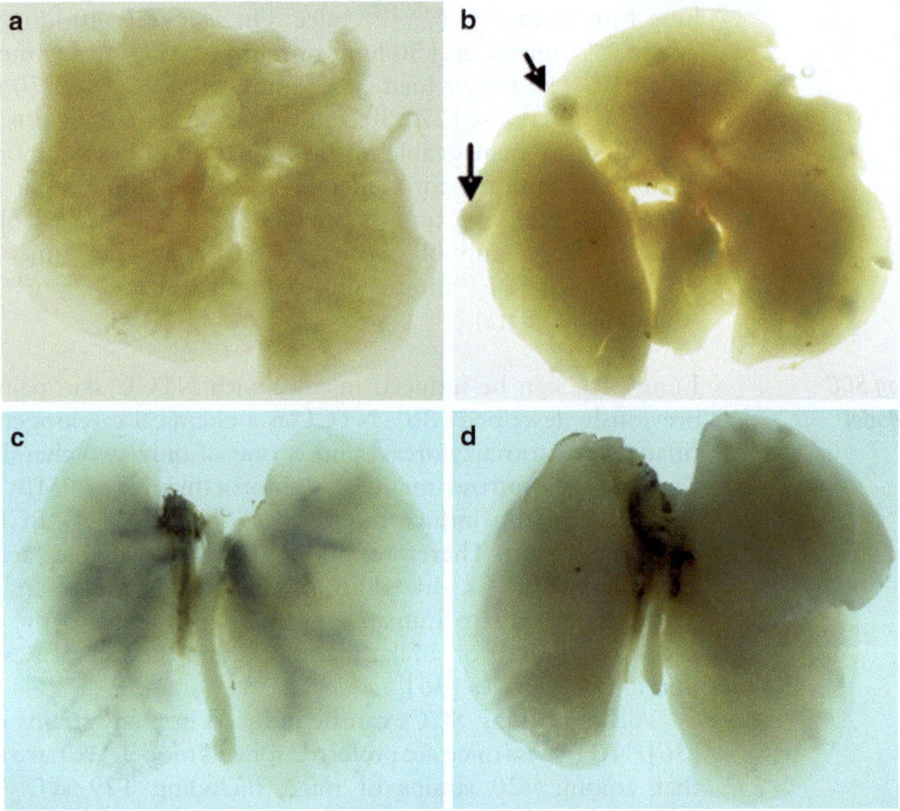

Fig. 4 Unlike the lungs with adenomas/adenocarcinomas (indicated with *arrows* in *panel b* (comparing to *panel a*), no countable individual tumors can be observed. Instead, the lungs with SCC become denser and less transparent (*panel d*) compared to the normal lung (*panel c*)

acetone-treated control lung without SCC; d, NTCU-treated lung with SCC). Also, SCCs from both MRI and micro-CT showed continuous lesions, whereas adenomas or adenocarcinomas are more discreet [26]. Distinctive histopathologic features in early (hyperplasia, squamous metaplasia), intermediate (dysplasia), and late (in situ, SCC) stages of human lung SCCs are also observed in NTCU-induced mouse lung SCC.

Several pathological microscopic features of NTCU-induced SCC are observed in the lung. SCC originates from the bronchial epithelial cells (Fig. 5a). The carcinogenesis process of SCC begins with normal epithelium in the bronchus and progresses through hyperplasia, metaplasia, dysplasia, and carcinoma in situ to invasive cancer. When hyperplasia occurs (Fig. 5b), although the cells maintain their normal appearance, a single layer of bronchiolar epithelial cells becomes multiple layers. Mitosis is rare. In bronchiolar metaplasia (Fig. 5c), the normal columnar epithelium is replaced by flattened squamous epithelium with increased keratin production. Bronchiolar dysplasia can be seen (Fig. 5d) with anisocytosis

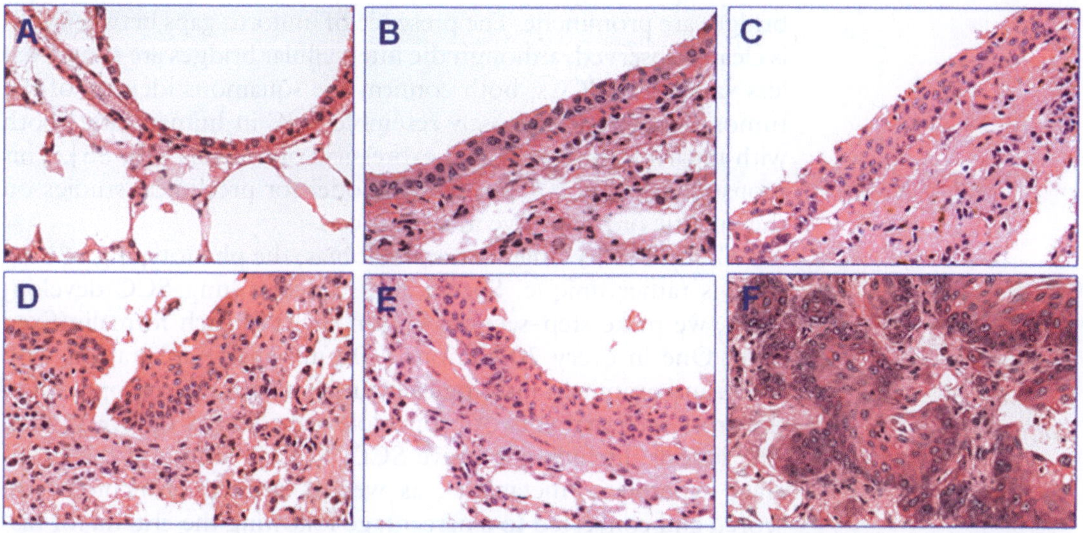

Fig. 5 Typical squamous lesions in the NTCU-treated lung of p53 transgenic mice. These lesions include SCC, CIS, bronchial metaplasia, and bronchial hyperplasia. When hyperplasia occurs, a single layer of bronchiolar epithelial cells (**a**) becomes multiple layers (**b**). The cells maintain their normal appearance. Mitosis is rare. In bronchiolar metaplasia (**c**)/dysplasia (**d**), a relatively rare event, the normal columnar epithelium is replaced by flattened squamous cells with increased keratin production. In CIS (**e**), also a relatively rare event, atypical cells (e.g., irregular shape, increased nucleus–cytoplasm ratio) with mitosis and loss of orderly differentiation replace the entire thickened epithelium. The bronchiole base membrane is intact. No tumor cells are found in the surrounding stroma. In SCC (**f**), general features of SCC such as keratin pearls, multiple nuclei, and increasing mitotic index can be seen. The normal architecture of the lung is disrupted. Nests of tumors can be seen in the subepithelial stroma. The shape and size of the neoplastic cells are pleomorphic, from polygonal to round, showing keratinization. The nuclei are irregularly shaped with coarsely clumped chromatin. The presence of gaps between the cancer, intercellular bridges, and keratin pearls are occasionally clearly observed

(cells of unequal size), poikilocytosis (abnormally shaped cells), and mitotic figures. Layers and cell number are increased. Dysplasia is often indicative of an early neoplastic process. In carcinoma in situ (Fig. 5e; meaning "cancer in place"), atypical cells replace the entire thickened epithelium. These cells have irregular shapes with mitosis, an increased nucleus–cytoplasm ratio, and loss of orderly differentiation. However, cancer cells remain localized, and the bronchiole base membrane is intact; and no tumor cells are found in the surrounding stroma. In invasive carcinoma (Fig. 5f), general features of SCC such as keratin pearls, multiple nuclei, and increasing mitotic index can be seen. The normal architecture of the lung is disrupted. Cords and nests of tumors can be seen in the subepithelial stroma. The tumor growth pattern is usually firm non-encapsulated masses formed with irregularly shaped sheets and nests of cells. The shape and size of the neoplastic cells are polygonal to round with reduced amounts of cytoplasm. The nuclei are hyperchromatic and irregular in shape with coarsely clumped chromatin. The squamous cells exhibiting loss of polarity and intercellular bridges are prominent. The presence of uniform gaps between cells is clearly observed, although the intercellular bridges are somewhat less variable in SCCs, both confirm the squamous identity of the tumor. These lesions closely resemble SCC in human lungs both with regard to histology and expression of keratins [26, 36]. This mouse lung SCC is a promising model for preclinical studies on therapeutic or preventive investigations.

Compared to lung adenocarcinomas, the phenotyping of lung SCC is rather unique. Specifically, to access lung SCC development, we make step–sections (5 μm each) of each formalin-fixed lung. One in every 20 sections (100 μm apart) are stained with H&E and examined histologically under a light microscope. All of the cross-sectional cuts of bronchiole are counted on every slide. The lesions, including invasive SCC, SCC in situ, and the bronchial hyperplasia/metaplasia, as well as normal bronchioles are scored and converted to a percentage following the criteria for histopathologic examination described above.

3.4 SCLC Mouse Model

One mouse SCLC model was developed with conditionally targeted alleles for both *Rb1* and *p53* [30]. Both *Rb1* and *p53* alleles are conditionally inactivated in the lung epithelium by using adenovirus-mediated somatic gene transfer of Cre recombinase [30]. We successfully used this SCLC mouse model to determine the efficacy of bexarotene and budesonide [29].

Mice carrying conditional alleles for *Rb1* (floxed at exon 19) and *p53* (floxed at exons 2–10) can be obtained from Dr. Anton Berns' laboratory (Division of Molecular Genetics, Netherlands Cancer Institute, Amsterdam, The Netherlands) [30]. Adeno-Cre virus (Ad5-CMV-Cre virus) is purchased from the University of Iowa Gene Transfer Vector Core (Iowa City, IA). For intratracheal Adeno-Cre virus administration, the Adeno-Cre virus is suspended in 3 % sucrose in PBS at a concentration of 1×10^{12} particles/ml and stored at −80 °C until used. The Ad-Cre virus is administered by intratracheal injection to somatically inactivate *p53* and *Rb1* in pulmonary bronchial epithelial cells of B5 (AJ × $Trp53^{F2\text{-}10/F2\text{-}10}$;$Rb1^{F19/F19}$) mice. For each mouse, 5×10^{10} particles of virus are delivered through the trachea. A cocktail is made with 1 ml of ketamine, 0.15 ml of xylazine, and 4 ml of PBS. Mice are anesthetized with 100 μL of the cocktail per 20-g mouse by i.p. injection and placed in a supine position with a rubber "pillow" under its neck to ensure that the airway was straight. A catheter [26-gauge × 19 mm (3/4-in., Venisystems, Abbocath-T, Abbott Ireland)] is inserted slowly into the trachea, a 1 ml syringe is attached, and the virus is delivered slowly. The mouse is held with two hands by the investigator at its forearms and a soft rub is given to the mouse's chest gently for about 15 s to facilitate the movement of the virus down into the lung and to prevent death by bronchus blockage [29, 38].

For a typical chemoprevention study using an SCLC mouse model, 7-week-old mice are randomized into control and treatment groups. Chemopreventive agents are given to mice 2 weeks before intratracheal administration of the Adeno-Cre virus. The mice are given AIN-76A Purified Diet no. 100,000 (Dyets, Inc.) continuously with or without chemopreventive agent until the end of the experiment. The mice in the control group are fed the AIN-76A-purified diet. The mice in the treatment group are fed AIN-76A-purified diet containing the test agent. Food and water are available ad libitum. Lung tissue is fixed in Tellyesniczky's solution and stored in 70 % ethanol. Lung tumor number is counted and the tumor diameter measured. For spherical tumors, the radius is used to calculate volume by the formula $V = (4/3)\ \pi r^3$. For irregular tumors, three measurements are taken as height (H), width (W), and length (L). The volume is calculated using the formula $V = (4/3)\ \pi \times L/2 \times W/2 \times H/2$.

In summary, this chapter highlighted mouse models of lung adenocarcinoma, SCC, and small-cell lung cancer, most of which we helped to develop. For conducting a successful preclinical chemoprevention study, it is essential to select the most appropriate mouse models and the specific protocols to identify agents which may prevent lung cancer development. Although most chemopreventive studies have been performed using mouse models of lung adenomas or adenocarcinomas, with several compounds have been identified as potentially effective chemopreventive agents, models of squamous cell lung cancer and small-cell lung cancer are becoming more widely used in lung cancer chemoprevention studies.

References

1. Siegel R, Naishadham D, Jemal A (2013) Cancer statistics, 2013. CA Cancer J Clin 63(1):11–30. doi:10.3322/caac.21166
2. Doll R, Hill AB (1952) A study of the aetiology of carcinoma of the lung. Br Med J 2(4797): 1271–1286
3. Herzog CR, Lubet RA, You M (1997) Genetic alterations in mouse lung tumors: implications for cancer chemoprevention. J Cell Biochem Suppl 28–29:49–63
4. Shopland DR, Eyre HJ, Pechacek TF (1991) Smoking-attributable cancer mortality in 1991: is lung cancer now the leading cause of death among smokers in the United States? J Natl Cancer Inst 83(16):1142–1148
5. Minna JD (1993) The molecular biology of lung cancer pathogenesis. Chest 103(4 Suppl): 449S–456S
6. Jemal A, Siegel R, Xu J, Ward E (2010) Cancer statistics, 2010. CA Cancer J Clin 60(5):277–300. doi:10.3322/caac.20073
7. Herbst RS, Heymach JV, Lippman SM (2008) Lung cancer. N Engl J Med 359(13):1367–1380. doi:10.1056/NEJMra0802714
8. Goldstraw P, Crowley J, Chansky K, Giroux DJ, Groome PA, Rami-Porta R, Postmus PE, Rusch V, Sobin L (2007) The IASLC Lung Cancer Staging Project: proposals for the revision of the TNM stage groupings in the forthcoming (seventh) edition of the TNM Classification of malignant tumours. J Thorac Oncol 2(8):706–714. doi:10.1097/JTO.0b013e31812f3c1a
9. Mountain CF, Dresler CM (1997) Regional lymph node classification for lung cancer staging. Chest 111(6):1718–1723
10. Mountain CF (1997) Revisions in the international system for staging lung cancer. Chest 111(6):1710–1717
11. Alifano M, Souaze F, Dupouy S, Camilleri-Broet S, Younes M, Ahmed-Zaid SM, Takahashi T, Cancellieri A, Damiani S, Boaron M, Broet P, Miller LD, Gespach C, Regnard JF, Forgez P

(2010) Neurotensin receptor 1 determines the outcome of non-small cell lung cancer. Clin Cancer Res 16(17):4401–4410. doi:10.1158/1078-0432.CCR-10-0659

12. Lovly CM, Carbone DP (2011) Lung cancer in 2010: one size does not fit all. Nat Rev Clin Oncol 8(2):68–70. doi:10.1038/nrclinonc.2010.224
13. (2012) Comprehensive genomic characterization of squamous cell lung cancers. Nature 489(7417):519–525. doi:10.1038/nature11404
14. Lockwood WW, Wilson IM, Coe BP, Chari R, Pikor LA, Thu KL, Solis LM, Nunez MI, Behrens C, Yee J, English J, Murray N, Tsao MS, Minna JD, Gazdar AF, Wistuba II, MacAulay CE, Lam S, Lam WL (2012) Divergent genomic and epigenomic landscapes of lung cancer subtypes underscore the selection of different oncogenic pathways during tumor development. PLoS One 7(5):e37775. doi:10.1371/journal.pone.0037775
15. Hainsworth JD, Cebotaru CL, Kanarev V, Ciuleanu TE, Damyanov D, Stella P, Ganchev H, Pover G, Morris C, Tzekova V (2010) A phase II, open-label, randomized study to assess the efficacy and safety of AZD6244 (ARRY-142886) versus pemetrexed in patients with non-small cell lung cancer who have failed one or two prior chemotherapeutic regimens. J Thorac Oncol 5(10):1630–1636. doi:10.1097/JTO.0b013e3181e8b3a3
16. Huynh H, Soo KC, Chow PK, Tran E (2007) Targeted inhibition of the extracellular signal-regulated kinase kinase pathway with AZD6244 (ARRY-142886) in the treatment of hepatocellular carcinoma. Mol Cancer Ther 6(1):138–146. doi:10.1158/1535-7163.MCT-06-0436
17. Ball DW, Jin N, Rosen DM, Dackiw A, Sidransky D, Xing M, Nelkin BD (2007) Selective growth inhibition in BRAF mutant thyroid cancer by the mitogen-activated protein kinase kinase 1/2 inhibitor AZD6244. J Clin Endocrinol Metab 92(12):4712–4718. doi:10.1210/jc.2007-1184
18. Haass NK, Sproesser K, Nguyen TK, Contractor R, Medina CA, Nathanson KL, Herlyn M, Smalley KS (2008) The mitogen-activated protein/extracellular signal-regulated kinase kinase inhibitor AZD6244 (ARRY-142886) induces growth arrest in melanoma cells and tumor regression when combined with docetaxel. Clin Cancer Res 14(1):230–239. doi:10.1158/1078-0432.CCR-07-1440
19. Ammoun S, Ristic N, Matthies C, Hilton DA, Hanemann CO (2010) Targeting ERK1/2 activation and proliferation in human primary schwannoma cells with MEK1/2 inhibitor AZD6244. Neurobiol Dis 37(1):141–146. doi:10.1016/j.nbd.2009.09.017
20. Estensen RD, Wattenberg LW (1993) Studies of chemopreventive effects of myo-inositol on benzo[a]pyrene-induced neoplasia of the lung and forestomach of female A/J mice. Carcinogenesis 14(9):1975–1977
21. Wattenberg LW, Wiedmann TS, Estensen RD, Zimmerman CL, Steele VE, Kelloff GJ (1997) Chemoprevention of pulmonary carcinogenesis by aerosolized budesonide in female A/J mice. Cancer Res 57(24):5489–5492
22. Wang Y, Zhang Z, Kastens E, Lubet RA, You M (2003) Mice with alterations in both p53 and Ink4a/Arf display a striking increase in lung tumor multiplicity and progression: differential chemopreventive effect of budesonide in wild-type and mutant A/J mice. Cancer Res 63(15):4389–4395
23. Zhang Z, Liu Q, Lantry LE, Wang Y, Kelloff GJ, Anderson MW, Wiseman RW, Lubet RA, You M (2000) A germ-line p53 mutation accelerates pulmonary tumorigenesis: p53-independent efficacy of chemopreventive agents green tea or dexamethasone/myo-inositol and chemotherapeutic agents taxol or adriamycin. Cancer Res 60(4):901–907
24. Anderson MW, Goodin C, Zhang Y, Kim S, Estensen RD, Wiedmann TS, Sekar P, Buncher CR, Khoury JC, Garbow JR, You M, Tichelaar JW (2008) Effect of dietary green tea extract and aerosolized difluoromethylornithine during lung tumor progression in A/J strain mice. Carcinogenesis 29(8):1594–1600. doi:10.1093/carcin/bgn129
25. Fu H, He J, Mei F, Zhang Q, Hara Y, Ryota S, Lubet RA, Chen R, Chen DR, You M (2009) Lung cancer inhibitory effect of epigallocatechin-3-gallate is dependent on its presence in a complex mixture (polyphenon E). Cancer Prev Res (Phila) 2(6):531–537. doi:10.1158/1940-6207.CAPR-08-0185
26. Wang Y, Zhang Z, Garbow JR, Rowland DJ, Lubet RA, Sit D, Law F, You M (2009) Chemoprevention of lung squamous cell carcinoma in mice by a mixture of Chinese herbs. Cancer Prev Res (Phila) 2(7):634–640. doi:10.1158/1940-6207.CAPR-09-0052
27. Wang Y, James M, Wen W, Lu Y, Szabo E, Lubet RA, You M (2010) Chemopreventive effects of pioglitazone on chemically induced lung carcinogenesis in mice. Mol Cancer Ther 9(11):3074–3082. doi:10.1158/1535-7163.MCT-10-0510
28. Khan N, Afaq F, Kweon MH, Kim K, Mukhtar H (2007) Oral consumption of pomegranate fruit extract inhibits growth and progression of primary lung tumors in mice. Cancer Res

67(7):3475–3482. doi:10.1158/0008-5472.CAN-06-3941

29. Wang Y, Wen W, Yi Y, Zhang Z, Lubet RA, You M (2009) Preventive effects of bexarotene and budesonide in a genetically engineered mouse model of small cell lung cancer. Cancer Prev Res (Phila) 2(12):1059–1064. doi:10.1158/1940-6207.CAPR-09-0221
30. Meuwissen R, Linn SC, Linnoila RI, Zevenhoven J, Mooi WJ, Berns A (2003) Induction of small cell lung cancer by somatic inactivation of both Trp53 and Rb1 in a conditional mouse model. Cancer Cell 4(3):181–189
31. Lavigueur A, Maltby V, Mock D, Rossant J, Pawson T, Bernstein A (1989) High incidence of lung, bone, and lymphoid tumors in transgenic mice overexpressing mutant alleles of the p53 oncogene. Mol Cell Biol 9(9):3982–3991
32. Wang Y, Zhang Z, Yao R, Jia D, Wang D, Lubet RA, You M (2006) Prevention of lung cancer progression by bexarotene in mouse models. Oncogene 25(9):1320–1329. doi:10.1038/sj.onc.1209180
33. Hecht SS (1999) Tobacco smoke carcinogens and lung cancer. J Natl Cancer Inst 91(14):1194–1210
34. Kassie F, Melkamu T, Endalew A, Upadhyaya P, Luo X, Hecht SS (2010) Inhibition of lung carcinogenesis and critical cancer-related signaling pathways by N-acetyl-S-(N-2-phenethylthiocarbamoyl)-l-cysteine, indole-3-carbinol and myo-inositol, alone and in combination. Carcinogenesis 31(9):1634–1641. doi:10.1093/carcin/bgq139
35. Zhang Z, Wang Y, Lantry LE, Kastens E, Liu G, Hamilton AD, Sebti SM, Lubet RA, You M (2003) Farnesyltransferase inhibitors are potent lung cancer chemopreventive agents in A/J mice with a dominant-negative p53 and/or heterozygous deletion of Ink4a/Arf. Oncogene 22(40):6257–6265. doi:10.1038/sj.onc.1206630
36. Wang Y, Zhang Z, Yan Y, Lemon WJ, LaRegina M, Morrison C, Lubet R, You M (2004) A chemically induced model for squamous cell carcinoma of the lung in mice: histopathology and strain susceptibility. Cancer Res 64(5):1647–1654
37. Rehm S, Lijinsky W, Singh G, Katyal SL (1991) Mouse bronchiolar cell carcinogenesis. Histologic characterization and expression of Clara cell antigen in lesions induced by N-nitrosobis-(2-chloroethyl) ureas. Am J Pathol 139(2):413–422
38. DuPage M, Dooley AL, Jacks T (2009) Conditional mouse lung cancer models using adenoviral or lentiviral delivery of Cre recombinase. Nat Protoc 4(7):1064–1072. doi:10.1038/nprot.2009.95

Chapter 7

The Azoxymethane Plus Dextran Sulfate Sodium-Induced Mouse Colon Cancer Model for the Study of Dietary Chemoprevention of Inflammation-Associated Carcinogenesis

Ha-Na Lee, Hye-Won Yum, and Young-Joon Surh

Abstract

The azoxymethane (AOM) plus dextran sulfate sodium (DSS)-induced mouse colon carcinogenesis model is a fascinating tool for investigating the pathogenesis and chemoprevention of colitis-associated colorectal cancer. In this two-stage mouse colon cancer model, tumorigenesis is initiated by a single intraperitoneal administration of the carcinogen AOM and promoted by DSS-induced inflammation. The successful induction of AOM plus DSS-induced colorectal cancer relies on several critical factors, such as the molecular weight and the dosage of DSS, the strain, age, and sex of animals, and other experimental conditions. Here, we provide the optimized protocol for effective induction of colon tumors in mice by treatment with AOM plus DSS. Inflammation-induced colon carcinogenesis is accompanied by a series of histopathological and molecular changes. In this chapter, we also describe the step-by-step protocols for macroscopic examination, hematoxylin and eosin (H & E) staining, immunohistochemical analysis, immunoblot analysis, and the electrophoretic mobility shift assay, all of which are used for investigating the inflammation-associated colon carcinogenesis and the chemopreventive effect of dietary phytochemicals.

Key words DSS-induced colitis, AOM plus DSS-induced colon carcinogenesis, H & E staining, IHC analysis, Immunoblot analysis, EMSA

1 Introduction

Inflammation is a well-known risk factor for colorectal cancer. Several molecular events involved in the chronic inflammatory process may contribute to multistep carcinogenesis of human colorectal cancer. For understanding the pathogenesis of inflammation-induced colon cancer, a two-stage mouse colon carcinogenesis model has been developed, in which initiation is achieved with azoxymethane (AOM) and promotion with dextran sodium sulfate (DSS) [1]. This model is based on a single intraperitoneal (i.p.) injection of AOM (10 mg/kg body weight) and subsequent administration of DSS (2.5 %) in drinking water for 1 week. Colon

Ann M. Bode and Zigang Dong (eds.), *Cancer Prevention: Dietary Factors and Pharmacology*, Methods in Pharmacology and Toxicology, DOI 10.1007/978-1-4614-9227-6_7, © Springer Science+Business Media New York 2014

cancer development following DSS-induced colitis provides supporting evidence showing that chronic inflammation in inflammatory bowel diseases plays a crucial role in epithelial neoplasia in the colon [2].

AOM is a potent carcinogen resulting in colorectal cancer in rodents. AOM does not interact with DNA directly, but instead a metabolite of AOM causes DNA mutations by changing the nucleotides from G–C to A–T. Cytochrome P450, especially isoform CYP2E1, has been reported to catalyze the conversion of AOM into methylazoxymethanol, which then breaks down into formaldehyde and reactive alkylating species, such as methyldiazonium. This reactive chemical causes DNA mutation through the alkylation of guanine to O^6-methylguanine and to O^4-methylthymine [3].

DSS is a sulfate polysaccharide with highly variable molecular weights, ranging from 5 kDa to up to 1,400 kDa. It is widely used to induce colitis, characterized by severe infiltration of inflammatory cells and epithelial damage in the colon, a reduced colon length, increased weight of the colon, and body weight loss [4]. However, the mechanism underlying DSS-induced colitis remains unclear. The proposed mechanism is that DSS is toxic to colonic epithelial cells and causes defects in the epithelial barrier integrity, thereby allowing the entry of luminal antigens and microorganisms into the mucosa and subsequently resulting in overwhelming inflammatory responses [5]. The molecular weight of DSS is the most important factor in the induction of murine colitis. DSS at 30–50 kDa has been proven to induce severe colitis in the distal part of the colon. However, DSS with a low molecular weight (5 kDa) causes less activity, and DSS with a high molecular weight (500 kDa) cannot induce colitis [6].

The successful induction of AOM plus DSS-induced colorectal cancer is dependent on several key factors, including concentration, duration, and frequency of DSS exposure and genetic background, sex, age, and body weight of the animals. In a dose–response study to assess the ability of DSS to stimulate colon carcinogenesis in mice initiated with AOM, the tumor-promoting activity of DSS was not observed at a concentration of 0.1 or 0.25 %. Higher doses of DSS increased the incidence and the multiplicity of colonic tubular adenoma and adenocarcinoma. In addition, the severity of colonic inflammation, determined by the histological inflammation score and the nitrotyrosine-positive score, was much greater in mice that received higher doses of DSS after AOM administration. Tanaka et al. conducted a time-course study on AOM plus DSS-induced colorectal carcinogenesis, demonstrating that the tumor incidence increased gradually with time and reached 100 % with a multiplicity of 6.20 ± 2.48 at week 6 after AOM exposure. At week 14, the multiplicity of adenocarcinoma was further increased to 9.75 ± 2.49 [7, 8].

The different susceptibility to DSS-induced colitis can be caused by genetic differences in the ability of the mucosa to withstand inflammatory damage. Melgar et al. have demonstrated the differences in the susceptibility to DSS-induced colitis between two commonly used strains, BALB/c and C57BL/6. After DSS withdrawal (one cycle), the severity of colitis was reduced in BALB/c mice, whereas colitis progressed into the chronic phase in C57BL/6 mice [9]. Different strains of mice are known to have variable sensitivities to either AOM or DSS. For example, the BALB/c strain is known to be susceptible to AOM, whereas the C3H, C57BL/6, and DBA/2 strains are less sensitive. Therefore, the differences in genetic background of the mice could possibly affect the frequency of AOM plus DSS-induced colon adenocarcinoma. Crj:CD-1 (ICR) mice (outbreed strain), receiving a single i.p. injection of AOM (10 mg/kg body weight) followed by DSS (2 %) in drinking water for 7 days (1 week after the AOM injection), showed an 100 % incidence of adenocarcinomas at week 6 after AOM exposure [7, 8]. In general, the younger the animal the greater the success rate of induction, with the optimal range being between 5 and 6 weeks. Animals <4 weeks of age suffer a great deal of toxicity of the reagents, whereas animals >8 weeks have a diminished sensitivity. As a rule, induction colitis and adenoma formation should be performed at 5–6 weeks of age or between 25 and 30 g body weight. In relation to gender, although both males and females develop colitis, males develop more significant and chronic colitis [8].

In conclusion, the AOM plus DSS-induced mouse colon carcinogenesis model is a powerful tool for investigating the pathogenesis and chemoprevention of colitis-associated colorectal cancer. In this chapter, we comprehensively describe the step-by-step protocols, from the induction of colitis and colitis-associated adenocarcinoma to the examination of histological and molecular changes in the colon.

2 Materials

2.1 Equipment

For specific equipment described in the experimental protocols below, any model of comparable capability can be substituted.

1. A balance (AND, Seoul, South Korea) for measuring body weight.
2. Micromesh cassettes (Thermo Fisher Scientific, Rockford, IL), rack (Ted Pella Inc., Redding, CA), jar (Ted Pella Inc.), probe-on-plus slides (Thermo Fisher Scientific), cover glass (Ted Pella, Inc.), light microscopy (Nikon, Tokyo, Japan), and a PAP pen (Abcam Inc., Cambridge, MA) for staining and microscopic examination of colonic section.

3. Homogenizer (IKA, Seoul, South Korea), vortex mixer (Scientific Industries, Bochemia, NY), centrifuge (Eppendorf, Hamburg, Germany), Thermo bath (FINEPCR, Seoul, South Korea) and UV–visible spectrophotometer (GE Healthcare, Beverly, MA) for protein extraction and sample preparation from colonic tissue.
4. Hoefer SE 600 ruby (Amersham Biosciences, Uppsala, Sweden), Hoefer transphor tank transfer unit (Amersham Biosciences), PowerPac™ basic power supply (Bio-Rad, Hercules, CA), SH30 Orbital Shaker (FINEPCR, Seoul, South Korea), and LAS-4000 image reader (Fuji Film, Tokyo, Japan) for immunoblot analysis of protein expression.
5. Scintillation counter (PerkinElmer, Waltham, MA), vacuum gel dryer (Amersham Biosciences), and X-ray film cassette (Amersham Biosciences) for gel shift analysis of protein–nucleic acid interaction.

2.2 Reagents and Solutions

1. DSS (36–50 kDa; MP Biomedicals, Solon, OH).
2. AOM (Sigma Chemical Co., St. Louis, MO).
3. Phosphate-buffered saline (PBS): 8 g of NaCl, 0.2 g of KCl, 1.14 g of Na_2HPO_4, and 0.24 g of KH_2PO_4 in 800 mL of double-distilled water (DDW). Adjust the pH to 7.4 with HCl. Add DDW to 1 L.
4. Mayer's hematoxylin (Sigma).
5. 0.25 % acid alcohol: 2,578 mL of 95 % ethanol (Merck Millipore, Nottingham, UK), 950 mL of DDW, and 9 mL of HCl (Sigma).
6. 1.36 % Lithium carbonate: 47 g of lithium carbonate (Sigma) in 3,500 mL of DDW.
7. Eosin: 1 % aqueous eosin-Y (Sigma), 0.01 % aqueous phloxin B (Sigma), 780 mL of 95 % ethanol (Merck Millipore, Nottingham, UK), and 4 mL of glacial acetic acid.
8. 3 % H_2O_2: 30 mL of H_2O_2 (Sigma) and 970 mL of DDW.
9. 10 mM sodium citrate buffer: 2.94 g of sodium citrate in 800 mL of DDW. Adjust the pH to 6.0 and add DDW to 1 L.
10. 1 % DAB: 0.1 g of 3,3′-diaminobenzidine (DAB; Sigma) in 10 mL of DDW. Add 10N HCl three to five drops and solution turns light brown color. Shake for 10 min and DAB should dissolve completely. Aliquot and store at −20 °C.
11. 1× Cell lysis buffer: 20 mM Tris–HCl (Amresco LLC, MA, USA; pH 7.5), 150 mM NaCl, 1 mM disodium ethylenediaminetetraacetate (Na_2EDTA; Sigma), 1 mM ethylene glycol tetraacetic acid (EGTA; Sigma), 1 % Triton (Sigma), 2.5 mM sodium pyrophosphate (Sigma), 1 mM β-glycerophosphate (Sigma), 1 mM Na_3VO_4 (Sigma), and 1 μg/mL leupeptin (Sigma).

Table 1
Preparation of separating gels for SDS-polyacrylamide gel electrophoresis (for one large format gel)

Acrylamide concentration (%)	6	8	10	12	15
Range of separation (kDa)	**57–212**	**36–94**	**20–80**	**12–60**	**10–43**
DDW	11.6	10.6	9.6	8.6	7.1
40 % acrylamide-bis solution	3	4	5	6	7.5
1.5 M Tris (pH 8.8)	5	5	5	5	5
10 % SDS	0.2	0.2	0.2	0.2	0.2
10 % APS	0.2	0.2	0.2	0.2	0.2
TEMED	0.016	0.012	0.008	0.008	0.008
Total volume	20 mL				

12. EDTA-free cocktail tablet (Roche, Penzberg, Germany).
13. Hypotonic buffer A: 10 mM 4-(2-hydroxyethyl)-1-piperazineethanesulfonic acid (HEPES; Sigma; pH 7.8), 1.5 mM $MgCl_2$, 10 mM KCl, 0.5 mM dithiothreitol (DTT; Sigma), 0.2 mM phenylmethylsulfonyl fluoride (PMSF; Sigma) and 0.1 % Nonidet P-40 (Sigma).
14. Hypertonic Buffer C: 20 mM HEPES, 420 mM NaCl, 1.5 mM $MgCl_2$, 0.2 mM EDTA, 0.5 mM DTT, 0.2 mM PMSF, and 20 % glycerol (Amresco LLC).
15. Bicinchoninic acid assay (BCA) protein assay kit (Pierce, Rockford, IL).
16. 5× SDS gel-loading buffer: 0.3 M Tris–HCl (pH 6.8), 25 % 2-mercapto-ethanol (Sigma), 12 % sodium dodecyl sulfate (SDS; Amresco LLC), 25 mM EDTA, 20 % glycerol, and 0.1 % bromophenol blue (Sigma).
17. SDS-polyacrylamide gel for immunoblot analysis (Tables 1 and 2): 40 % acrylamide-bis solution (LPS solution, Daejeon, South Korea), 1.5 M Tris–HCl (pH 8.8), 1.0 M Tris–HCl (pH 6.8), SDS, ammonium persulfate (APS; Amresco LLC), and tetramethylethylenediamine (TEMED; Amresco LLC).
18. Transfer buffer: 25 mM Tris–HCl (pH 8.9), 192 mM glycine (Amresco LLC), and 20 % methanol.
19. Tris-buffered saline with Tween 20 (TBST): 20 mM Tris–HCl (pH 7.5), 150 mM NaCl, and 0.1 % Tween 20 (Amresco LLC).
20. Enhanced chemiluminescence (ECL) detection kit (Amersham Pharmacia Biotech, Buckinghamshire, UK).

Table 2
Preparation of 5 % stacking gel for SDS-polyacrylamide gel electrophoresis (for one large format gel)

5 % Stacking gel	
DDW	2.9
40 % acrylamide-bis solution	0.5
1.0 M Tris (pH 6.8)	0.5
10 % SDS	0.04
10 % APS	0.04
TEMED	0.004
Total volume	4 mL

21. 5× Tris/Borate/EDTA (TBE) buffer: 27 g of Tris base (Amresco LLC), 13.75 g of Boric acid, 10 mL of 0.5 M EDTA (pH 8.0), and 450 mL of DDW.
22. Incubation buffer: 10 mM Tris–HCl (pH 7.5), 100 mM NaCl, 1 mM DTT, 1 mM EDTA (pH 8.0), 4 % glycerol, and 0.1 mg/mL sonicated salmon sperm DNA (Sigma).
23. 1× Tris/EDTA (TE) buffer: 0.01 M Tris–HCl (pH 7.5) and 1 mM EDTA (pH 8.0).
24. Bromophenol blue dye: 0.1 % bromophenol blue in 1× TE buffer.
25. Non-denaturing gel for gel shift analysis: 31.43 mL of DDW, 6 mL of 40 % acrylamide-bis solution, 2 mL of 5× TBE, 400 μL of 10 % APS, and 20 μL of TEMED for one large gel.

3 Methods

3.1 Animal Care

Transportation unavoidably causes stress in animals. Therefore, when animals first arrive at the animal facility, a period of acclimation is necessary to allow the animals to recover from transport stress. Also, during acclimation, animals become accustomed to new husbandry environment including food, water, handlers, cage mates, noises, smells, light cycle, and other variables and regain homeostasis.

1. Obtain 5-week-old ICR male mice.
2. Acclimate ICR mice to the facility for 1 week.
3. After 1 week of acclimation, distribute ICR mice randomly into control and experimental groups.
4. House ICR mice in plastic cages under controlled temperature conditions (23 ± 2 °C), humidity (50 ± 10 %) and light (12–12 h light–dark cycle).

3.2 Short-Term Experiment to Induce Colitis

DSS-induced colitis is an easy and highly reproducible animal model mimicking human intestinal inflammation, such as inflammatory bowel disease. DSS is toxic to the epithelial lining of the colon and induces severe colitis, which is characterized by loss of body weight and bloody diarrhea. These symptoms appear during 4–7 days after DSS administration in drinking water.

3.2.1 Prepare Reagents and Treat Mice

1. Prepare an appropriate amount of dietary chemopreventive agents before treatment.
2. Treat mice with fresh dietary chemopreventive agents every day before DSS administration and thereafter until the end of the experiment (**Note 1**).
3. On experimental day 7, prepare 2.5 % (w/v) DSS mixture by dissolving 5 g of DSS in 200 mL of tap water (per cage). Stir overnight.
4. From experimental day 8, allow the mice free access to the 2.5 % DSS mixture for 1 week with continuous treatment of fresh dietary chemopreventive agents. Replenish water bottles with fresh 2.5 % DSS mixture three times a week.
5. After 1 week on DSS administration, sacrifice mice by CO_2 asphyxiation (Fig. 1).

3.2.2 Assess Colitis Severity

1. Measure the weight of mice everyday during DSS administration. Calculate the weight loss in percentage from starting weight.
2. Evaluate disease severity daily using the disease activity index (DAI). Score macroscopic assessment of the disease grade from 0 to 4 in a modified design depending on the severity of diarrhea and blood physical appearance daily [10] (Fig. 2).

3.3 Long-Term Experiment to Induce Adenocarcinomas

The AOM plus DSS-induced mouse colorectal carcinogenesis model is based on a single i.p. injection of AOM (10 mg/kg body weight) and 1 week administration with DSS (2.5 %) in drinking water. With this model, multistep tumor development can be efficiently reproduced in the outbred ICR susceptible murine strain. Time-course observation revealed that dysplasia is observed at 4 weeks after AOM administration, and colorectal adenoma and adenocarcinoma develop 6 weeks after AOM administration (Fig. 3).

1. Prepare an appropriate amount of dietary chemopreventive agents and AOM (1 mg/mL dissolved in PBS).
2. Give mice a single i.p. injection of AOM (10 mg/kg body weight) using 1 mL disposable syringes.
3. Starting from the day of AOM injection, treat mice with fresh dietary chemopreventive agents every day until the end of the experiment.

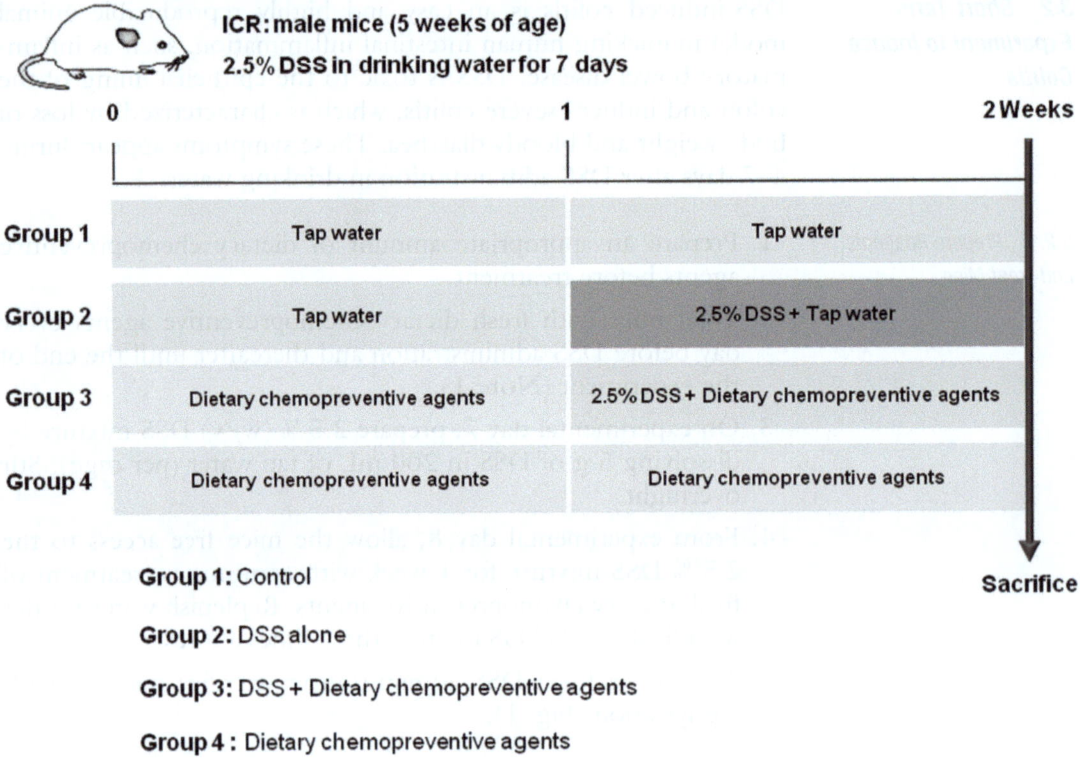

Fig. 1 A scheme for a short-term experiment to induce colitis. After 1 week of acclimation, animals are randomly distributed into control and experimental groups. The animals are treated with 2.5 % DSS (molecular weight of 36,000–50,000) in drinking water for 7 days. To determine the protective effect of dietary factors on DSS-induced colitis, candidate phytochemicals are usually administered to mice before and during DSS administration (total of 2 weeks). After DSS administration for 7 days, all animals are harvested to examine the histological and molecular changes in colon

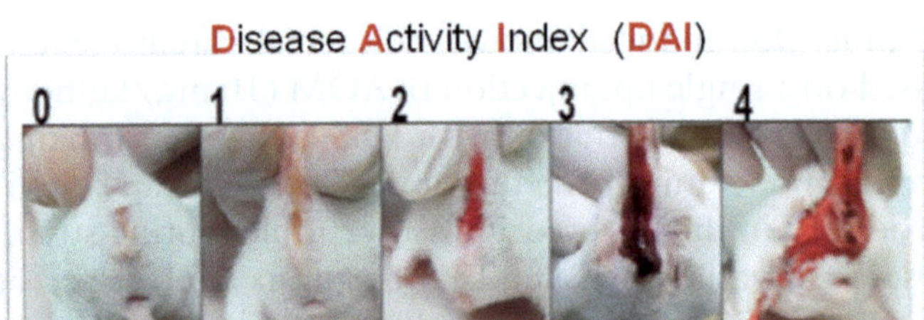

DAI score	Stool consistency	Rectal bleeding
0	Normal stool	Negative
1	Loose stool	Negative
2	Loose stool	Positive
3	Diarrhea	Positive
4	Diarrhea	Gross bleeding

Fig. 2 The disease activity Index (DAI) scoring. Based on the severity of rectal bleeding and stool consistency, fecal blood and diarrhea are scored from 0 to 4, respectively. The sum is given in a form of the disease activity index

4. On experimental day 7, prepare 2.5 % (w/v) DSS mixture by dissolving 5 g of DSS in 200 mL of tap water (per cage). Stir overnight.
5. From experimental day 8, allow the mice free access to the 2.5 % DSS mixture for 1 week with continuous treatment of

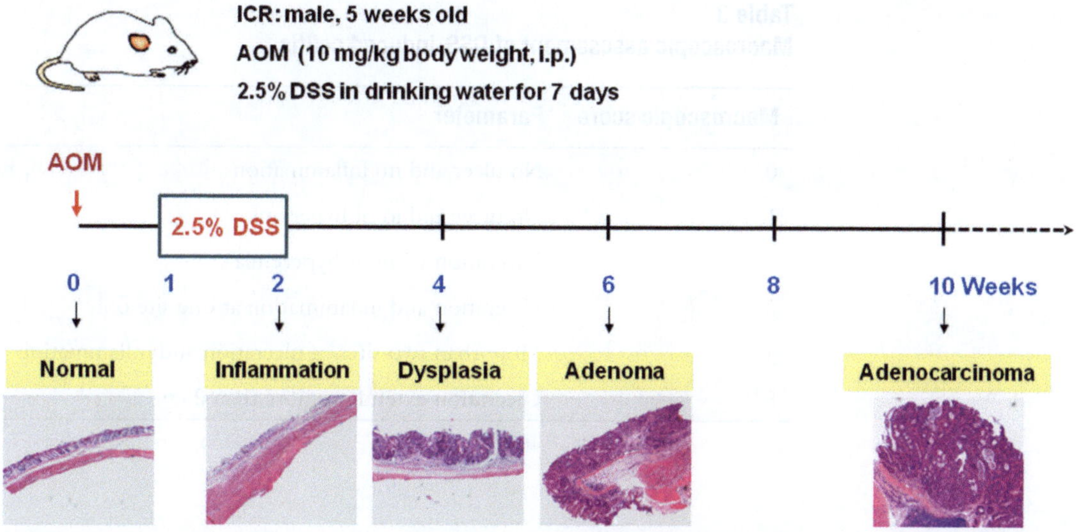

Fig. 3 Time-course observation of AOM plus DSS-induced colorectal cancer development

fresh dietary chemopreventive agents. Replenish water bottles with fresh 2.5 % DSS mixture three times a week.

6. At the time of harvest, sacrifice mice by CO_2 asphyxiation.

3.4 Preparation of the Colon for Macroscopic Examination

Mice are subjected to a gross examination at the time of euthanasia by CO_2 asphyxiation. The entire colon is excised, cut longitudinally and washed with PBS to remove feces. After macroscopic analysis, each specimen is divided into three pieces; one is fixed in 10 % buffered formalin for hematoxylin and eosin (H & E) staining and immunohistochemistry, and the remaining two pieces are flash frozen in lipid nitrogen and kept at −70 °C for Western blot analysis and electrophoretic mobility gel-shift assay (EMSA).

1. Sacrifice mice by CO_2 asphyxiation.
2. Fix the feet of the mouse with thumbtacks on the plate to ensure a stable position of the animal during the operation.
3. Apply 70 % ethanol on the abdomen to wet the fur.
4. Open the abdomen using surgical scissors.
5. Find the colon, hold carefully the middle part of the colon using forceps and cut the pelvic bones.
6. Carefully excise the entire colon from the anus to below the cecum using scissors.
7. Place the colon on a piece of 3MM Whatman paper (Whatman, Maidstone, UK) and measure its length (**Note 2**).
8. Cut the colon longitudinally along the main axis to open it and remove feces gently using forceps.

Table 3
Macroscopic assessment of DSS-induced colitis

Macroscopic score	Parameter
0	No ulcer and no inflammation
1	No ulcer and local hyperemia
2	Ulceration without hyperemia
3	Ulceration and inflammation at one site only
4	More than two sites of ulceration and inflammation
5	Ulceration extending more than 2 cm

9. After washing with PBS, spread the colon on a new piece of 3MM Whatman paper and remove fecal materials completely. Take care not to damage the tissue.
10. Repeat **step 9**.
11. After macroscopic examination (Table 3) and polyp counting, cut the distal section of the colon (0.5 cm from the anus) and transfer a piece of tissue to a micromesh cassette. Immerse the tissue cassette in 10 % buffered formalin (Sigma) and allow it to be fixed for at least 24 h at room temperature prior to paraffin embedding.
12. Divide another portion of the colon longitudinally into two pieces and transfer them into 1.7 mL tubes separately. Colon tissues are flash frozen in lipid nitrogen and kept at –70 °C for Western blot analysis and EMSA.

3.5 Hematoxylin and Eosin (H & E) Staining for Microscopic Examination

H & E staining is the most widely used staining method in medical diagnosis. It gives an overview of the structure of the tissue, enabling differentiation of the structures as normal, inflamed or degeneratively changed. Hematoxylin has a deep blue-purple color and stains the nucleus by binding to the negatively charged phosphate of nucleic acids. Eosin is pink and binds to proteins, thereby used for cytoplasmic staining in histology. Nuclei show varying cell-type- and cancer-type-specific patterns of condensation of heterochromatin (stained by hematoxylin) that are diagnostically very important [11].

3.5.1 Prepare the Paraffin-Embedded Tissue Sections

1. Embed specimens of the colon fixed with 10 % buffered formalin in paraffin according to standard protocols.
2. Section the paraffin-embedded tissues in a cross-sectional manner (4 μm).
3. Mount three sections on a glass slide.

3.5.2 De-Paraffinize and Hydrate the Tissue Section

1. Put the slides into a rack.
2. Dip the rack into a jar containing xylene (Sigma) to remove paraffin twice for 5 min each.
3. Put the rack in ethanol to remove xylene
   (a) 100 % ethanol for 5 min
   (b) 95 % ethanol for 5 min
   (c) 80 % ethanol for 5 min
   (d) 70 % ethanol for 5 min

3.5.3 Stain Nucleus with Hematoxylin

1. Put the rack into a jar containing filtered hematoxylin for 5 min (**Note 3**).
2. Rinse the slides with tap water to remove hematoxylin for 10 min.
3. For decolorization, dip the rack into a jar containing 0.25 % acid alcohol three times (each 1 s).
4. Rinse the slides with tap water for 5 min.
5. Dip the rack into a jar containing 1.36 % lithium carbonate three times (each 3 s).
6. Rinse the slides with tap water for 5 min.

3.5.4 Stain the Cytoplasm with Eosin and Dehydrate the Tissue Section

1. Put the rack into a jar containing eosin for 3 min.
2. Dip the rack into a jar containing 95 % ethanol twice for 3 min each.
3. Dip the rack into a jar containing 100 % ethanol twice for 3 min each.
4. Dip the rack into a jar containing xylene twice for 3 min each.
5. Mount two to three drops of mountant onto the slide, place a cover glass on the slide and dry the slide.

3.5.5 Microscopic Examination

1. Examine the H & E-stained tissue sections by light microscopy.
2. Evaluate the severity of inflammation and epithelial damage using a scoring system (Table 4) and diagnose tumors by a pathologist blinded to experimental manipulation (Table 5).

3.6 Immunohistochemical Analysis

Immunohistochemistry (IHC) makes detecting the expression and distribution of specific cellular components within cells and in the proper tissue context by the use of antibodies possible. In this regard, the prompt and adequate fixation of tissues is essential for preservation of tissue architecture and cell morphology. Most antigens reportedly can be successfully preserved in formalin-fixed paraffin-embedded tissue sections [12]. Endogenous peroxidase activity is frequently observed in tissues, and can be detected by reacting with DAB substrate. Therefore, eliminating endogenous peroxidase activity by treating tissue sections with hydrogen peroxide prior to primary antibody incubation is necessary.

Table 4
Microscopic score of inflammation and epithelial damage in DSS-induced colitis and AOM plus DSS-induced colorectal cancer models

Microscopic score	Parameter
0	Normal appearance with intact epithelial crypts in the mucosa
1	Loss or disruption of the basal 1/3 of the crypts with mild inflammation in the mucosa
2	Loss or disruption of the basal 2/3 of the crypts with moderate inflammation in the mucosa
3	Loss or disruption of entire crypts with severe inflammation in the mucosa and submucosa, but retaining of the surface epithelium
4	Presence of mucosal ulcer with severe inflammation (infiltration of neutrophils and lymphocytes) in the mucosa, submucosa, and/or lamina propria

Table 5
Microscopic assessment of tumors in the AOM plus DSS-induced colorectal cancer model

Diagnosis	Incidence	Score
Normal (with or without inflammation)		0
Adenoma (noninvasive neoplasms)	Focal Multiple foci	1 2
Adenoma (invasive into submucosa)	Focal Multiple foci	3 4
Adenocarcinoma (invasive into muscularis propria)	Focal Multiple foci	5 6
Adenocarcinoma (invasive through muscularis propria)	Focal Multiple foci	7 8

3.6.1 Quench the Peroxidase

1. Deparaffinize and hydrate the paraffin-embedded tissue sections (See Sects. 3.5.1 and 3.5.2).
2. Dip the rack into a jar containing 3 % H_2O_2 for 10 min.
3. Rinse the slides with tap water for 15 min.

3.6.2 Antigen Unmasking

1. Put the rack into the cooker containing boiled 10 mM sodium citrate buffer (pH 6.0).
2. Put a lid on the cooker and heat the cooker in the microwave for 10–15 min.
3. Cool the rack on the bench top for 30 min at room temperature.
4. Rinse the slides with tap water for 5 min.
5. Dip the rack into a jar containing PBS for 10 min

3.6.3 Staining (**Note 4**)

1. Put a wet tissue on the chamber with the lid.
2. Encircle the tissue sample with a PAP pen, put the slide on the wet tissue and add 100–400 μL of the blocking solution. Incubate for 30 min at room temperature.
3. Remove the blocking solution from the slide (not washing).
4. Add 100–400 μL of primary antibody (e.g., cyclooxygenase-2), diluted in TBST, to each section. Incubate overnight at 4 °C.
5. Remove the antibody solution and place the slides into a rack.
6. Dip the rack into a jar containing PBS twice for 5 min each.
7. Put the slides in the chamber again.
8. Add 100–400 μL of horseradish peroxidase (HRP)-conjugated secondary antibody, diluted in TBST, to the slide. Incubate 30 min at room temperature.
9. Repeat **steps 5–7**.
10. Add 100–400 μL of 1 % DAB to the slide. Incubate 5 min at room temperature.
11. Rinse the slides with tap water for 3 min.
12. If desired, counterstain the section using hematoxylin (see Sect. 3.5.3).
13. Dehydrate the section
    (a) Dip the rack into a jar containing 95 % ethanol twice for 3 min each.
    (b) Dip the rack into a jar containing 100 % ethanol twice for 3 min each.
    (c) Dip the rack into a jar containing xylene twice for 3 min each.
14. Mount two to three drops of mountant onto the slide, place a cover glass onto the slide and dry the slide.
15. Examine the IHC-stained tissue sections by light microscopy.

3.7 Immunoblot Analysis of Protein Expression

Immunoblot analysis is a method used to separate proteins in tissue homogenates by molecular weight and to detect target proteins using specific antibodies. The term "blotting" refers to the transfer of proteins from the gel to the membrane and their subsequent detection on the surface of the membrane. Three types of membranes are used for immunoblotting: nitrocellulose, nylon and polyvinylidene fluoride (PVDF). The first step in the immunoblotting procedure is to separate proteins using gel electrophoresis. After electrophoresis, the separated proteins are transferred or blotted onto the membrane, generally a PVDF membrane. Transfer can be conducted under wet or semidry conditions. Semidry transfer is faster, but wet transfer is better to transfer large proteins, >100 kDa [13]. Next, the membrane is blocked to prevent any nonspecific binding of antibodies to the surface of the membrane. Most commonly, the transferred protein is complexed with an enzyme-labeled antibody as a probe. The most sensitive detection methods use a chemiluminescent substrate that, when combined with the enzyme, produces light as a by-product. The light signals can be captured with X-ray film, CCD camera imaging devices, and phosphorimagers.

3.7.1 Tissue Lysis for Protein Extraction

1. Prepare 50 mL of 1× lysis buffer containing one tablet of protease inhibitor cocktail.
2. Transfer the snap-frozen colon tissues to 14 mL round-bottom tubes (SPL Life Sciences, Pocheon, Korea).
3. Add 1 mL of 1× lysis buffer to 14 mL round-bottom tubes.
4. Homogenize tissues on ice 30 times for 1 s each (**Note 5**).
5. Transfer homogenates into 1.7 mL tubes (Axygen, Union city, CA).
6. Incubate for 1 h with vortex in every 10 min on ice.
7. Centrifuge at 14,000 rpm for 15 min at 4 °C.
8. Remove supernatant fractions to new 1.7 mL tubes.
9. Store at –70 °C until analysis (**Note 5**).

3.7.2 Fractionation of Cytosolic and Nuclear Extracts

1. Transfer the snap-frozen colon tissues to 14 mL round-bottom tubes.
2. Add 1 mL hypotonic buffer A to 14 mL round-bottom tubes.
3. Homogenize tissues 20 times for 1 s each.
4. Transfer homogenates into 1.7 mL tubes.
5. Incubate for 1 h with vortex in every 10 min on ice.
6. Centrifugation at 14,000 rpm for 15 min at 4 °C.
7. Collect and store supernatant fractions (cytosolic extracts) at –70 °C until needed.
8. Wash precipitated pellets three times using 500 μL of the buffer A containing 0.1 % NP-40.
9. Centrifuge them at 14,000 rpm for 15 min and discard the supernatant fractions.
10. Resuspend the pellets in 100–150 μL buffer C with pipetting.
11. Incubate for 3 h with vortex in every 10 min on ice.
12. After centrifugation at 14,000 rpm for 15 min at 4 °C, collect and store supernatant fractions (nuclear extracts) at –70 °C until analysis (**Note 6**).

3.7.3 Immunoblot Analysis

1. Thaw samples to be assayed on ice.
2. Determine the protein concentration of samples using the BCA protein assay kit according to manufacturer's protocol.

3. Transfer 30–50 μg of lysates to 0.75 mL tubes.
4. Add 3 μL of 5× SDS gel-loading buffer and make up to a total volume of 15 μL with DDW.
5. Boil the samples at 99 °C for 5 min to denature the proteins.
6. Load samples into the bottom of the wells of the stacking gel.
7. Run the gel at 8 V/cm. After the dye reaches the resolving gel, increase the voltage to 15 V/cm and run the gel until the bromophenol blue reaches the bottom of the resolving gel.
8. Remove the glass plates from the gel.
9. Soak the PVDF membrane (Gelman Laboratory, Ann Arbor, MI) in methanol for 1 min.
10. Electrotransfer the proteins in the gel to PVDF membrane for 12 h at a constant current of 100 mA according to manufacturer's protocol (Bio-Rad) (**Note** 7).
11. Block the membrane with 5 % fat-free dry milk in TBST for 1 h at room temperature.
12. Incubate with the specific antibody for COX-2 (Cayman Chemical, Ann Arbor, MI), diluted 1:1,000 in 3 % fat-free dry milk in TBST, overnight at 4 °C on the shaker.
13. Wash the membranes with TBST at 10 min intervals for 30 min.
14. Incubate with 1:5,000 dilution of an HRP-conjugated anti-rabbit IgG antibody (Zymed Laboratories, San Francisco, CA) in 3 % fat-free dry milk in TBST for 2 h at room temperature.
15. Wash the membranes with TBST at 10 min intervals for 30 min.
16. Visualize the protein expression with an ECL detection kit and LAS-4000 image reader according to the manufacturer's instructions.

3.8 EMSA

An electrophoretic mobility shift assay (EMSA), also referred to as a gel shift assay, is a common affinity electrophoresis technique to detect protein–DNA interactions. The nucleic acid bound to protein has less mobility through a gel than the free unbound nucleic acid. Depending on the size and charge, protein–nucleic acid complexes are separated on the gel. The classical EMSA protocol has three major steps: (1) Manufacture and radiolabelling of the DNA probe; (2) Binding of nuclear extracts with radiolabelled DNA probes; and (3) Separation of the protein–DNA complexes from the free DNA probes. The control lane (the nucleic acid probe without proteins) will contain a single band corresponding to the free DNA probe. Also, to unambiguously identify the target protein–DNA complex, specific antibodies against target proteins can be added during the nucleic acid protein binding reaction (referred to as a supershift assay). Here, the method for checking DNA binding activity of NF-κB is described.

*3.8.1 Preparation of Radiolabelled DNA Probes (**Note 8**)*

1. Mix 3 μL of oligonucleotide containing the NF-κB binding domains (Promega), 2 μL of 5× T4 polynucleotide buffer (Promega), 1 μL of T4 kinase (10 unit/μL; Promega) and 11 μL of DDW.
2. Incubate for 10 min on ice.
3. Add 3 μL of ^{32}P-γATP (3,000 Ci/mmol at 10 mCi/mL) to the mixture.
4. Incubate for 15 min at 37 °C.
5. During the incubation period, prepare a Sephadex G-25 Column (GE healthcare). Spin the Sephadex G-25 Column at 7,500 rpm for 1 min to remove the buffer.
6. Load the probe mixture onto the resin in the Sephadex G-25 Column.
7. Collect purified probe by spinning the loaded column at 7,500 rpm for 2 min. Use 1.7 mL tubes to collect purified probe.
8. Check probe activity with scintillation counter and dilute the labeled probe to 100,000–400,000 cpm in TE buffer.

3.8.2 The Nucleic Acid Protein Binding Reaction

1. Transfer 8–12 μg of nuclear extracts to 1.7 mL tubes containing 1× incubation buffer and DDW. Add unlabeled probes to the competition tube. If conducting a supershift assay, add 1 μg of NF-κB p65 antibody to an additional tube containing nuclear extracts/1× incubation buffer/DDW mixture (**Note 9**).
2. Incubate for 15 min on ice.
3. Incubate for 30 min at room temperature.
4. Add 3 μL of diluted radiolabelled probe to tubes.
5. Incubate for 50 min at room temperature.
6. Add 2 μL of bromophenol blue dye to tubes.
7. Load samples onto the gel, and run gel at a constant 10 V/cm until the bromophenol blue is near the bottom of the gel (**Note 10**).
8. Remove the glass plates from the gel and overlay one side of the gel with a piece of 3MM Whatman paper. Peel the paper/gel from the glass plate and place it on a vacuum gel dryer. Place a cover or wrap on top of the gel.
9. Dry the gel for 90 min at 80 °C (**Note 11**).
10. Remove the dried gel from the vacuum dryer and place in an X-ray film cassette with three to four films (Agfa, Maharashtra, India).

11. Incubate at −80 °C to achieve the maximum signal (**Note 12**).
12. Develop the film.

4 Notes

1. Treat mice with dietary chemopreventive agents by diet or oral administration.
2. Measure the colon length from ileocecal junction to the anal verge.
3. Hematoxylin must be protected from light and filtered before use to remove oxidized particles.
4. The slide should not be dried.
5. Samples should not be heated.
6. To avoid repeated thawing and freezing samples, dividing the protein sample into several individual aliquots is recommended.
7. Ensure that no air bubbles have formed between the gel and the PVDF membrane.
8. To achieve high activity of labeled probes, labeling DNA probes with ^{32}P-γATP the day before the experiment is recommended.
9. For competition and supershift assays, use the nuclear extract that is expected to show the strongest DNA binding affinity.
10. To obtain results from EMSA at high resolution, the gel should be pre-run for at least 30 min prior to loading samples.
11. Over-drying of the gel will result in large cracks, whereas insufficient-drying will induce the appearance of blurry bands.
12. The incubation time may range from hours to days depending on the activity of radiolabelled probe.

References

1. Tanaka T, Kohno H, Suzuki R, Yamada Y, Sugie S, Mori H (2003) A novel inflammation-related mouse colon carcinogenesis model induced by azoxymethane and dextran sodium sulfate. Cancer Sci 94(11):965–973
2. Seril DN, Liao J, Yang GY, Yang CS (2003) Oxidative stress and ulcerative colitis-associated carcinogenesis: studies in humans and animal models. Carcinogenesis 24(3):353–362
3. Chen J, Huang XF (2009) The signal pathways in azoxymethane-induced colon cancer and preventive implications. Cancer Biol Ther 8(14):1313–1317
4. Domenech E (2006) Inflammatory bowel disease: current therapeutic options. Digestion 73(Suppl 1):67–76. doi:10.1159/000089781
5. Perse M, Cerar A (2012) Dextran sodium sulphate colitis mouse model: traps and tricks. J Biomed Biotechnol 2012:718617. doi:10.1155/2012/718617
6. Kitajima S, Takuma S, Morimoto M (2000) Histological analysis of murine colitis induced by dextran sulfate sodium of different molecular weights. Exp Anim 49(1):9–15
7. Tanaka T (2012) Development of an inflammation-associated colorectal cancer

model and its application for research on carcinogenesis and chemoprevention. Int J Inflam 2012:658786. doi:10.1155/2012/658786

8. Rosenberg DW, Giardina C, Tanaka T (2009) Mouse models for the study of colon carcinogenesis. Carcinogenesis 30(2):183–196. doi:10.1093/carcin/bgn267
9. Melgar S, Karlsson A, Michaelsson E (2005) Acute colitis induced by dextran sulfate sodium progresses to chronicity in C57BL/6 but not in BALB/c mice: correlation between symptoms and inflammation. Am J Physiol Gastrointest Liver Physiol 288(6):G1328–G1338. doi:10.1152/ajpgi.00467.2004
10. Yomogida S, Kojima Y, Tsutsumi-Ishii Y, Hua J, Sakamoto K, Nagaoka I (2008) Glucosamine, a naturally occurring amino monosaccharide, suppresses dextran sulfate sodium-induced colitis in rats. Int J Mol Med 22(3):317–323
11. Fischer AH, Jacobson KA, Rose J, Zeller R (2008) Hematoxylin and eosin staining of tissue and cell sections. CSH Protoc 2008: pdb prot4986. doi:10.1101/pdb.prot4986
12. Taylor CR, Levenson RM (2006) Quantification of immunohistochemistry—issues concerning methods, utility and semiquantitative assessment II. Histopathology 49(4):411–424. doi:10.1111/j.1365-2559.2006.02513.x
13. Sambrook J, Russell DW (2001) Molecular cloning: a laboratory manual, 3rd edn. Cold Spring Harbor Laboratory Press, Cold Spring Harbor, NY

Chapter 8

The Use of Seahorse Extracellular Flux Analyzer in Mechanistic Studies of Naturally Occurring Cancer Chemopreventive Agents

Michelle B. Moura, Eun-Ryeong Hahm, Bennett Van Houten, and Shivendra V. Singh

Abstract

Metabolic pathways and bioenergetics were described in great detail over half a century ago, and during the past decade a resurgence in integrating these cellular processes with other biological properties of the cell, including growth control, protein kinase cascade signaling, cell cycle division, and autophagy, has occurred. Because many chronic pathological conditions, including cancer, are associated with altered metabolism and production of energy, developing new approaches to measure these cellular parameters is important. Recent studies also indicate that many naturally occurring cancer chemopreventive agents, such as watercress constituent phenethyl isothiocyanate and *Withania somnifera* component withaferin A, alter mitochondrial bioenergetics to elicit death of cancer cells. This chapter summarizes a relatively new and exciting approach based on the Seahorse Extracellular Flux Analyzer, which takes real-time measurements of oxidative phosphorylation and glycolysis in living cells. These bioenergetic profiles are then compared with steady-state levels of cellular adenosine triphosphate as measured by a luciferase assay.

Key words Oxidative phosphorylation, Glycolysis, ATP, Chemoprevention, Bioenergetics profile

1 Introduction

Edible as well as medicinal plants continue to draw attention for identification of potential cancer chemopreventive agents. Bioactive phytochemicals with cancer chemopreventive activity have now been cataloged in numerous edible plants (e.g., isothiocyanates from cruciferous vegetables and organosulfides from garlic) as well as in alternative medicine constituents (e.g., ingredients of Ayurvedic medicine practiced in India) [1, 2]. A mechanistic model applicable to many structurally diverse cancer chemopreventive phytochemicals implicates altered mitochondrial bioenergetics in their cancer chemopreventive activity [3–5]. For example, the molecular circuitry of cancer cell apoptosis triggered by some of these phytochemicals [e.g., watercress constituent phenethyl

Ann M. Bode and Zigang Dong (eds.), *Cancer Prevention: Dietary Factors and Pharmacology*, Methods in Pharmacology and Toxicology, DOI 10.1007/978-1-4614-9227-6_8, © Springer Science+Business Media New York 2014

isothiocyanate (PEITC) and *Withania somnifera* component withaferin A (WA)] is characterized by inhibition of mitochondrial oxidative phosphorylation (OXPHOS) leading to production of reactive oxygen species and ensuing cell death (apoptotic and/or autophagic cell death) [3, 5]. Likewise, mammary cancer prevention by PEITC in a transgenic mouse model is accompanied by changes in expression of glycolysis-related proteins [4]. Development of a technique for real-time and simultaneous measurement of OXPHOS and glycolysis rates involving the Seahorse Extracellular Flux Analyzer has facilitated mechanistic studies of cancer chemopreventive agents exemplified by PEITC and WA [3, 5]. Renewed interest in the ability to measure cellular bioenergetics stems with the realization that changes in OXPHOS and glycolysis are associated with a large number of human conditions such as aging, cardiovascular diseases, and neurodegenerative diseases [6–9]. The newly emerged technology, the Seahorse Extracellular Flux Analyzer, developed by Seahorse *Bioscience*, allows for precise quantitation of oxygen consumption and pH changes in the media of living cells providing accurate assessments of OXPHOS and glycolysis, respectively [10]. After briefly describing the technology behind the Seahorse Extracellular Flux Analyzer, this chapter provides a step-by-step overview of how to use this instrument in conjunction with steady-state adenosine triphosphate (ATP) measurements to determine the bioenergetics of cells grown in culture.

1.1 Principle of the Assays

The Seahorse Extracellular Flux Analyzer is a novel instrument that is capable of measuring up to 20 wells of cells (XF24 format) or 92 wells (XF96 format) at a density of $4–10 \times 10^4$ cells per well in a 96-well format size. The instrument employs a disposable cartridge that contains dual fluorescent probes, which through excitation and emission of light, simultaneously measures oxygen and pH in a small sealed volume (~7 μL) over the cells in the well. OXPHOS consumes oxygen to produce water through a four-electron reduction at complex IV. The major source of proton production in the media of cells grown in culture is lactate generated by glycolysis. In addition to the fluorescent probe, each well of cells can be treated with four different conditions. Once the disposable cartridge is lowered down into the wells for a typical measurement period of 2–3 min, the instrument makes continuous measurements of oxygen concentrations and proton flux. These continuous measurements are converted into two rates: the rate of oxygen consumption (OCR) and the rate of proton production, or extracellular acidification rate (ECAR), which are indicative of OXPHOS and glycolysis, respectively. After making a measurement, the cartridge is lifted to allow mixing of the reserve media above the cells. After a period of waiting, the cartridge is again lowered and another series of rate measurements are made. Experiments providing a metabolic bioenergetic profile are performed by simultaneously measuring three to ten replicates of cell wells, for three to four rates under five different conditions: basal, and after addition of oligomycin, FCCP (carbonyl cyanide *p*-trifluoromethoxyphenylhydrazone), 2-deoxyglucose (2-DG), and rotenone as described below, in each of 20 wells of cells.

In a typical experiment, basal levels of OCR and ECAR are initially measured. The next measurement condition occurs during inhibition of ATP synthesis at complex V by oligomycin. This causes a buildup of protons across the inner matrix with subsequent loss of electron flow, a decrease in oxygen consumption, and an ensuing rise in proton production due to the cell's sole dependence upon glycolysis for ATP. The addition of the uncoupling molecule, FCCP, causes the protons on the outside of the inner mitochondrial membrane to be carried across to the basic matrix, allowing the electron flow to proceed. In some cells, such as neurons, this causes a large increase in oxygen consumption, which David G. Nicholls has called "spare respiration capacity" [11, 12]. The third injection of 2-DG inhibits glucose uptake into glycolysis and the tricarboxylic acid (TCA) cycle. In some cells, this is accompanied by an even further increase in oxygen consumption and loss of proton production due to inhibition of glycolysis. The fourth and final injection of rotenone, a complex I inhibitor, causes cessation of both electron flow and oxygen consumption.

In a separate experiment, steady-state ATP is measured by quantifying the amount of light produced by an ATP-dependent luciferase in a luminometer. Together, these two experimental methods give a clear indication of how the cell is generating ATP. These measurements can be made within about 3 h and allow fairly rapid throughput.

1.2 Advantages and Disadvantages of the Assays

The Seahorse technology offers several advantages, including a convenient microtiter plate format, the ability to use a relatively low number of intact cells, and the ability to make real-time measurements of both glycolysis and OXPHOS after injection of up to four different metabolic inhibitors or agonists. Another advantage of the microplate format is the possibility of running many biological replicates in the same plate, as well as to compare controls with different treatments.

The Seahorse Extracellular Flux Analyzer also allows the user to observe the immediate effect of up to four compounds (e.g., inhibitors, uncouplers, and agonists) in different orders on both OXPHOS and glycolysis in the same experiment. Cells can also be pretreated with inhibitors and the effect on basal OXPHOS and glycolysis can be measured.

Another nice feature of the Seahorse Extracellular Flux Analyzer is its ease of operation. Users just need to set up the protocol and place the calibration and experimental plate in the machine. All the measurements, injection of compounds and mixing of the samples are fully automated.

One particularly nice feature is the ability to measure cellular bioenergetics in non-adherent cells. Using products such as BD Cell-Tak Cell and Tissue Adhesive (BD Biosciences, San Jose, CA) or poly-D-lysine (Sigma-Aldrich, St. Louis, MO) it is possible to attach non-adherent cells, isolated mitochondria, or parasites to the plate [13].

Finally, the results are monitored in real-time and the data can be used directly from the machine with the Seahorse software, which allows for immediate analysis of the observed rates. The software is very flexible in allowing the investigator to look at graph and/or data in different ways and also can combine results, and optimize data output for several applications. The main disadvantage of this technology is that the instrument is designed to only work at 37 °C and at ambient levels of oxygen. However, some laboratories have overcome this problem by placing the entire instrument inside an environmental chamber.

The major advantages of the ATP luciferase assay are the simplicity, high sensitivity and linearity of the protocol, and the lack of cell harvesting or separation steps. In addition, the ATPLite lysis buffer is able to irreversibly inactivate the endogenous ATPases, overcoming the problem presented by other kits.

2 Materials

2.1 Equipment

1. Seahorse XF24 Extracellular Flux Analyzer (Seahorse *Bioscience*, North Billerica, MA).
2. Two types of incubators: a CO_2 incubator is necessary for growing cells in an atmosphere of 5–10 % CO_2 and a non-CO_2 incubator is necessary for pH and temperature stabilization.
3. CASY cell counter (Roche Diagnostics, Indianapolis, IN).
4. Innova 2000 platform shaker (New Brunswick Scientific, Enfiled, CT).
5. Synergy 2 plate reader (BioTek, Winooski, VT).
6. Except for the Seahorse XF24 Extracellular Flux Analyzer, other piece of equipment can be replaced with a comparable capability instrument.

2.2 Reagents and Solutions

1. XF24 FluxPak (Seahorse *Bioscience*, 100850-001). The kit includes XF24 V7 cell culture microplates, calibration plates, disposable sensor cartridges and XF calibrant necessary for 18 assays.
2. Dulbecco's Modified Eagle's Medium (DMEM) Base 8.3 g/L (Sigma-Aldrich, D5030) supplemented with 2 mM GlutaMax™-1 (Life Technologies, 35050-061), 1 mM sodium pyruvate (Sigma-Aldrich, S8636), 25 mM glucose (Sigma-Aldrich, G8270), 32 mM sodium chloride (Sigma-Aldrich,

S3014), and 15 mg phenol red (Sigma-Aldrich, P5530) was used for the XF assay. Unbuffered media is necessary for measuring fluctuations in pH during glycolysis.

3. Oligomycin (Sigma-Aldrich, O4876). 50 mM solution: Diluted in 1 mL of dimethyl sulfoxide (DMSO) (Fisher Biotech, Wembley, WA, Australia). Store in 100 μL aliquots at −20 °C. Dilute the 50 mM stock to 1 mM with DMSO. Aliquots in use are kept at 4 °C.
4. FCCP (Sigma-Aldrich, C2920). Prepare a 30 mM stock: 10 mg FCCP diluted in 1.31 mL of DMSO. Store in 100 μL aliquots at −20 °C. Dilute the 30 mM stock to 300 μM with DMSO. Aliquots in use are kept at 4 °C.
5. 2-Deoxy-D-glucose (2-DG) (Sigma-Aldrich, D6134). The 2-DG solution is prepared fresh every time.
6. Rotenone (Sigma-Aldrich, R8875). A 50 mM stock solution: Diluted in 1 mL of DMSO. Store in 100 μL aliquots at −20 °C. Dilute the 50 mM stock to 1 mM with DMSO. Aliquots in use are kept at 4 °C.
7. ATPLite luminescence assay system kit (PerkinElmer, Waltham, MA, 6016941). The kit includes a mammalian cell lysis solution, substrate (Luciferase/Luciferin), substrate buffer solution and ATP standard. These reagents are stored at 4 °C. The diluted aliquots of the ATP standard are kept at −20 °C.
8. Culture Plate-96 Black (PerkinElmer, 6005660).

3 Methods

3.1 Bioenergetics Experiment

Day 1

3.1.1 Cell Culture

The success of the Seahorse XF assay is linked to good cell culture practices. We have observed high reproducibility and low variation between runs when a rigorous protocol of cell passaging (splitting and maintaining a specific cell density) is performed prior to the experiment. In addition, verifying that the cell lines to be used in these experiments are not contaminated with mycoplasma is imperative. Among other effects, mycoplasma contamination may induce changes in cell metabolism and cause increases in inhibitor efflux out of the cell, and thus can interfere with data interpretation. Further care needs to be placed on even cell seeding within the experimental plates.

1. *Cell density.* Because cells can differ in size, use of appropriate density is important to avoid a lower number or confluence of cells. In this way, before beginning metabolic experiments, we strongly recommend that a pilot run be used to determine the

optimum cell number. We suggest testing three or four different densities, varying from 2 to 10×10^4 cells per well. In our experiment with the MDA-MB-231 human breast cancer cell line, cells were seeded at a density of 4×10^4 cells per well [3].

2. *Cell seeding*. Starting from a non-confluent culture (80–90 % confluence), harvest cells by trypsinizing from flasks. Resuspend the cells in growth media to obtain a desired density and add 100 μL per well in the Seahorse XF24 plates. Keep the plate at 37 °C, 5–10 % CO_2 for 1–5 h allowing cells to adhere. Gently add 150 μL of growth media to each well (**Note 1**). Place the plate back in the CO_2 incubator at 37 °C, 5–10 % CO_2 until the following day. If using non-adherent cells, seeding cells on the day before the experiment is not necessary (see **Note 2**).

3.1.2 Cartridge Preparation

The Seahorse XF24 cartridge has two fluorophores for analyte detection at the end of each sensor sleeve, which need to be hydrated before the experiment. Remove the green lid of the cartridge and add 1 mL of Seahorse XF24 calibrating solution per well on a Seahorse XF24 cartridge plate. Put the green lid back on the plate and place the cartridge overnight at 37 °C on a non-CO_2 incubator (**Note 3**).

Day 2

3.1.3 Preparing the XF24 Cell Plate for the Seahorse XF24 Assay

1. Warm the unbuffered DMEM media to 37 °C.
2. Using an aspirator pipette, remove approximately 150 μL of the growth media (**Note 4**).
3. Wash cells (including the temperature correction wells A1, B4, C3, and D6) with 1 mL of unbuffered DMEM.
4. Remove all but ~50 μL of media from the wells (**Note 4**).
5. Add 675 μL of unbuffered DMEM to the wells and keep the plate at 37 °C in a non-CO_2 incubator for 1 h.

3.1.4 Preparing the Injection Compounds and Loading the Sensor Cartridge

While the cells are equilibrating in unbuffered media, start to prepare the injection compounds (**Note 5**).

1. Oligomycin. 10× solution (10 μM): Add 30 μL of 1 mM stock solution to 3 mL of unbuffered DMEM. Add 75 μL of this solution to port A of the calibrated cartridge. The final concentration inside the well will be 1 μM.
2. FCCP. 11× solution (3.3 μM): Add 33 μL of 300 μM stock solution into 3 mL of unbuffered DMEM. Add 75 μL of this solution to port B of the calibrated cartridge. The final concentration inside the well will be 0.3 μM (**Note 6**).
3. 2-DG. 1.2 M solution: 0.542 g of 2-DG diluted in 2.7 mL of unbuffered DMEM. Adjust the pH to 7.4 by adding 4–8 μL of 0.1 M NaOH. Add 75 μL of this solution to port C of the

calibrated cartridge. The final concentration inside the well will be 100 mM.

4. Rotenone. 13× solution (13 μM): Add 39 μL of 1 mM stock solution into 3 mL of unbuffered DMEM. Add 75 μL of this solution to port D of the calibrated cartridge. The final concentration inside the well will be 1 μM.

3.1.5 Calibrating the Sensors and Running the Experiment

Before starting the bioenergetics measurements, calibrating the sensor cartridge is necessary. Login to the XF24 software and set up an experimental template by using the "Assay Wizard" option. Carefully add information about media, cells, compounds and their concentrations. Save the template and be sure that the "Save Directory" and "Save Name" fields contain the proper information (**Note 7**).

Begin the calibration step by clicking on the "Start" button. When the loading door opens, place the sensor cartridge with the calibration plate on the tray. Be careful with the position of the cartridge (**Note 5**). Click the "Continue" button. The calibration step will take approximately 30 min. When the calibration is complete, replace the calibration plate with the experimental cell plate. The duration of the run can vary from experiment to experiment. The protocol commands used in our experiments are as follows:

calibrate probes→loop 4× (points 1–4)→mix for 3 min→time delay of 2 min→measure for 3 min→loop end→inject port A→loop 3× (points 5–7)→mix for 2 min→time delay of 2 min→measure for 4 min→loop end→inject port B→loop 3× (points 8–10)→mix for 4 min→time delay of 2 min→measure for 2 min→loop end→inject port C→loop 3× (points 11–13)→mix for 4 min→time delay of 2 min→measure for 2 min→loop end→inject port D→loop 3× (points 14–16)→mix for 2 min→time delay of 2 min→measure for 4 min→loop end→program end.

3.1.6 Normalization of Results by Cell Number

Cells are known to have different growth rates. Sometimes calculating the cell number before the bioenergetics experiment might be difficult especially when working with primary or stem cells. In order to mitigate this problem, we strongly suggest normalizing every run by cell number, protein concentration, or another method. In our laboratory for adherent cells, we measure the total number of cells in each well after the bioenergetics assay using a CASY cell counter, and then normalize data per cell number. For non-adherent cells, we measure the cell number directly before plating onto Cell-Tak.

3.1.7 Data Analysis

The data obtained from the bioenergetics experiment can be analyzed using the area under the curve (AUC) ANOVA tool available with the Seahorse software (**Note 8**). The software also allows for the combination and analyses of different runs when the plate

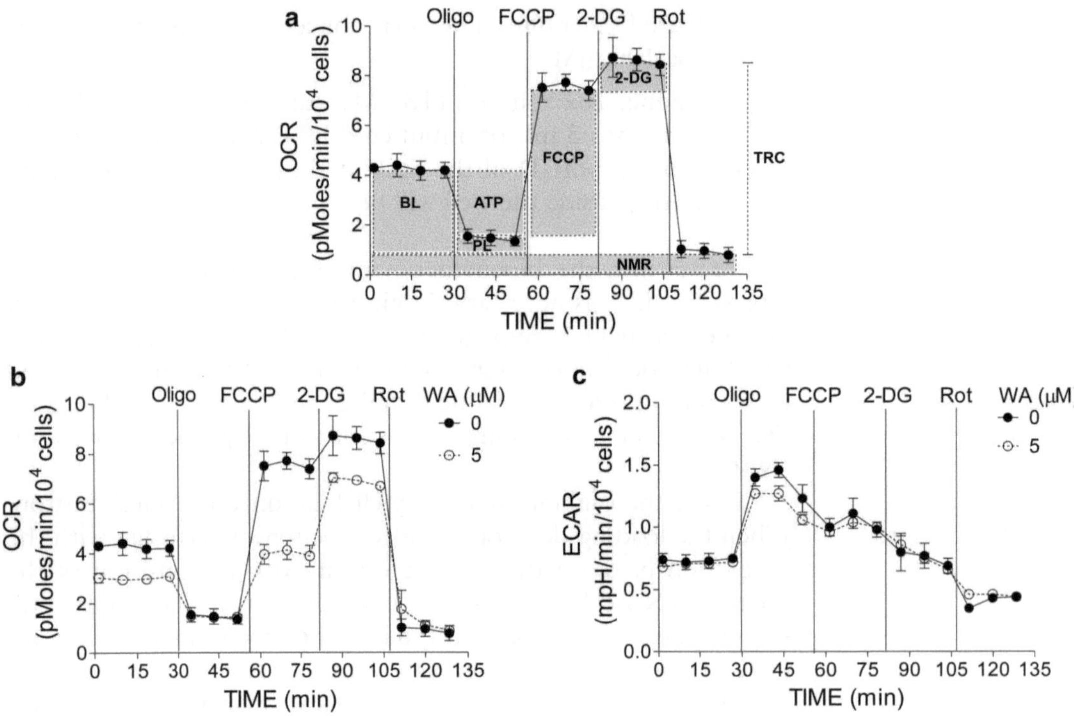

Fig. 1 (**a**) Detailed description of pharmacological profiling of oxygen consumption, indicative of OXPHOS. Oxygen consumption rate (OCR) was determined through real-time measurements using the Seahorse XF24 Extracellular Flux analyzer. The basal level (BL) is calculated by the difference between the mean of rates at points #1–4 and the mean of rates at points #14–16. The proton leak (PL) is calculated by the difference between the mean rates at points #5–7 and the mean of rates at points #14–16. The ATP-coupled (ATP) rate is calculated by the difference between the basal level and the proton leak. The FCCP-activated (FCCP) effect is calculated by the difference between the mean of rates at points #8–10 and the mean of rates at points #5–7. The 2-DG activated (2-DG) effect is calculated by the difference between the mean of rates at points #11–13 and the mean of rates at points #8–10. Total reserve capacity (TRC) obtains all these parameters. Non-mitochondrial respiration (NMR) is calculated by the mean of rates at points #14–16. (**b**) OCR profile elucidated through the use of metabolic inhibitors in MDA-MB-231 cells after 4 h treatment with DMSO and 5 μM withaferin A (WA). Oligomycin (1 μM), FCCP (300 nM), 2-DG (100 mM), and Rotenone (1 μM) were injected sequentially at the indicated time points after the basal level measurements. (**c**) ECAR profile elucidated through the use of metabolic inhibitors. Results are expressed as the mean of three different experiments ± S.E.M

templates are identical. A step-by-step analysis using the Seahorse software can be found in the Seahorse XF24 training course workbook. Another approach to data analysis is to extract the Seahorse data to a Microsoft Excel spreadsheet and analyze it manually. Six fundamental parameters can be calculated from the Seahorse output.

The OCR basal level is calculated by the difference between the mean of the four measurements, prior to injection A (oligomycin), and the mean rates 14–16, after injection D (rotenone) (Fig. 1). This basal OCR represents the normal amount of oxygen that is being consumed to maintain OXPHOS at a level to supply

ATP for the growing cells. For ECAR, the basal level is calculated by the mean of rates 1–4, prior to injection A.

The proton leak is calculated by the difference between the mean of rates points 5–7, prior to injection B (FCCP), and the mean of the rates 14–16, after injection D (Fig. 1).

The FCCP-activated rate is a measure of the maximum rate at which the electron transport chain can supply electrons to complex IV, and is calculated by the difference between the mean rates 8–10, prior to injection C (2-DG), and the mean rates 5–7 (Fig. 1). The 2-DG activated rate is an indication of the total respiration capacity that the cells can achieve and is calculated by the difference between the mean of rates 11–13, prior to injection D, and the mean rates 8–10 (Fig. 1). These parameters together represent the total reserve capacity (TRC).

The non-mitochondrial respiration represents the cellular process that consumes oxygen without ATP generation, and it can be calculated by the mean rates 14–16 (Fig. 1). An example of this phenomenon is the activity of the NADPH oxidase complex.

The oligomycin-induced ECAR represents the mean of rates at 5–7.

3.2 ATP Luciferase Assay

The steady-state ATP measurements can be finished in just 1 day. However, as for the bioenergetics experiments, a good cell culture practice is critical to obtain high reproducibility. We also strongly recommend running a pilot experiment to determine the optimum cell density, varying from 2 to 10×10^4 cells per well. Usually, the same cell density used for the Seahorse XF assay is ideal for the steady-state ATP measurements.

3.2.1 Preparing the Plate for the Steady-State ATP Measurements

1. *Seeding cells.* Starting from a non-confluent culture (80–90 % confluence), harvest cells by trypsinizing from flasks. Resuspend cells in unbuffered DMEM (same media used for the Seahorse XF24 assay) in appropriate volume, enough for 50 μL per well, to obtain the desired concentration of cell per well in the ATP plates. Plate cells in quadruplicate. In our experiment with the MDA-MB-231 human breast cancer cell line, cells were seeded at a density of 4×10^4 cells/well [5].
2. *Preparing the inhibitors.* The inhibitors must be 2× concentrated and diluted in appropriate volume of unbuffered DMEM, enough for 50 μL per well. Final concentrations inside the well: Oligomycin—1 μM; FCCP—0.3 μM; 2-DG—100 mM; and Rotenone—1 μM.
3. *Preparing the ATP standard.* Reconstitute a vial of lyophilized ATP (included in the kit) with 1,170 μL of water to obtain a 10 mM stock solution. From the stock solution, mix 10 μL with 990 μL of water to obtain a 100 μM solution. Vortex the microcentrifuge tube. Prepare a set of dilutions that most

Table 1
Preparation of ATP standards

Concentration (μM)	From stock solution (100 μM)	μL H_2O
1	1 μL	99 μL
2	2 μL	98 μL
4	4 μL	96 μL
8	8 μL	92 μL
16	16 μL	84 μL
32	32 μL	68 μL
64	64 μL	36 μL

closely corresponds to the expected concentration. Standard samples should be tested in triplicate and the results averaged. Use Table 1 to prepare a set of ATP standards to make a standard solution.

3.2.2 Assay Protocol for Measurement of Steady-State ATP

1. After seeding the cells, add the inhibitors and place the plate in an incubator (37 °C without CO_2 if using unbuffered DMEM) for 45 min.
2. Remove the ATPLite reagents from the refrigerator and allow them to equilibrate to room temperature (around 30 min).
3. After incubation, add 10 μL of the ATP standards to the appropriate wells. Add 10 μL of unbuffered DMEM to the blank wells.
4. Using a multichannel pipette, add 50 μL of mammalian cell lysis solution to 100 μL of cell suspension/inhibitors per well, including the standards and blanks, and shake the plate for 5 min in a platform shaker at 300 rpm.
5. Reconstitute one lyophilized substrate solution bottle by adding 5 mL of substrate buffer solution. Agitate gently until the solution is homogeneous.
6. Using a multichannel pipette, add 50 μL of reconstituted substrate solution to the wells, including the standards and blanks.
7. Wrap the plate in aluminum foil and shake it in a platform shaker at 270 rpm for 5 min.
8. Dark adapt the plate for 10 min and measure the luminescence.

3.2.3 Data Analysis

Analysis of data obtained by the luciferase ATP assay is performed using a Microsoft Excel spreadsheet. The luminescence readings of the replicates are averaged. The data presented as Fig. 2 are a combination of three different experiments and the error bars represent the standard error of the mean.

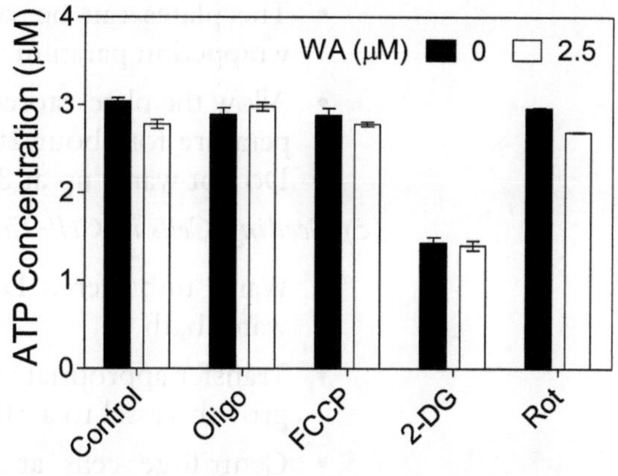

Fig. 2 ATP steady-state levels evaluated in the absence or presence of the oligomycin (1 μM), FCCP (300 nM), 2-DG (100 mM), and Rotenone (1 μM). MDA-MB-231 cells were treated for 4 h with DMSO or 2.5 μM withaferin A (WA). Steady-state level of ATP was measured using ATPLite Luminescence Assay kit. Results shown are mean of three different experiments ± S.E.M

4 Notes

1. Do not seed cells in temperature correction wells (A1, B4, C3, and D6). Gently tap the plate on all sides to assure even cell seeding. If cells are clumped in the middle or edge of the well, a large amount of variation is observed. Use a multichannel pipette to minimize sampling error.
2. Our protocol for coating XF24 plates with BD Cell-Tak Cells and Tissue Adhesive is as follows:

(a) *Reagents*

- BD Cell-Tak Cells and Tissue Adhesive (BD Biosciences, CN 354240)
- $NaHCO_3$ (Sigma-Aldrich, S5761)
- Tissue Culture (TC) Grade Sterile Water (Invitrogen-Life Technologies, CN 15230)

(b) *Preparation*

- Dissolve 420 mg $NaHCO_3$ in 50 mL of TC water and pH to 8.0 (should be very close) for 0.1 M solution. Filter-sterilize; use or store at 4 °C.
- For one XF24 plate, prepare 1.5 mL of Cell-Tak solution by adding 17 μL of Cell-Tak stock to 1.5 mL of 0.1 M $NaHCO_3$, mix, and pipette immediately onto XF24 plate, 50 μL/well.
- Allow to sit in hood about 20 min, then siphon off solution, add 200 μL of TC water and siphon off to wash off $NaHCO_3$, and let sit in hood for 20 min to dry with lids open.

- The plates can be saved for 1 week at 4 °C with rim wrapped in parafilm to avoid condensation.
- Allow the plates stored at 4 °C to warm up to room temperature for about 20 min in the hood before seeding. Do not warm up at 37 °C, Cell-Tak will lose activity.

(c) *Seeding Cells in Cell-Tak Coated Plates for XF Assay*

- Warm unbuffered DMEM (assay medium) in a 37 °C water bath.
- Transfer appropriate volume of cell suspension from the growth vessel to a 50 mL conical tube.
- Centrifuge cells at room temperature, 12,000 rpm, 5 min.
- While cells are being centrifuged, pipette 100 μL unbuffered DMEM into temperature control wells of a room-temperature Cell-Tak-coated XF24 tissue cultured plates.
- Remove supernatant fraction and gently flick the bottom of the tube with finger to loosen the pellet.
- Resuspend cells in 5 mL of warm unbuffered DMEM to make a cell suspension.
- Change centrifuge settings to settings used for seeding: set centrifuge to slow acceleration (4 on scale of 9 for Eppendorf 5810R) and zero braking.
- Transfer the cell suspension to a tissue culture reservoir.
- With a multipipettor, pipette 100 μL of cell suspension to the side of each well.
  - Centrifuge the cells down to the bottom of the well as follows.
  - Transfer plates to centrifuge plate carriers immediately after seeding.
  - Spin centrifuge up to 450 rpm (about 40 × *g*) and hit stop as soon as it reaches 450 rpm; let centrifuge spin slowly to a stop.
  - Reverse the orientation of the plates on the plate carriers (now column 1 should point out to the rim of the centrifuge).
- Spin centrifuge up to 650 rpm (about 80 × *g*) and stop.
- Transfer plates to a 37 °C incubator NOT supplemented with CO_2 and let sit for 25–30 min. Most of the cells should be stably adhered to the cultured surface in 25–30 min.
  - *NOTE: sensor cartridge calibration should be started at this time on the XF analyzer to streamline the assay process.*

- After 25–30 min incubation, slowly and gently add 500 μL of warm unbuffered DMEM to the top of each well along the side of the wall. Use manual P1000 pipette only and add medium carefully and gradually to avoid disturbing cells.
- Return the cell plates to incubator for 15–25 min.
- After 15–25 min, cell plates are ready for assay. Total time following centrifugation should be no greater than 1 h for best results.
- Place cell plate on XF Analyzer, and proceed following XF assay protocol.

3. Seahorse *Bioscience* recommends hydrating the sensor cartridge overnight. However, a minimum incubation time of 4 h is acceptable. A hydrated cartridge can be stored for up to 72 h at 37 °C. Wrap parafilm around the edges to prevent evaporation.
4. Be careful not to remove all media and do not touch the bottom of the wells.
5. Be aware of the orientation of the cartridge when loading compounds and when placing in the machine. If the cartridge is loaded in a backwards position, only the basal level can be measured. The sensor cartridge is loaded into the instrument with the bar code facing the back and the lot number facing the front. The temperature correction well should be loaded with media or injection compounds. Different compounds and combinations can be used for bioenergetics experiments depending on the assay type.
6. We strongly suggest optimizing the FCCP dose to be used in the bioenergetics experiments. In our laboratory for cancer cell lines, we have found that 300 nM is optimal, but this concentration can differ from cell line to cell line.
7. The template can be prepared in advance and saved. The protocol commands that have not yet been executed can be changed during the experiment. Be sure that the cartridge and the experimental plate are firmly attached to the bottom of the tray. If not, it can damage the Seahorse instrument.
8. A new XF^e Extracellular Flux Analyzers (XF^e96 and XF^e24 formats) is now available where the main difference from the old version is the simplified user-friendly software. In addition, the AUC ANOVA statistics package is not available on the new Seahorse machines.

5 Summary

The Seahorse Extracellular Flux Analyzer has been used by a number of researchers to measure cellular bioenergetics under a number of conditions. Many of these references are listed at the Seahorse

Bioscience web site under the XF resources button (http://www.seahorsebio.com). This technology should help make measurements of mitochondrial function and glycolysis more accessible to a larger group of investigators. Using the technology described herein, we were able to decipher inhibition of OXPHOS in apoptosis induction by PEITC and WA [3, 5]. This technology should be highly useful for mechanistic evaluations of other naturally occurring or synthetic anticancer agents. For example, cancer cell apoptosis by D,L-sulforaphane, which is a synthetic racemic analogue of broccoli constituent L-sulforaphane, garlic constituent diallyl trisulfide, garden cress constituent benzyl isothiocyanate, and oriental medicine component plumbagin is intimately linked to production of reactive oxygen species [14–17]; however, whether inhibition of mitochondrial OXPHOS is the primary driver for their pro-oxidant and pro-apoptotic effect is not yet clear.

Acknowledgement

The work cited from the authors' laboratories on the phytochemicals listed in this article was supported by United States Public Health Service grants CA101753, CA113363, CA115498, CA129347, and CA142604 awarded by the National Cancer Institute. The Seahorse instrument was partly funded by a grant from the National Cancer Institute at the National Institutes of Health (P30 CA047904).

References

1. Stan SD, Kar S, Stoner GD, Singh SV (2008) Bioactive food components and cancer risk reduction. J Cell Biochem 104(1):339–356. doi:10.1002/jcb.21623
2. Garodia P, Ichikawa H, Malani N, Sethi G, Aggarwal BB (2007) From ancient medicine to modern medicine: ayurvedic concepts of health and their role in inflammation and cancer. J Soc Integr Oncol 5(1):25–37
3. Hahm ER, Moura MB, Kelley EE, Van Houten B, Shiva S, Singh SV (2011) Withaferin A-induced apoptosis in human breast cancer cells is mediated by reactive oxygen species. PLoS One 6(8):e23354. doi:10.1371/journal.pone.0023354
4. Singh SV, Kim SH, Sehrawat A, Arlotti JA, Hahm ER, Sakao K, Beumer JH, Jankowitz RC, Chandra-Kuntal K, Lee J, Powolny AA, Dhir R (2012) Biomarkers of phenethyl isothiocyanate-mediated mammary cancer chemoprevention in a clinically relevant mouse model. J Natl Cancer Inst 104(16):1228–1239. doi:10.1093/jnci/djs321
5. Xiao D, Powolny AA, Moura MB, Kelley EE, Bommareddy A, Kim SH, Hahm ER, Normolle D, Van Houten B, Singh SV (2010) Phenethyl isothiocyanate inhibits oxidative phosphorylation to trigger reactive oxygen species-mediated death of human prostate cancer cells. J Biol Chem 285(34):26558–26569. doi:10.1074/jbc.M109.063255
6. Hill BG, Dranka BP, Zou L, Chatham JC, Darley-Usmar VM (2009) Importance of the bioenergetic reserve capacity in response to cardiomyocyte stress induced by 4-hydroxynonenal. Biochem J 424(1):99–107. doi:10.1042/BJ20090934
7. Perez J, Hill BG, Benavides GA, Dranka BP, Darley-Usmar VM (2010) Role of cellular bioenergetics in smooth muscle cell proliferation induced by platelet-derived growth factor. Biochem J 428(2):255–267. doi:10.1042/BJ20100090
8. Wu JJ, Quijano C, Chen E, Liu H, Cao L, Fergusson MM, Rovira II, Gutkind S, Daniels MP, Komatsu M, Finkel T (2009)

Mitochondrial dysfunction and oxidative stress mediate the physiological impairment induced by the disruption of autophagy. Aging (Albany NY) 1(4):425–437

9. Yao J, Irwin RW, Zhao L, Nilsen J, Hamilton RT, Brinton RD (2009) Mitochondrial bioenergetic deficit precedes Alzheimer's pathology in female mouse model of Alzheimer's disease. Proc Natl Acad Sci U S A 106(34):14670–14675. doi:10.1073/pnas.0903563106
10. Wu M, Neilson A, Swift AL, Moran R, Tamagnine J, Parslow D, Armistead S, Lemire K, Orrell J, Teich J, Chomicz S, Ferrick DA (2007) Multiparameter metabolic analysis reveals a close link between attenuated mitochondrial bioenergetic function and enhanced glycolysis dependency in human tumor cells. Am J Physiol Cell Physiol 292(1):C125–C136. doi:10.1152/ajpcell.00247.2006
11. Nicholls DG, Johnson-Cadwell L, Vesce S, Jekabsons M, Yadava N (2007) Bioenergetics of mitochondria in cultured neurons and their role in glutamate excitotoxicity. J Neurosci Res 85(15):3206–3212. doi:10.1002/jnr.21290
12. Yadava N, Nicholls DG (2007) Spare respiratory capacity rather than oxidative stress regulates glutamate excitotoxicity after partial respiratory inhibition of mitochondrial complex I with rotenone. J Neurosci 27(27):7310–7317. doi:10.1523/JNEUROSCI.0212-07.2007
13. Furtado C, Kunrath-Lima M, Rajao MA, Mendes IC, de Moura MB, Campos PC, Macedo AM, Franco GR, Pena SD, Teixeira SM, Van Houten B, Machado CR (2012) Functional characterization of 8-oxoguanine DNA glycosylase of *Trypanosoma cruzi*. PLoS One 7(8):e42484. doi:10.1371/journal.pone.0042484
14. Powolny AA, Singh SV (2008) Plumbagin-induced apoptosis in human prostate cancer cells is associated with modulation of cellular redox status and generation of reactive oxygen species. Pharm Res 25(9):2171–2180. doi:10.1007/s11095-008-9533-3
15. Singh SV, Srivastava SK, Choi S, Lew KL, Antosiewicz J, Xiao D, Zeng Y, Watkins SC, Johnson CS, Trump DL, Lee YJ, Xiao H, Herman-Antosiewicz A (2005) Sulforaphane-induced cell death in human prostate cancer cells is initiated by reactive oxygen species. J Biol Chem 280(20):19911–19924. doi:10.1074/jbc.M412443200
16. Xiao D, Choi S, Johnson DE, Vogel VG, Johnson CS, Trump DL, Lee YJ, Singh SV (2004) Diallyl trisulfide-induced apoptosis in human prostate cancer cells involves c-Jun N-terminal kinase and extracellular-signal regulated kinase-mediated phosphorylation of Bcl-2. Oncogene 23(33):5594–5606. doi:10.1038/sj.onc.1207747
17. Xiao D, Powolny AA, Singh SV (2008) Benzyl isothiocyanate targets mitochondrial respiratory chain to trigger reactive oxygen species-dependent apoptosis in human breast cancer cells. J Biol Chem 283(44):30151–30163. doi:10.1074/jbc.M802529200

Chapter 9

Utilizing RNA-Seq to Define Phytochemical-Induced Alterations in Insulin and IGF-Regulated Transcriptomes

Heather Beckwith and Douglas Yee

Abstract

Cancer at its root is a genetic disease brought on by genomic alterations that lead to uncontrolled cell division, metastasis, and enhanced cell survival. The study of genomics can address many of the genetic abnormalities associated with cancer and represents a rapidly progressing field. Our knowledge base regarding specific gene mutations and alterations leading to cancer and the development of subsequent gene-targeted therapies is being rapidly transformed by the application of new RNA and DNA sequencing technology, including a number of high-throughput sequencing methods. In contrast to older Sanger sequencing methods, next-generation high-throughput sequencing methods enable the sequencing of thousands to millions of molecules at once. Here we review how the specific high-throughput sequencing method, RNA sequencing (RNA seq), can be utilized to study the impact of phytochemicals on growth factors, such as insulin-like growth factor, that have been shown to play a primary role in both cancer development and progression. RNA seq is a method of high-throughput sequencing of cDNA in order to gain information about a sample's RNA content. In addition to determining an RNA sequence of a specific sample, RNA-seq provides information regarding an organism's transcriptome, including information regarding abundances of transcripts, mutations, fusion transcripts, noncoding RNA, transcriptional modification, gene regulation, and protein information.

Key words RNA-seq, High-throughput, IGF, Phytochemical, Cancer

1 Introduction

Researchers and cancer advocates have long been interested in the study of natural compounds that have anticancer properties. Specifically, the effect of various phytochemicals on growth factor stimulation of cancer has been of particular interest. The insulin-like growth factors (IGFs) are proteins with high sequence similarity to insulin. Elevated IGF and insulin levels have long been associated with a number of pathological states including cancer. Growth hormone secretion from the pituitary gland stimulates release of IGF-1 from the liver. IGF-II is a related molecule produced by many tissues and is not dependent on growth hormone action. IGFs bind the insulin-like growth factor tyrosine kinase receptor

Ann M. Bode and Zigang Dong (eds.), *Cancer Prevention: Dietary Factors and Pharmacology*, Methods in Pharmacology and Toxicology, DOI 10.1007/978-1-4614-9227-6_9, © Springer Science+Business Media New York 2014

(IGF-1R) to trigger downstream cascades of signaling. IGF signaling through the IGF receptor is a well-established key regulator of tumor cell growth, proliferation, survival, and metastasis.

The effect of various lifestyle factors on the IGF pathway has been studied in recent years. Observational human studies have reported increased cancer mortality in those with obesity and type 2 diabetes, which may be attributed to elevated levels of IGF, hyperinsulinemia, or both [1, 2]. The Women's Intervention Nutrition Study tested the hypothesis that dietary fat reduction would increase the relapse-free survival rate of breast cancer. The study found that low-fat dietary interventions could influence body weight and decrease breast cancer recurrence. After 5-year follow-up, relapse-free survival was 24 % higher in the low-fat diet group. In subgroup analysis the effect was found to be greatest in estrogen receptor-negative cancer, suggesting that pathways other than estrogen receptor signaling, such as IGF or insulin signaling, are important [3]. Multiple studies have identified diabetes and its associated insulin resistance as a risk factor for breast cancer. Both preclinical and clinical data suggest that insulin resistance activates a cascade that promotes cell proliferation and inhibits programmed cell death. The risk of breast cancer in women with type II diabetes is increased by 27 %, a figure that decreases to 16 % after adjustment for body mass index (BMI) [4]. Diet and physical activity can reverse insulin resistance and potentially insulin's tumorigenic effect.

In addition to the influence of lifestyle factors such as obesity, exercise, and diabetes on IGF signaling, a number of phytochemicals have been identified that interact with the IGF pathway and have therefore been studied in regard to both cancer treatment and prevention. Green tea catechins have been studied extensively as chemopreventive agents against cancer. Epigallocatechin-3-gallate (EGCG), the major catechin in green tea, appears to inhibit proliferation and apoptosis in cancer cells [5]. EGCG is thought to inhibit carcinogenesis by a number of mechanisms. One such mechanism is inhibition of a number of receptor tyrosine kinases including the IGF-1R. Its inhibition of the IGF-1R has been demonstrated in a number of cell lines including colorectal, hepatocellular, and breast cancer cell lines [6, 7]. In these studies, EGCG causes a decrease in expression levels of IGF. In addition, through activation of AP-1 and NF-κB, EGCG modulates the expression of target genes, which are associated with apoptosis and cell cycle arrest in cancer cells [8].

The effect of ginseng on the IGF signaling pathway has also been studied. Ginseng is traditionally used in parts of the world for treatment of a number of diseases including cancer. Treatment of breast cancer cell lines with ginsenoside Rp1, a component of ginseng, inhibits breast cancer cell proliferation and breast cancer cell colony formation. Ginsenoside Rp1 decreases the stability of the IGF-1R protein and is thought to account for its inhibition of cancer [9].

Another phytochemical that has been demonstrated to have an inhibitory effect on the IGF-1R signaling pathway is silibinin, also known as silybin. Silibinin is a polyphenolic flavonoid from the milk thistle plant. Silibinin has been shown to have anticancer activity against numerous in vitro cancer cell lines including prostate and breast carcinoma. Silibinin-treated cells have been shown to down-regulate proteins involved in proliferation and up-regulate a number of proteins involved in apoptosis. In prostate cancer PC-3 cells, treatment with silibinin resulted in increased insulin-like growth factor-binding protein-3 (IGFBP3) levels [10]. IGFBP3 binds IGFs and inhibits their interaction with cell surface receptors. In addition, silibinin treatment of these cells also demonstrated reduced phosphorylation of insulin receptor substrate-1, a protein immediately downstream of the IGF-1R [10]. Silibinin treatment of MCF-7 breast cancer cells has been shown to induce apoptosis. When treatment with an inhibitor of the IGF-1R was combined with silibinin, the pro-apoptotic effect was enhanced and synergistic inhibition of growth was demonstrated [11].

Certain phytochemicals have been shown to induce IGF activity and are therefore thought to enhance carcinogenesis. One such phytochemical is the phytoestrogen, soy. A study examining whether diet modification with a soy supplement affected circulating levels of IGF-1 in postmenopausal women at high risk for developing breast cancer found that a soy-rich diet was associated with increased concentrations of both IGF-1 and IGF-binding protein [12]. Soy has also been shown in mouse xenograft models to stimulate MCF-7 human breast tumor growth. After only 2 weeks of a high-soy-protein-isolate diet, tumors had higher IGF-1R and cyclin D1. Interestingly, tumor growth and proliferation after prolonged exposure to soy protein isolate could be attenuated with a diet high in flax seed, suggesting that flax seed may have a tumor inhibitory effect [13]. Furthermore, dietary flaxseed enhanced the effectiveness of tamoxifen (a medication used in the treatment of estrogen receptor-positive breast cancer) in athymic mice with low estrogen levels [14]. Another phytoestrogen, formononetin, one of the main components of red clover plants, has also been found to have an effect on IGF signaling. In vitro and in vivo studies have demonstrated that formononetin causes cell cycle arrest in breast cancer cells both by inactivating the IGF-1/IGF-1R-PI3-K/Akt pathways and decreasing cyclin D1 mRNA and protein expression [15].

In order to study the potential impact of phytochemicals on cancer prevention and treatment, the changes that phytochemicals induce in the gene expression and genetic character of cancer must be examined. Cancer at its root is a genetic disease. Cancer has been known for decades to be caused by a series of mutations occurring in normal cell division. Each mutation drives a wave of cellular multiplication associated with gradual increases in tumor size, disorientation, and malignancy [16]. Therefore, to best characterize the multiple factors that account for the malignant

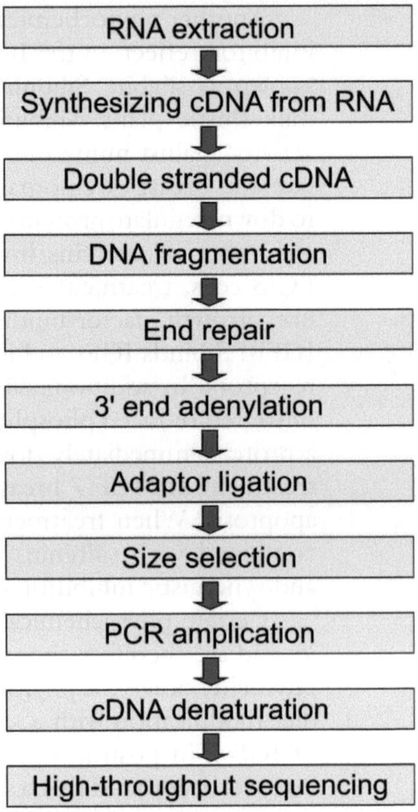

Fig. 1 Standard stepwise protocol for RNA seq

phenotype, a detailed analysis of the genetic abnormalities associated with cancer cells is necessary.

This chapter describes a specific laboratory technique, RNA sequencing (RNA seq), which sequences DNA molecules reverse transcribed from RNAs (Fig. 1). Sequenced reads are then mapped to the reference genome or transcriptome. The mapping locations reflect where the RNAs are transcribed, and the abundances of cDNAs reflect abundances of their corresponding transcripts in cells [17]. Mutations and fusion transcripts can also be detected by this technique.

2 Materials

2.1 Equipment

Equipment required is standard equipment found in most laboratories:

1. Heat block
2. Thermal cycler

3. Spectrophotometer
4. Microcentrifuge

2.2 Plastics

1. 10 cm^2 culture dishes
2. 1.5 mL Eppendorf tubes
3. PCR tubes
4. Collection tubes
5. Collection tubes with spin columns

2.3 Reagents and Solutions

Most of the reagents required are available in kits from commercial sources:

1. Cultured cells
2. Tripure reagent (Roche, USA)
3. Isopropanol
4. 75 % ethanol
5. Diethylpyrocarbonate-treated RNase-free water
6. First Strand cDNA synthesis kit (ThermoScientific, USA):

   M-MuLV reverse transcriptase

   RiboLock RNase inhibitor

   5× Reaction buffer

   dNTP mix, 10 mM each

   Oligo (dT)18 primer

   Random hexamer primer

   Control *GAPDH* RNA

   Forward *GAPDH* primer, 10 μM (5′-CAAGGTCATCCATGACAACTTTG-3′)

   Reverse *GAPDH* primer, 10 μM (5′-GTCCACCACCCTGTTGCTGTAG-3′)

   Water, nuclease free
7. 5× second-strand buffer (Invitrogen, Grand Island, NY)
8. 10 U/μL *E. coli* DNA ligase (Invitrogen)
9. 10 U/μL *E. coli* DNA polymerase I (Invitrogen)
10. 2 U/μL *E. coli* RNase H (Invitrogen)
11. 5 U/μL T4 DNA polymerase (Promega, Madison, WI)
12. QIAquick PCR Purification Kit (Qiagen, Valencia, CA):

    QIAquick spin columns

    Buffer PB

    Buffer PE (concentrate)

    Buffer EB

pH indicator I

Collection tubes (2 mL)

Loading dye

13. DNase I buffer (New England Biolabs, Ipswich, MA)
14. DNase I enzyme (New England Biolabs)
15. End-It DNA End-Repair Kit (Epicentre Biotechnologies, Madison, WI):

    10× end-repair buffer (1× final)

    2.5 mM dNTP mix (0.25 mM final)

    10 mM ATP (1 mM final)

    End-repair enzyme mix
16. Klenow buffer (NEB buffer 2; New England Biolabs)
17. Klenow fragment (3′–5′ exo-; New England Biolabs)
18. 1 mM dATP (prepare from 100 mM dATP; New England Biolabs; store in 25 μL single-use aliquots at −20 °C)
19. QIAquick MinElute PCR Purification Kit including Buffer EB (Qiagen):

    MinElute spin columns

    Buffer PB

    Buffer PE (concentrate)

    Buffer EB

    pH indicator

    Collection tubes (2 mL)

    Loading dye
20. T4 DNA ligase buffer (Promega)
21. 2× Phusion High Fidelity Master Mix (Finnzymes, Cat. No. F-531)
22. 1.5–2 % agarose gel in Tris–acetate–EDTA (TAE) buffer
23. Qiagen gel extraction kit including buffer EB:

    QIAquick spin columns

    Buffer QG

    Buffer PE (concentrate)

    Buffer EB

    Collection tubes (2 mL)

    Loading dye
24. MicroPoly(A)Purist Kit (Invitrogen):

    Lysis solution

Lysate wash
Dilution solution
2× Binding solution
Wash solution 1
Wash solution 2
THE RNA storage solution
Olido(dT) cellulose
5 M ammonium acetate
Glycogen (5 mg/mL)
25. 100 % ethanol

3 Methods

3.1 Cell Culture

A variety of cell lines can be utilized for cancer research. Some examples of common cell lines include A549 cells for the study of non-small-cell lung cancer, THP-1 cells for the study of acute myeloid leukemia, and FM3 cells for the study of melanoma. Cancer cell lines are grown in a cell incubator with conditions ideal for growth (e.g., typically 37 °C, 5 % CO_2). Cells are maintained in sterile flasks containing growth media specific to the cell line utilized. In breast cancer research, the most common cell line utilized is the MCF-7 cell line. The MCF-7 cell line was derived in 1970 from a patient with metastatic breast cancer [18]. MCF-7 breast cancer cells are maintained in Eagle's minimum essential medium supplemented with 0.01 mg/mL insulin and 10 % fetal bovine serum. Cells should be passaged every 4–5 days to maintain culture stability and avoid overgrowth. Cells are passaged by washing with phosphate-buffered saline, trypsinization, centrifugation, resuspension in fresh media, and transfer of a portion of the resuspension to a new flask containing fresh media.

To plate cells for experiments, cells can be counted utilizing a hemacytometer. Aspirate media from cell culture. Wash cells with phosphate-buffered saline, trypsinize cells, centrifuge the cells, aspirate media, and re-suspend the cells in fresh media. Add 10 μL of the cell suspension to a hemacytometer for counting. Calculate the volume of cells needed to plate at approximately $1–3 \times 10^6$ cells (depending on the cell line) per 10 cm^2 plate.

3.2 Cell Treatments

Once cells have reached approximately 70 % confluency, they are ready for serum starvation. Cells must be starved prior to use in order to synchronize cells in a quiescent (G0 state) growth state. To starve cells, aspirate culture media, wash the cells twice with phosphate-buffered saline, and replace the media with serum-free media and incubate under normal culture conditions for 24–48 h [19].

Cells are now ready for treatment and can be treated with any number of treatments. For example, to study the effect of insulin and IGF-1 on MCF-7 cells, cells are stimulated with 5 nM insulin and 5 nM IGF-1, respectively [20]. Cells should be treated in serum-free media for a minimum of 4 h for RNA/transcriptome analysis.

3.3 Preparation of RNA for RNA seq

RNA seq involves the direct sequencing of complementary DNAs (cDNAs) using high-throughput DNA sequencing technologies that are followed by mapping of the sequencing reads to the genome. The cDNA is made from polyadenylated RNA, then fragmented by DNase I, and ligated to adapters. The adapter-ligated cDNA fragments are then amplified and sequenced in a high-throughput manner to obtain short sequence reads (Fig. 1) [21].

3.4 Extracting RNA

The following protocol is taken directly from the Roche TriPure Isolation Reagent protocol (version June 2008, www.roche-applied-science.com).

1. Aspirate media from cells.
2. At room temperature add 1 mL of TriPure Isolation Reagent for each 10-cm^2 area covered by cells (**Note 1**).
3. Pass the cell lysate through a pipette several times. Transfer the cell lysate to a polypropylene centrifuge tube. Let lysate and tripure solution sit for 5 min at 15–25 °C to ensure complete dissociation of nucleoprotein complexes.
4. To each sample, add 0.2 mL chloroform for each 1 mL TriPure Isolation Reagent required in the initial homogenization. Cap tube securely and shake vigorously for 15 s. Incubate tube at 15–25 °C for 2–15 min.
5. To separate the solution into three phases (RNA, DNA, protein), centrifuge the tube at 12,000 × *g* for 15 min at 2–8 °C. RNA will be isolated from the upper aqueous phase.
6. Transfer the colorless upper aqueous phase obtained to a new polypropylene tube. Add isopropanol to the aqueous phase. Use 0.5 mL isopropanol for each 1 mL TriPure Isolation Reagent required in the initial homogenization procedure. Cap the tube, and then invert it several times to mix it thoroughly. Incubate at 15–25 °C for 5–10 min to allow the RNA precipitate to form.
7. Centrifuge the sample at 12,000 × *g* for 10 min at 2–8 °C. Discard the supernatant fraction.
8. Add at least 1 mL of 75 % ethanol to each centrifuge tube for each 1 mL TriPure Isolation Reagent required in the initial homogenization procedure. Wash the RNA pellet in the ethanol by vortexing.

9. Centrifuge the samples at 7,500 × *g* for 5 min at 2–8 °C. Discard the supernatant fraction.
10. Remove the excess ethanol from the RNA pellet by air-drying. Resuspend the RNA pellet in diethylpyrocarbonate (DEPC)-treated RNase-free water.
11. Dissolve the RNA pellet by passing the solution through a pipette tip several times and then incubating the solution for 10–15 min at 55–60 °C.
12. Measure the RNA concentration by spectrophotometry with DEPC water as a reference (**Note 2**).
13. RNase, an enzyme known to degrade RNA, is commonly found in the laboratory environment. In order to ensure the purity and integrity of the RNA being used, the laboratory environment and materials must be free of RNases (**Note 3**).

3.5 Preparation of Poly(A) + RNA

Total RNA is composed of messenger RNA (mRNA), ribosomal RNA (rRNA), and transfer RNA (tRNA). Messenger RNA in eukaryotes is marked by polyadenylation at the 3′ end. In order to separate the mRNA, the RNA that is being transcribed, polyadenylated RNA must be separated out from the total RNA. The following protocol is directly from the Invitrogen MicroPoly(A) Purist Kit protocol (Part Number AM1919, 2008, www.invitrogen.com). A number of other commercially available kits for separation of polyadenylated RNA from total RNA are also available.

1. Preparation of total RNA
   (a) Add the following to the RNA previously collected.
   - 0.1 volume 5 M ammonium acetate or 3 M sodium acetate.
   - 1 μL glycogen (**Note 4**).
   - 2.5 volumes 100 % ethanol.
   - Mix thoroughly by vortexing.

   (b) Precipitate at −20 °C overnight, or quick freeze the solution in ethanol and dry ice or place in a −70 °C freezer for 30 min.

   (c) Recover the RNA by centrifugation at 12,000 × *g* for 20–30 min at 4 °C.

   (d) Carefully remove and discard the supernatant fraction (**Note 5**).

   (e) Centrifuge the tube briefly a second time, and aspirate away any additional fluid that collects with a fine-tipped pipette.

(f) Add 1 mL 70 % ethanol, and vortex the tube a few times. Re-pellet the RNA by centrifuging for 10 min at 4 °C. Carefully remove the supernatant fraction.

(g) Re-suspend 2–400 μg RNA in 250 μL of nuclease-free water. Vortex vigorously to completely re-suspend the pellet.

(h) Add 250 μL 2× binding solution (i.e., an equal volume) and mix thoroughly.

2. Bind to oligo(dT) cellulose.

(a) Add each RNA sample to one tube oligo(dT) cellulose and mix well (**Note 6**).

(b) Heat the mixture for 5 min at 65–75 °C.

(c) Rock the tube gently for 30–60 min at room temperature.

(d) Pellet the oligo(dT) cellulose by centrifuging at 4,000 × *g* for 3 min at room temperature.

(e) Remove the supernatant fraction by aspiration, and save it on ice until the recovery of poly(A) RNA has been verified.

(f) Preheat the THE RNA storage solution to 68–75 °C (**Note 7**).

3. Wash the oligo(dT) cellulose:

(a) Add 500 μL wash solution 1 to the oligo(dT) cellulose pellet and vortex briefly to mix well.

(b) Place a spin column for each RNA prep into a collection tube, and transfer the oligo(dT) cellulose suspension to the spin column.

(c) Centrifuge at 4,000 × *g* for 3 min at room temperature to pass the wash solution 1 through the oligo(dT) cellulose. Discard the flow-through from the collection tube, and put the spin column back in the tube.

(d) Add a second aliquot of 500 μL wash solution 1 to the oligo(dT) cellulose, close the tube, and vortex briefly to thoroughly mix the wash solution with the cellulose.

(e) Repeat step c (above).

(f) Repeat steps a–d with wash solution 2. Wash the oligo(dT) cellulose twice with 500 μL wash solution 2.

4. Recover the poly(A) RNA.

(a) Place the spin column into a new collection tube.

(b) Add 200 μL preheated (68–75 °C) THE RNA storage solution to the oligo(dT) cellulose. Close the tube over the spin column and vortex briefly to mix.

(c) Immediately centrifuge at 5,000 × *g* for 2 min. The poly(A) RNA should now be at the bottom of the microfuge tube.

(d) Discard the spin column.

(e) Add the following to the eluted poly(A) RNA:
- 20 μL of 5 M ammonium acetate.
- 1 μL glycogen.
- 550 μL 100 % ethanol.

(f) Leave the precipitation mixture at −20 °C overnight, or quick freeze the mixture in either ethanol and dry ice or place in a −70 °C freezer for 30 min.

(g) Recover the RNA by centrifugation at 12,000 × *g* for 20–30 min at 4 °C.

(h) Carefully remove and discard the supernatant fraction.

(i) Centrifuge the tube briefly a second time, and use a fine-tipped pipette to aspirate away any additional fluid that collects.

(j) Resuspend the poly(A) RNA in the THE RNA storage solution by dissolving the poly(A) RNA pellet in 5–50 μL of the THE RNA storage solution. If necessary, heat the mixture to 60–80 °C to get the RNA into solution.

3.6 Creating cDNA from RNA

The following is directly from the Thermoscientific First Strand cDNA synthesis kit protocol (www.thermoscientific.com). A number of other commercially available kits are also available for production of cDNA from RNA.

1. RNA samples should be thawed and stored on ice. Add the following reagents into a sterile, nuclease-free tube on ice in the indicated order:

Template RNA	Total RNA	0.1–5 μg
	Or poly(A) mRNA	10 ng to 0.5 μg
	Or specific RNA	0.01 pg to 0.5 μg
Primer	Oligo(dT) 18 primer	1 μL
	Or random hexamer primer	1 μL
	Or gene-specific primer	15–20 pmol
Water, nuclease-free		To 11 μL
Total volume		11 μL

2. Mix gently and centrifuge.
3. For oligo (dT)18 or gene-specific primed cDNA synthesis, incubate for 60 min at 37 °C. For random hexamer primed synthesis, incubate for 5 min at 25 °C followed by 60 min at 37 °C.
4. Terminate the reaction by heating at 70 °C for 5 min.

5. The reverse transcription reaction product can be directly used in PCR applications or stored at –20 °C for less than 1 week. For longer storage –70 °C is recommended.

3.7 Synthesizing Double-Stranded cDNA

The remainder of this protocol, from "synthesizing double-stranded cDNA" through "size-select PCR-amplified cDNA library products," is directly from Current Protocols in Molecular Biology (**Note 8**).

1. Add the following reagents, in order, to the first-strand reaction tube:
   (a) 91 μL nuclease-free H_2O
   (b) 30 μL 5× second-strand buffer (1× final)
   (c) 3 μL 10 mM dNTP mix (0.2 mM final)
   (d) 1 μL 10 U/μL *E. coli* DNA ligase
   (e) 4 μL 10 U/μL *E. coli* DNA polymerase I
   (f) 1 μL 2 U/μL *E. coli* RNase H
2. Mix well by pipetting up and down, and incubate for 2 h at 16 °C in a thermal cycler (**Note 9**).
3. Add 2 μL of 5 U/μL T4 DNA polymerase, mix by pipetting up and down, and incubate at 16 °C for an additional 5 min.
4. Add 10 μL of 0.5 M EDTA, microcentrifuge briefly to collect solution at bottoms of tubes, and place tubes on ice.
5. Purify the double-stranded cDNA product using Qiagen's QIAquick PCR Purification Kit (**Note 10**).

3.8 Fragment Double-Stranded cDNA

1. Mix 8 μL of water, 1 μL of DNase I buffer, and 1 μL of DNase I enzyme (2 U/μL) in a microcentrifuge tube.
2. Add 2 μL of this mixture to 25 μL of cDNA.
3. Add nuclease-free water to bring the total volume to 34 μL.
4. Incubate for 10 min at 37 °C, immediately transfer to a 100 °C heat block, and incubate for 10 min to terminate the DNase I reaction.
5. Purify the fragmented cDNA using the QIAquick PCR Purification Kit (**Note 11**).
6. Place the tube on ice until ready for library preparation.

3.9 Perform End Repair of cDNA Fragments

1. Add the following reagents to fragmented cDNA (total volume should be 50 μL) and mix by pipetting up and down:
   (a) 5 μL 10× end-repair buffer (1× final)
   (b) 5 μL 2.5 mM dNTP mix (0.25 mM final)
   (c) 5 μL 10 mM ATP (1 mM final)
   (d) 1 μL end-repair enzyme mix

2. Incubate for 45 min at room temperature.
3. Purify the end-repaired cDNA fragments using the QIAquick PCR Purification Kit (**Note 11**).

3.10 Add Deoxyadenine Base to 3′ Ends

This step is performed to aid the ligation of the Illumina adapters, which have a single thymine (T) base overhang at their 3′ ends.

1. Combine and mix the following components in a clean microcentrifuge tube:
   (a) 34 μL end-repaired DNA
   (b) 5 μL of Klenow buffer (NEB buffer 2)
   (c) 10 μL of 1 mM dATP
   (d) 1 μL of Klenow fragment (3′–5′ exo-) (**Note 12**)
2. Incubate for 30 min at 37 °C in a water bath or heat block.
3. Purify using Qiagen's QIAquick MinElute PCR Purification Kit (**Note 13**).

3.11 Ligate Illumina Adapters

1. Combine and mix the following components in a clean microcentrifuge tube (total volume should be 30 μL):
   (a) 10 μL purified DNA
   (b) 15 μL of T4 DNA ligase buffer
   (c) 1 μL Illumina adapter mix (diluted 1:10 to 1:50 in H_2O)
   (d) 2 μL of nuclease-free water
   (e) 2 μL of 3 U/μL T4 DNA ligase
2. Incubate for 15 min at room temperature.
3. Purify 150- to 350-bp DNA fragments using agarose gel electrophoresis.
4. Elute in a final volume of 23 μL buffer EB.

3.12 PCR Amplification

1. For each reaction, add the following components to a PCR tube (**Note 14**):
   (a) 23 μL DNA
   (b) 1 μL Illumina PCR primer 1.1
   (c) 1 μL Illumina PCR primer 2.1
   (d) 25 μL of 2× Phusion DNA polymerase master mix
2. Mix gently by pipetting up and down (**Note 15**).
3. Place the tubes in the thermal cycler and perform the following thermal cycling program:
   (a) One cycle: 30 s 98 °C, initial denaturation
   (b) Five cycles: 10 s 98 °C, denaturation
   30 s 65 °C, annealing
   30 s 72 °C, extension

(c) One cycle: 5 min 72 °C, final extension

4. Purify the PCR product using the QIAquick MinElute PCR Purification Kit (**Note 16**).

3.13 Size-Select PCR-Amplified cDNA Library Products

1. Separate 15 μL of PCR-amplified product by electrophoresis on a 1.5–2 % TAE agarose gel.
2. Excise the bands in a range of 150–350 bp with a clean, disposable scalpel.
3. Recover the cDNA library product from the gel slices using Qiagen's Gel Extraction Kit (**Note 17**).
4. Check the concentration of the cDNA library using a spectrophotometer (**Note 18**).

3.14 DNA Sequencing and Data Analysis

For most laboratories, the actual sequencing is performed by a core facility. Data are typically received in FASTA format. Analysis of RNA-seq data is by far the most time-consuming component of the process because a huge amount of data is produced. This requires substantial storage and backup capacity. Analysis of these data can be performed on a number of computational programs. The process can take weeks to months and is best performed with the aid of an expert in bioinformatics. Analysis of the data involves matching the reads to the reference genome, defining transcribed regions, identifying novel introns and genes, and comparing sequence expression scores between growth conditions [22].

4 Notes

1. Caution: Not using enough TriPure Isolation Reagent may contaminate RNA with DNA requiring an additional RNA purification procedure.
2. If concerned for residual organics (low 260:230 ratio), further purify RNA on an RNeasy spin column according to the manufacturer's instructions.
3. All tubes and pipette tips should be certified nuclease-free or treated with DEPC. Gloves should be worn at all times and changed frequently. All reagents should be RNase-free, including RNase-free water. An RNase inhibitor, such as Ribolock, can be used to clean equipment of RNases. Keep all kit components tightly sealed when not in use.
4. The glycogen acts as a carrier to increase precipitation efficiency from dilute RNA solutions; it is necessary for solutions with >200 μg RNA/mL.
5. The RNA pellet may not adhere tightly to the walls of the tubes, so remove supernatant fraction by gentle aspiration with a fine-tipped pipette.

6. Mix by inversion to thoroughly re-suspend the resin. If necessary, clumps can be broken up by pipetting up and down.
7. This will be used to elute the poly(A) RNA from the oligo(dT) cellulose near the end of the procedure.
8. Unit 4.11, RNA-Seq: A Method for Comprehensive Transcriptome Analysis by Ugrappa Nagalakshmi, Karl Waern, and Michael Snyder, Wiley Interscience.
9. Do not allow the temperature to rise above 16 °C.
10. Follow the manufacturer's recommended protocol, but elute to a final volume of 25 μL of buffer EB.
11. Follow the manufacturer's recommended protocol, but elute in a final volume of 34 μL of buffer EB.
12. Total volume should be 50 μL.
13. Follow the manufacturer's recommended protocol, and elute in a final volume of 10 μL of buffer EB.
14. Total volume should be 50 μL.
15. Try to avoid creation of bubbles, and centrifuge briefly to collect the solution in the bottom of the tube.
16. Follow the manufacturer's recommended protocol, but elute in a final volume of 15 μL of buffer EB.
17. Follow the manufacturer's recommended protocol, and include all optional steps, but elute in a final volume of 15 μL of buffer EB.
18. The ideal concentration is 15–25 ng/μL. If the cDNA concentration is lower, the sequencing efficiency will be low.

References

1. Giovannucci E, Harlan DM, Archer MC, Bergenstal RM, Gapstur SM, Habel LA, Pollak M, Regensteiner JG, Yee D (2010) Diabetes and cancer: a consensus report. CA Cancer J Clin 60(4):207–221. doi:10.3322/caac.20078
2. Gallagher EJ, LeRoith D (2011) Minireview: IGF, insulin, and cancer. Endocrinology 152(7):2546–2551. doi:10.1210/en.2011-0231
3. Blackburn GL, Wang KA (2007) Dietary fat reduction and breast cancer outcome: results from the Women's Intervention Nutrition Study (WINS). Am J Clin Nutr 86(3): s878–s881
4. Boyle P, Boniol M, Koechlin A, Robertson C, Valentini F, Coppens K, Fairley LL, Zheng T, Zhang Y, Pasterk M, Smans M, Curado MP, Mullie P, Gandini S, Bota M, Bolli GB, Rosenstock J, Autier P (2012) Diabetes and breast cancer risk: a meta-analysis. Br J Cancer 107(9):1608–1617. doi:10.1038/bjc.2012.414
5. Khan N, Afaq F, Saleem M, Ahmad N, Mukhtar H (2006) Targeting multiple signaling pathways by green tea polyphenol (-)-epigallocatechin-3-gallate. Cancer Res 66(5): 2500–2505.doi:10.1158/0008-5472.CAN-05-3636
6. Shimizu M, Deguchi A, Hara Y, Moriwaki H, Weinstein IB (2005) EGCG inhibits activation of the insulin-like growth factor-1 receptor in human colon cancer cells. Biochem Biophys Res Commun 334(3):947–953. doi:10.1016/j.bbrc.2005.06.182
7. Shimizu M, Shirakami Y, Sakai H, Tatebe H, Nakagawa T, Hara Y, Weinstein IB, Moriwaki H (2008) EGCG inhibits activation of the insulin-like growth factor (IGF)/IGF-1 receptor axis

in human hepatocellular carcinoma cells. Cancer Lett 262(1):10–18. doi:10.1016/j.canlet.2007.11.026

8. Masuda M, Suzui M, Lim JT, Deguchi A, Soh JW, Weinstein IB (2002) Epigallocatechin-3-gallate decreases VEGF production in head and neck and breast carcinoma cells by inhibiting EGFR-related pathways of signal transduction. J Exp Ther Oncol 2(6):350–359
9. Kang JH, Song KH, Woo JK, Park MH, Rhee MH, Choi C, Oh SH (2011) Ginsenoside Rp1 from Panax ginseng exhibits anti-cancer activity by down-regulation of the IGF-1R/Akt pathway in breast cancer cells. Plant Foods Hum Nutr 66:298–305
10. Zi X, Zhang J, Agarwal R, Pollak M (2000) Silibinin up-regulates insulin-like growth factor-binding protein 3 expression and inhibits proliferation of androgen-independent prostate cancer cells. Cancer Res 60(20):5617–5620
11. Wang HJ, Tashiro S, Onodera S, Ikejima T (2008) Inhibition of insulin-like growth factor 1 receptor signaling enhanced silibinin-induced activation of death receptor and mitochondrial apoptotic pathways in human breast cancer MCF-7 cells. J Pharmacol Sci 107(3): 260–269
12. McLaughlin JM, Olivo-Marston S, Vitolins MZ, Bittoni M, Reeves KW, Degraffinreid CR, Schwartz SJ, Clinton SK, Paskett ED (2011) Effects of tomato- and soy-rich diets on the IGF-I hormonal network: a crossover study of postmenopausal women at high risk for breast cancer. Cancer Prev Res (Phila) 4(5):702–710. doi:10.1158/1940-6207.CAPR-10-0329
13. Power KA, Chen JM, Saarinen NM, Thompson LU (2008) Changes in biomarkers of estrogen receptor and growth factor signaling pathways in MCF-7 tumors after short- and long-term treatment with soy and flaxseed. J Steroid Biochem Mol Biol 112(1–3):13–19. doi:10.1016/j.jsbmb.2008.07.003
14. Chen J, Saggar JK, Corey P, Thompson LU (2011) Flaxseed cotyledon fraction reduces tumour growth and sensitises tamoxifen treatment of human breast cancer xenograft (MCF-7) in athymic mice. Br J Nutr 105(3):339–347. doi:10.1017/S0007114510003557
15. Chen J, Zeng J, Xin M, Huang W, Chen X (2011) Formononetin induces cell cycle arrest of human breast cancer cells via IGF1/PI3K/Akt pathways in vitro and in vivo. Horm Metab Res 43(10):681–686. doi:10.1055/s-0031-1286306
16. Vogelstein B, Kinzler KW (1993) The multistep nature of cancer. Trends Genet 9(4):138–141
17. Feng H, Qin Z, Zhang X (in press) Opportunities and methods for studying alternative splicing in cancer with RNA-Seq. Cancer Lett. doi:10.1016/j.canlet.2012.11.010
18. Soule HD, Vazguez J, Long A, Albert S, Brennan M (1973) A human cell line from a pleural effusion derived from a breast carcinoma. J Natl Cancer Inst 51(5):1409–1416
19. Jackson JG, White MF, Yee D (1998) Insulin receptor substrate-1 is the predominant signaling molecule activated by insulin-like growth factor-I, insulin, and interleukin-4 in estrogen receptor-positive human breast cancer cells. J Biol Chem 273(16):9994–10003
20. Zhang H, Fagan DH, Zeng X, Freeman KT, Sachdev D, Yee D (2010) Inhibition of cancer cell proliferation and metastasis by insulin receptor downregulation. Oncogene 29(17): 2517–2527. doi:10.1038/onc.2010.17
21. Nagalakshmi U, Waern K, Snyder M (2010) RNA-Seq: a method for comprehensive transcriptome analysis. Curr Protoc Mol Biol 4.11.1–4.11.13. doi:10:1002/0471142727.mb0411s89
22. Wilhelm BT, Marguerat S, Goodhead I, Bahler J (2010) Defining transcribed regions using RNA-seq. Nat Protoc 5(2):255–266. doi:10.1038/nprot.2009.229

Chapter 10

The Ex Vivo Use of Keratinocytes from Adult Mice to Define Stem Cell Activities in Cancer Research

Rebecca J. Morris, Nyssa Readio, Kelly M. Johnson, Anupama Singh, Heuijoon Park, Ashok Singh, and Todd F. Schuster

Abstract

Primary keratinocytes are harvested from the dorsal skin of 7-week-old mice. Euthanized mice are clipped and cleaned with serial washes in povidone iodine and ethanol solutions. The dorsal skin is removed and treated with a mild 32 °C trypsinization to detach the dermis from the epidermis. Keratinocytes harvested by this method can be used for molecular biology, biochemistry, or numerous ex vivo procedures relevant to cancer research such as clonal culture or fluorescence-activated cell sorting (FACS). FACS, a type of flow cytometry, is a quantitative means of sorting cell mixtures using diameter, fluorescent dye, and the molecular charge of each cell type in the sample suspension. This technique is performed using specialized shared instruments at The Hormel Institute, including the BD FACSAria II for cell sorting and the BD FACSCalibur for analysis only. The equipment and techniques presented here are useful as an ex vivo readout of in vivo experiments on skin and for preparation of enriched stem cells for further study in molecular biology and other applications.

Key words Keratinocytes, Cell culture, Stem cells, Adult mice, Flow cytometry

1 Introduction

The skin is the largest organ of the body and serves a multitude of roles, including protection through thermal regulation as well as immune and barrier functions. Over the last 50 years, research on the skin of mice has yielded new information on the structure and function of the skin as well as the mechanisms of carcinogenesis. Because of their usefulness in studies of hair follicle growth and carcinogenesis experiments, isolating and culturing primary epidermal keratinocytes from adult mice to use in conjunction with in vivo studies are highly desirable. The procedures presented here are documented and successful methods of harvesting primary keratinocytes from adult mice for downstream applications such as clonal culture [1–4], enrichment of hair follicle stem cells by FACS [5–7], preparation of RNA for quantitative real-time polymerase

Ann M. Bode and Zigang Dong (eds.), *Cancer Prevention: Dietary Factors and Pharmacology*, Methods in Pharmacology and Toxicology, DOI 10.1007/978-1-4614-9227-6_10, © Springer Science+Business Media New York 2014

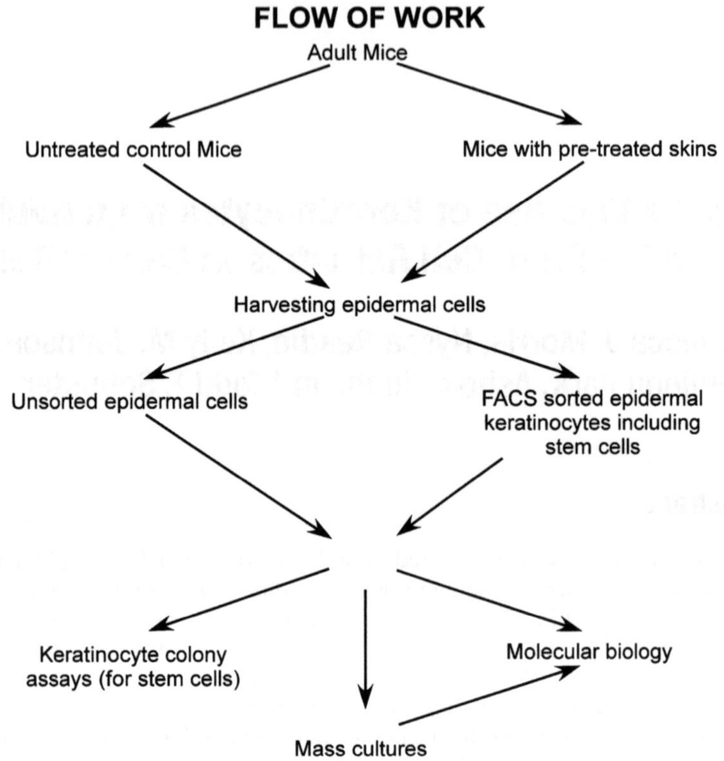

Fig. 1 Typical flow of work for the ex vivo applications of epidermal keratinocytes from adult mice. Epidermal cells are harvested from either untreated mice or from those pretreated with modifiers or treatments used in carcinogenesis studies. The harvested epidermal cells may be used for cell culture of molecular biology with or without FACS sorting to enrich for hair follicle stem cells

chain reaction or gene expression arrays [6–8], or preparation of DNA for adduct analysis following carcinogen treatment [9]. Figure 1 illustrates the typical workflow of ex vivo studies within the context of in vivo studies on cancer prevention.

2 Materials

2.1 Cells and Tissues

1. Epidermal keratinocytes: Four to five adult female mice approx 6–8 weeks of age should be obtained. Mice older than 8 weeks will have entered into anagen (i.e., have growing hair follicles), and the viability of cells from the preparation is reduced. Additionally, epidermal trypsinization is more difficult if the mice are in the anagen stage of the hair growth cycle. The harvesting procedure has been optimized for the thinner skin of female mice (**Note 1**).
2. Swiss mouse 3T3 fibroblasts (ATCC, Rockville, MD; cat. number CCL-92).

3. Mouse dorsal skin may also be obtained through Jackson Laboratories or Charles River. Mice are euthanized by CO_2 inhalation. Dorsal skin is clipped, removed, and packaged in 39 ml DMEM + 10 ml fetal bovine serum (FBS) + 1 ml penicillin (Jackson) or RPMI medium (Charles River). The skins are packaged on wet ice or in a "NanoCool" box and shipped overnight. Skins must not freeze during shipping because freezing will damage the cells. Obtaining skin rather than mice is sometimes useful when harvesting keratinocytes from mutant mice is required or when housing additional mice is problematic.

2.2 Supplies

2.2.1 Keratinocyte Harvesting Supplies

1. Oster Pro-Cord/Cordless Trimmer with number 40 blade (Jarden Consumer Solutions/Oster, Boca Raton, FL; cat. number 78997-010).
2. Nalgene PC Straight-Side Wide-Mouth Jars, 16 oz (Thermo Fisher Scientific, Waltham, MA; cat. number 2116-0500).
3. Triadine; 10 % Povidone-Iodine Prep Topical Solution, 16 oz (Triad Group, Hartland, WI; cat. number 10-8216).
4. Twice-distilled water (ddH_2O) (made fresh; from distilled reverse osmosis water).
5. 70 % ethanol (non-denatured) in water (trace chemicals in denatured ethanol will kill the cells).
6. Autoclaved harvesting instruments put into a beaker of 70 % ethanol:
   (a) One pair of scissors (Biomedical Research Instruments, Silver Spring, MD; cat. number 25-1050).
   (b) One pair of full-curve eye dressing forceps (Miltex, Bethpage, NY; cat. number 18-784).
   (c) One pair of "thumb" dressing forceps (Miltex, Bethpage, NY; cat. number 6-4).
   (d) Number 4 scalpel handles (Biomedical Research Instruments, Rockville, MD; cat. number 26-1200).
7. Number 22 sterile stainless-steel blades (BD Biosciences, Franklin Lakes, NJ; cat. number 371222).
8. Fisherbrand 4 oz. Sterile Specimen Container (Thermo Fisher Scientific, Waltham, MA; cat. number 16-320-730).
9. VWR Plastic Petri dishes, sterile Space Saver 100 × 10 (VWR, Radnor, PA; cat. number 25384-324).
10. Sterile conical tube (15 and 50 ml, BD Falcon, Franklin Lakes, NJ; cat. number 15 ml tube 352097; 50 ml tube 352098).
11. Disposable pipets (5 and 10 ml, BD Falcon, Franklin Lakes, NJ; cat. number 5 ml pipet 357543; 10 ml pipet 357551).
12. Square sterile plastic Petri dishes (BD Falcon, Franklin Lakes, NJ; cat. number 351112).

13. 2 ml Screw Cap Micro Tube Conical (Sarstedt, Newton, NC; cat. number 72.608).
14. Pyrex Brand Plain Stemless Glass Funnel (Corning, Corning, NY; cat. number 6240-75).
15. 90 mm diameter Spectra Mesh filter, 74 micrometer pore size (Spectrum Laboratories, Inc., Rancho Dominguez, CA; cat. number 145956).
16. Cell Strainer, 70-micrometer sterile (BD Discovery Labware, Franklin Lakes, NJ; cat. number 352350).
17. 2 oz Nalgene jar (60 ml, Thermo Fisher Scientific, Waltham, MA; cat. number 2118-0002) with a 1.5 in magnetic stir bar with pivot ring (Bel-Art, Wayne, NJ; cat. number 371101128).
18. Plastic Petri dish 100 mm × 20 mm sterile (Corning, Corning, NY; cat. number 430167).
19. 32 oz Nalgene sterile Square Storage Bottles: PETG (1,000 ml, Thermo Fisher Scientific, Waltham, MA; cat. number 2019-1000).
20. Hemacytometer with octagon glass cover slip (Hausser Scientific, Horsham, PA; cat. number 1492).
21. Manostat Colony Counter System (Sigma-Aldrich Corp. Hybri-Max, St. Louis, MO; cat. number Z367885-1EA).
22. Fowler Xtra-value Electronic Calipers (Fred V. Fowler, Newton, MA; cat. number 54-101-150-2).

2.2.2 Keratinocyte Culturing Supplies

1. 35-mm sterile culture dish (Corning, Corning, NY; cat. number 430165).
2. 6-well plates (Corning, Corning, NY; cat. number 3516).
3. 60-mm sterile culture dish (Corning, Corning, NY; cat. number 430166).

2.2.3 3T3 Culturing Supplies

1. Corning 2 ml Polypropylene Cryogenic Vial, Self-Standing with Round Bottom (Corning, Corning, NY; cat. number 430659).
2. Nalgene “Mr. Frosty” cell freezer (Thermo Fisher Scientific, Waltham, MA; cat. number 5100-0001).
3. CoolCell Economical cell freezing container for 1 or 2 ml cryovials (Biocision, Larkspur, CA; cat. number BCS-136PK).
4. 225 cm^2 (T-225) culture flask (Corning, Corning, NY; cat. number 431082).
5. 150 cm^2 (T-150) culture flask (Corning, Corning, NY; cat. number 430825).

2.2.4 Media and Supplement Preparation Supplies

1. Corning filter flask (500 ml, Corning, Corning, NY; cat. number 431097).
2. PALL life sciences filters, Acrodisc syringe filter sterile, 0.2 μm, 25 mm HT Tuffryn Membrane (Pall Life Sciences, Port Washington, NY; cat. number 4192).

2.2.5 FACS Supplies

1. Falcon 15 ml conical tube (BD Biosciences, Franklin Lakes, NJ; cat. number 352096).
2. Falcon polystyrene tubes, sterile (BD Biosciences, Franklin Lakes, NJ; 12 × 75 mm, cat. number 352058).
3. Sterile transfer pipet (Thermo Fisher Scientific Samco, Waltham, MA; cat. number 1371121).
4. Samples are filtered (prior to sorting) through a cell strainer cap designed for flow cytometry over a 12 × 75 mm, 5 ml polystyrene round bottom test tube, 1,400 RCF rating (BD Biosciences, Franklin Lakes, NJ; cat. number 352235).
5. Falcon polystyrene 4-way sorting tube (for cell collection) (BD Biosciences, Franklin Lakes, NJ; 12 × 75 mm cat. number 352058). Tubes should contain no less than 500 μl of medium supplemented with 20 % FBS.

2.2.6 DNA and RNA Supplies

1. 1.5 ml centrifuge tubes, Eppendorf Flex Tubes (Eppendorf, Hauppage, NY; cat. number 022364120).
2. RNeasy Mini kit (50) (unsorted cells and tissues) (Qiagen Sciences, Germantown, MD; cat. number 74104).
3. RNeasy Micro Kit (50) (FACS sorted cells) (Qiagen Sciences, Germantown, MD; cat. number 74004).
4. Microcell, 50 μm cuvettes (Beckman Coulter, Indianapolis, IN; cat. number 523452).
5. PCR
   (a) MicroAmp 8-Tube Strip (0.2 ml) PCR Tubes (Life Technologies Applied Biosystems, Grand Island, NY; cat. number N8010580).
   (b) MicroAmp 8-cap Strip PCR Tube caps (Life Technologies Applied Biosystems, Grand Island, NY; cat. number N801-0535).
6. RT-PCR
   (a) MicroAmp Optical 8-Tube Strip (0.2 ml) PCR Tubes (Life Technologies Applied Biosystems, Grand Island, NY; cat. number 4316567).
   (b) MicroAmp Optical 8-cap Strip PCR Tube caps (Life Technologies Applied Biosystems, Grand Island, NY; cat. number 4323032).

2.2.7 Instruments

1. IEC Centra MP4R Centrifuge (International Equipment Company, Needham Heights, MA; cat. number 2438).
2. Zeiss AxioObserver.D1 Inverted light microscope with phase and brightfield optics; (Carl Zeiss Microscopy GmbH, Jena, Germany; cat. number 431006).
3. FACSCalibur flow cytometer by Becton Dickinson (BD Biosciences, San Jose, CA).
4. BD FACSAria II Special Order System (BD Biosciences, San Jose, CA).
5. Centrifuge 5415D (room temperature) (Eppendorf, Hauppauge, NY; cat. number for 5415R model 022621408).
6. DU800 Spectrophotometer (Beckman Coulter, Indianapolis, IN).
7. GeneAmp PCR System 7500 (Life Technologies Applied Biosystems, Grand Island, NY; cat. number N8050200).
8. 7500 Real-Time PCR System (Life Technologies Applied Biosystems, Grand Island, NY; cat. number 4351105).
9. Zeiss Axio Imager.Z1 upright microscope with bright field and fluorescence (Carl Zeiss Microscopy GmbH, Jena, Germany).

2.2.8 Software

1. BD FACSDIVA v6.1.2 (BD Biosciences, San Jose, CA).
2. ModFit LT software v3.2.1 (Verity Software House, Inc., Topsham, ME).
3. DU 800 UV/Vis software v3.0 (Beckman Coulter, Indianapolis, IN; cat. number 512984).
4. RT-PCR 7500 System Sequence Detection Software v 1.4 (Life Technologies Applied Biosystems, Grand Island, NY).
5. Microsoft Excel 2010 (Microsoft, Redmond, Washington).
6. AxioVision v4.7.1 image analysis software (Carl Zeiss Microscopy GmbH, Jena, Germany).

2.3 Reagents and Solutions

2.3.1 General Cell Culture Laboratory Reagents

1. Dulbecco's phosphate-buffered saline (DPBS, 1×) Ca^{2+} and Mg^{2+} free, sterile (Life Technologies GIBCO, Grand Island, NY; cat. number 14190-144).
2. 2.5 % Trypsin solution (10×), no phenol red (Life Technologies GIBCO, Grand Island, NY; cat. number 15090-046).
3. SMEM: Ca^{2+} and Mg^{2+} free minimal essential medium for suspension culture (Life Technologies GIBCO, Grand Island, NY; cat. number 11380-037).
4. Defined FBS (Thermo Fisher Scientific Hyclone, Logan, UT; cat. number SH 300070.03).
5. 0.4 % Trypan blue 1× in 0.9 % saline (Life Technologies GIBCO, Grand Island, NY; cat. number 15250-061).

6. Gentamicin 50 mg/ml 10 ml (Life Technologies GIBCO, Grand Island, NY; cat. number 15750-060).
7. Antibiotics: Penicillin–streptomycin (pen–strep), Liquid (10,000 units/ml penicillin, 10,000 μg/ml streptomycin) (Life Technologies GIBCO, Grand Island, NY; cat. number 15140-122).
8. Dimethyl sulfoxide (DMSO) (Sigma-Aldrich Corp. Hybri-Max, St. Louis, MO; cat. number D2650).
9. 10 % neutral buffered formalin (Fisher Scientific, Pittsburgh, PA; cat. number 23-305-510).
10. Rhodamine B (Sigma-Aldrich Corp., St. Louis, MO; cat. number R6626-25G).
11. Methanol (Sigma-Aldrich Corp., St. Louis, MO; cat. number 32213-1L).

2.3.2 Solutions for Keratinocyte Harvest

1. Phosphate-buffered saline (PBS) with 2× gentamicin: Dulbecco's PBS (500 ml) and gentamicin (2 ml).
2. Trypsin solution: PBS with 2× gentamicin (45 ml) and 2.5 % trypsin (5 ml).
3. Collagen dish-coating solution:
   (a) Cell culture medium (100 ml).
   (b) Fibronectin (1 mg); Fibronectin (Sigma-Aldrich Corp., St. Louis, MO; cat. number F1141-1MG).
   (c) 1.0 mg/ml stock bovine serum albumin stock (10 ml); bovine serum albumin (BD Biosciences, San Jose, CA; cat. number 354331).
   (d) Collagen (1 ml); Collagen, Bovine, Type I, 30 mg (BD Biosciences, San Jose, CA; cat. number 354231).
   (e) 1 M HEPES (1 ml); 1 M HEPES Buffer, sterile (Sigma-Aldrich Corp., St. Louis, MO; cat. number H0887).
   (f) 116 mM $CaCl_2$ (1 ml) (Sigma-Aldrich Corp., St. Louis, MO; cat. number C7902).
4. SMEM (Ca^{2+} and Mg^{2+} free) + 10 % FBS + 2× gentamicin.

2.3.3 Keratinocyte Media

1. Harvesting medium: SMEM (500 ml); FBS (50 ml); and 2× gentamicin (1 ml).
2. Medium used for mass culture is a low-calcium medium formulation (e.g., KGM). Commercial medium used is KGM-Gold Keratinocyte Growth Medium Ca^{2+} Free BulletKit (Lonza Inc., Allendale, NJ; cat. number 195769; please note that this kit contains the basal medium (cat. number 195130) and the supplement SingleQuot kit (cat. number 192152)). Prepare medium according to the manufacturer's instructions.

3. Medium used for clonogenic culture is a "high-calcium" Williams E medium formulation with the following additives:
   (a) Williams E Medium (500 ml) (Life Technologies GIBCO, Grand Island, NY; cat. number 12551-032).
   (b) Added supplements:
      - Epidermal growth factor (EGF) (1 ml of 5 μg/ml stock) (BD Biosciences Pharmingen, San Jose, CA; cat. number 354001).
      - Glutamine (14.5 ml) (Sigma-Aldrich Corp., St. Louis, MO; cat. number G8540-10MG).
      - Hydrocortisone (0.5 ml of 2.5 mg/ml stock; BD Biosciences Pharmingen, San Jose, CA; cat. number 354203).
      - Insulin from bovine pancreas (1 ml) (Sigma-Aldrich Corp., St. Louis, MO; cat. number I6634-50MG).
      - Linoleic acid:BSA (0.5 ml of 0.1 mg/ml stock) (BD Biosciences Pharmingen, San Jose, CA; cat. number 354227).
      - Pen–strep (5 ml).
      - Transferrin bovine (1 ml of 5 mg/ml stock) (Sigma-Aldrich Corp., St. Louis, MO; cat. number T1428-50MG).
      - Vitamin A (57.5 μl of 1 mg/1 ml stock) (Sigma-Aldrich Corp., St. Louis, MO; cat. number R0635-5MG).
      - Vitamin D2 (50 μl of 10 mg/ml stock) (Sigma-Aldrich Corp., St. Louis, MO; cat. number E8014-5MG).
   (c) Sterile filter, add 100 ml FBS, and store working medium at 4 °C. Pre-warm medium for 30 min in 37 °C water bath before changing medium on culture dishes.

2.3.4 Solutions for 3T3 Culture

1. ATCC Dulbecco's modified eagle's medium (DMEM) (ATCC, Manassas, VA, cat. number 30-2002).
2. Bovine calf serum (BCS) (Thermo Fisher Scientific Hyclone, Logan, UT; cat. number SH30073.03).
3. Trypsin solution: 1× DPBS + 2× gentamicin (45 ml) and 2.5 % trypsin (5 ml).

2.3.5 Medium for 3T3 Culture

1. 3T3 fibroblast complete growth medium (CGM): 900 ml DMEM; 100 ml BCS; and 10 ml pen–strep.
2. DMSO–CGM cell freezing solution: DMSO (2 ml) and CGM (18 ml).

2.4 Fluorescence-Activated Cell Sorting

2.4.1 Solutions for FACS

1. 10 % Clorox bleach, germicidal disinfectant (Legasse Inc., Deerfield, IL; cat. number CLO 02490).
2. If cells aggregate, may use DNAse or HBSS (w/o Ca^{2+} and Mg^{2+}) + 1 % BSA (or FCS).
3. Hanks balanced salt solution (HBSS), no calcium, no magnesium, no phenol red, with glucose (Life Technologies GIBCO, Grand Island, NY; cat. number 14175-145).

2.4.2 Antibodies

1. 0.2 mg/ml Rat IgG_{2a}, kappa PE isotype control, 0.1 mg clone R35-95 (BD Biosciences Pharmingen, San Jose, CA; cat. number 554689).
2. 0.5 mg/ml Rat IgG_{2a}, kappa FITC isotype control, 0.1 mg clone R35-95 (BD Biosciences Pharmingen, San Jose, CA; cat. number 554688).
3. 20 µl/test Rat IgG_{2a}, kappa PE CD49f integrin alpha 6 chain, 100 tests clone GoH3 (BD Biosciences Pharmingen, San Jose, CA; cat. number 555736).
4. 0.5 mg/ml Rat IgG_{2a}, kappa FITC CD34 (gp 105–120), 0.5 mg clone RAM34 (BD Biosciences Pharmingen, San Jose, CA; cat. number 553733).

2.4.3 Medium for FACS Sorting

1. SMEM (Ca^{2+} and Mg^{2+} free) + 10% FBS + 2× gentamicin.
2. SMEM (Ca^{2+} and Mg^{2+} free) + 20% FBS + 2× gentamicin.

2.5 Reagents for Isolation of DNA and RNA

2.5.1 Reagents for Preparing DNA and RNA from Epidermal Keratinocytes

1. RNA*later* RNA Stabilization Reagent (50 ml) (Qiagen Sciences, Germantown, MD; cat. number 76104).
2. Isolation of mRNA:
   (a) 2-Mercaptoethanol (Sigma-Aldrich Corp., St. Louis, MO; cat. number M6250-100ML).
   (b) 70 % ethanol.
   (c) 80 % ethanol.
   (d) RNase-free water, prepared without the use of diethyl-pyrocarbonate (DEPC) (Qiagen Sciences, Germantown, MD; cat. number 129112).
3. Master Mix for making cDNA; SuperScript First-Strand Synthesis System for RT-PCR (Life Technologies Invitrogen, Grand Island, NY; cat. number 11904-018).
4. Master mix for RT-PCR:
   (a) FastStart Universal SYBR Green Master (Rox) (Roche Applied Science, Indianapolis, IN; cat. number 04913850001).
   (b) Nuclease-free Water, PCR Grade (Roche Applied Science, Indianapolis, IN; cat. number 03315843001).

2.5.2 Medium for DNA and RNA Preparation

SMEM + 10 % FBS + 2× gentamicin: SMEM, Ca^{2+} and Mg^{2+} free minimal essential medium for suspension culture; FBS (Defined FBS; Hyclone, Logan, UT; cat. number SH 300070.03); and gentamicin (GIBCO, Grand Island, NY; cat. number 11380-037).

3 Methods

3.1 Pretreatment of Mice

1. In vivo studies are performed according to institutional animal use policies and approved IACUC protocols. In vivo treatments may include xenograft studies, carcinogenesis studies (e.g., chemical and UV), transplantation studies (e.g., bone marrow transplantation), models of disease (e.g., diabetes), and studies with application of pharmaceuticals.
2. Control mice are treated with solvent alone or are sham-irradiated. We typically include "normal" untreated controls that do not undergo any treatment and are usually the same age and sex as the experimentally treated mice. The control strains may vary but can include wild-type littermates, background strains, and known positive and/or negative control strains for the treatment of choice.
3. Bromodeoxyuridine (BrdU) can be used to identify proliferating cells. One hour prior to euthanasia, administer BrdU (BD Biosciences, San Jose, CA; cat. number 550891) at 50 mg/kg prepared in sterile saline via intraperitoneal (i.p.) injection.

3.2 Harvesting Epidermal Keratinocytes from Adult Mice

3.2.1 Keratinocyte Harvest and Seeding

1. Euthanize four to five mice with CO_2 inhalation followed by postmortem cervical dislocation according to institutional animal use facilities and IACUC standards (**Note 2**).
2. Clip approximately 15–18 cm^2 of the dorsal fur with an electric animal clipper, and place all mice into a 500 ml Nalgene jar with enough povidone iodine solution to cover them.
3. Shake the jar well to get even distribution of the solution over the mice. Pour off the solution and rinse with distilled water until liquid runs clear.
4. Repeat iodine wash followed by water rinse.
5. Rinse two times with 70 % ethanol accompanied with shaking.
6. After final rinse, add enough 70 % ethanol to cover the mice and soak for 5–10 min (**Note 3**).
7. Within a laminar flow hood or a biosafety cabinet, remove the dorsal skin (clipped portion only) using thumb forceps and scissors, and put skins into a cup filled with PBS/2× gentamicin. Do not remove skin along the sides to prevent contaminating the harvest with mammary cells.

8. With curved forceps and scalpel, place one skin at a time hairy side down onto a thin Petri dish. Scrape all subcutaneous tissue from the skin until the skin is semitranslucent. Attempt to remove all traces of subcutaneous tissue, but do not scrape so hard as to tear the skin or to remove the hair follicles through the dermis. Do this swiftly so that the skins do not dry out. Place the skin back into PBS until all other skins are processed.
9. Spread out a skin hairy side up on a thin Petri dish, bisect it lengthwise, and cut the skin into 0.5 × 1.5 cm strips.
10. Pipette 45 ml of PBS + 2× gentamicin into a 100 mm × 20 mm Petri dish and add 5 ml of 2.5 % trypsin. Use forceps to transfer and float the skins hairy side up on the surface of the 0.25 % trypsin solution. Place Petri dishes in 32 ° C incubator for 2 h (**Note 4**). During the incubation time, coat dishes to be seeded with collagen coating solution and place them in a 37 °C incubator for at least 1 h (**Note 5**); for clonogenic assays the dishes have already been coated 24 h prior to harvesting to allow the irradiated 3T3 feeder layer to attach and spread out.
11. Prepare a square Petri dish (bottom placed into and propped upon the inverted lid; this creates a surface at an incline of about 30° and is maintained by placing a microfuge cap in the lid where the lid and bottom meet) with 10–15 ml harvesting medium. Remove a strip of floating skin from the trypsin solution with forceps, and with a new scalpel blade, scrape off the epidermis into the medium. Special attention needs to be paid to scraping the epidermis (**Note 6**). Use sufficient force, but not excessive amounts, or the cell preparation will result in lower viability. Discard the dermis or retain it for histological confirmation of the full removal of the hair follicle with the epidermis.
12. Carefully pour the harvesting medium with the epidermis into a sterile 60 ml Nalgene jar with a 1.5 in stir bar. Rinse the Petri dish with additional harvesting medium, and bring the final volume in the jar to 30 ml. Screw the cap on. Stir at 100 rpm on a magnetic stirrer for 20 min at room temperature.
13. Place a sterile 70 micrometer mesh filter into a sterile glass funnel (70 μm cell strainer may be used as an alternative) and position on a 50 ml conical tube. Carefully remove the stir bar from the jar, and pour the contents into the filter that will strain out undesired hair and sheets of stratum corneum. Use curved forceps to press the materials within the mesh and manipulate them to free trapped cells and remove excess liquid. Rinse again with 5 ml of harvesting medium to allow additional cells to flow into the tube. If desired, material within mesh may be used for further histological analysis.

14. Cap tube and centrifuge for 7 min at 1,000 rpm at 4 °C. Aspirate the supernatant fraction, add 5 ml of refrigerated harvesting medium, and re-suspend the cells by triturating gently 20–25 times with a 5 ml pipet. Be sure to keep the cells at 4 °C to avoid their aggregation. Add 25 ml additional harvesting medium and triturate again 20–25 times with a 5 ml pipet. Remove 1 ml of this cell suspension and add to 19 ml of harvesting medium for a 1:20 dilution of the cells; triturate this dilution 20–25 times with a 5 ml pipet. This dilution helps ensure an accurate cell count.
15. Remove approximately 0.5 ml of the 1:20 dilution cell mixture and place into a small sterile microfuge tube. Remove 200 μl of the cell mixture to a clean centrifuge tube and add 200 μl of 0.4 % trypan blue solution. Gently pipet this mixture avoiding the creation of bubbles. Place cells within a hemacytometer, and count all nucleated cells. All dark or blue cells and large gold ones are scored as nonviable, whereas small gold and "pink" cells are scored as viable. Yields of cells should range on average from 15 to 25×10^6 viable cells per mouse. This yield also depends on the size of skin harvested.
16. Centrifuge original tube for 7 min at 1,000 rpm at 4 °C. Re-suspend cells in desired medium, and make appropriate dilutions for seeding cells.

3.2.2 Mass Cultures

Setup and Maintenance of Mass Cultures

1. For mass culture, cells are usually seeded at $2\text{–}4 \times 10^6$ viable cells per 35-mm dish in 2 ml of medium or 1.5×10^5 to 1.9×10^5 cells per cm^2 (KGM-type medium + supplements for monolayer cultures).
2. The cultures are incubated in a 32 °C, 95 % humidified incubator with 5 % CO_2.
3. For mass cultures, the medium is changed the day after initial seeding and three times weekly thereafter.

Ex Vivo Treatment of Mass Cultures

1. Mass cultures may be treated with biological or xenobiotic agents followed with appropriate analysis by biochemical or molecular biology methods.

Analysis of Mass Cultures

1. Mass culture dishes may be fixed with 10 % buffered formalin overnight at ambient temperature.
   (a) Dishes may then be stained with crystal violet for 1 h and rinsed with ddH_2O to observe morphology as illustrated in Fig. 2.
   (b) Alternatively, dishes may then be processed using standard immunohistochemistry (IHC) protocols with antibodies of interest (Table 1).

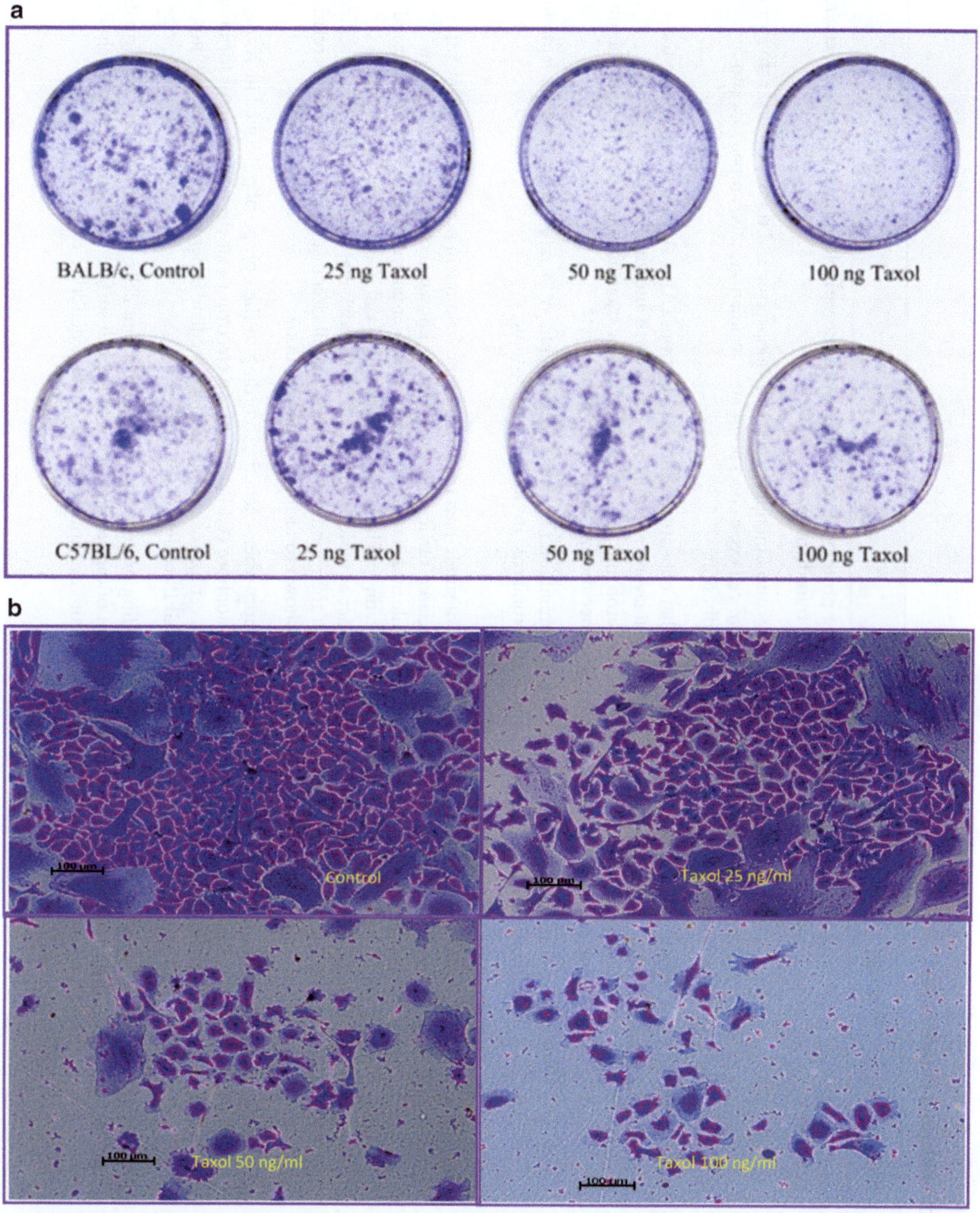

Fig. 2 An example of BALB/c and C57BL/6 keratinocyte mass cultures treated ex vivo with Taxol followed by formalin fixation and staining with crystal violet. The dosage effects of Taxol as well as the different responses of the two strains of mice are apparent in the dishes (**a**) as well as at the microscopic level (**b**). Scale bar = 100 μm

Table 1
Useful antibodies for epidermal keratinocytes

Antibody	Source	Purpose
CD3-Epsilon (48-2B)	Santa Cruz SC-1174	CD3 epsilon is one of at least three invariant proteins that associate with the variable antigen recognition chains of the T cell receptor and function in signal transduction.
Anti-p53 (PAb 240)	Abcam ab26	p53 is a 53 kDa protein that forms tetramers and functions as a tumor suppressor and transcriptional activator of genes that inhibit growth and/or invasion, cell cycle checkpoint after irradiation, DNA repair, apoptotic induction, signal transduction, and cell adhesion.
β-Catenin (14)	BD Bio 610153	β-Catenin is part of a complex of proteins that constitute adherens junctions (AJs). AJs are necessary for the creation and maintenance of epithelial cell layers by regulating cell growth and adhesion between cells. β-Catenin also anchors the actin cytoskeleton and may be responsible for transmitting the contact inhibition signal that causes cells to stop dividing once the epithelial sheet is complete.
α6-Integrin/ CD49F (clone GoH3)	BD Bio 555743	Integrin alpha-6/beta-1 is a receptor for laminin on platelets. Integrin alpha-6/beta-4 is a receptor for laminin in epithelial cells, and it plays a critical structural role in the hemidesmosome.
CD34 (RAM 34)	BD Bio 553731	The CD34 protein is a member of a family of single-pass transmembrane sialomucin proteins that show expression on early hematopoietic and vascular-associated tissue. However, little is known about its exact function. CD34 is also an important adhesion molecule and is required for T cells to enter lymph nodes. It is expressed on lymph node endothelia, whereas the L-selectin to which it binds is on the T cell. Conversely, under other circumstances CD34 has been shown to act as molecular "Teflon" and block mast cell adhesion or to facilitate opening of vascular lumens. Regardless of their mode of action, under all circumstances CD34 and its relatives, podocalyxin and endoglycan, have been shown to facilitate cell migration.
GFP	Ares Labs, Inc GFP-1020	Fluorescent proteins can act as electron donors when excited. According to their proposal published in *Nature Chemical Biology* the excited green chromophore (GFP) donates an electron to an electron acceptor forming a short-lived intermediate. If no electron acceptor is available the intermediate is permanently bleached; however, if it reacts with an electron acceptor the GFP reddens (GFP).
Langerin/CD207 (clone 929 F3.01)	Dendritics DDX 0362	Langerin is a transmembrane mannose-binding protein found on Langerhans cells. It is involved in the formation of Birbeck granules via the internalization of captured antigens at the cell surface. This antibody will help detect Langerin and distinguish between immature dendritic cells and mature dendritic cells.

K1 (AF-109)	Covance PRB-165P	The keratin 1 protein partners with another keratin protein, either keratin 9 or keratin 10, to form molecules called keratin intermediate filaments. These filaments assemble into strong networks that provide strength and resiliency to the skin and protect it from being damaged by friction and other everyday physical stresses.
Cytokeratin 8 (1E8)	Covance MMS-162P	Cytokeratin 8 is a simple epithelial keratin.
K10 (DE-k10)	Covance PRB-159p or MMS-1595	This antibody recognizes keratins in the high molecular weight range and labels squamous, ductal, and other complex epithelia and carcinomas arising from these tissues. It has also been reported to react with benign small-acinar lesions of the prostate. It generally does not react with simple epithelia and reacts variably with adenocarcinomas.
K10/13 (DE-K13)	Covance MMS-1575	The antibody DE-K13 reacts with cytokeratin 10 (56.5 kDa) and cytokeratin 13 (53 kDa). Cytokeratins are a member of intermediate filaments subfamily represented in epithelial tissues. DE-K13 recognizes only cytokeratin 13 on formalin-fixed, paraffin-embedded tissue sections.
K14 (AF-64)	Covance PRB-155P	Keratin 14 partners with a similar protein, keratin 5, to form molecules called keratin intermediate filaments. These filaments assemble into strong networks that help attach keratinocytes together and anchor the epidermis to underlying layers of skin. The network of keratin intermediate filaments provides strength and resiliency to the skin and protects it from being damaged by friction and other everyday physical stresses. Researchers believe that keratin 14 may also play a role in the formation of sweat glands and the development of patterned ridges on the skin of the hands and feet. These ridges, called dermatoglyphs, are the basis for each person's unique fingerprints.
CD11b m1170	BD Bio 553308	An alternative name for CD11b is integrin alpha M or ITGAM. It associates non-covalently with CD18 to form the CR3 integrin. CR3 is highly expressed on leukocytes of the innate immune system, including neutrophils, monocytes, and NK cells, but less so on macrophages. Antibody studies have shown CR3 to mediate inflammation by regulating leukocyte migration and adhesion and to be involved in cell-mediated cytotoxicity, chemotaxis, and other immune processes. It is known to be involved in the complement system and phagocytosis, being a receptor for inactivated complement component 3b (iC3b). Two genome-wide association studies conducted in 2008 showed single-nucleotide polymorphisms of ITGAM to have a strong link to systemic lupus erythematosus. Recent CD11b antibody studies have shown specific functions for the alpha and beta subunits of CR3, with CD11b being directly involved with adhesion and cell migration. However, CD11b expression and, therefore, leukocyte migration are dependent upon the presence of CD18.

(continued)

Table 1 (continued)

Antibody	Source	Purpose
CD11c HL3	BD Bio 553799	CD11c, a member of the leukointegrin family, is expressed prominently on tissue macrophages and dendritic cells and binds to complement fragment (iC3b), provisional matrix molecules (fibrinogen), and the Ig superfamily cell adhesion molecule, ICAM-1. CD11c has been proposed to function in phagocytosis, cell migration, and cytokine production by monocytes/macrophages as well as induction of T cell proliferation by Langerhans cells.
CD14 FMC5-3	BD Bio 55378	CD14 is a surface protein, which is primarily expressed by monocytes and macrophages. CD14 binds lipopolysaccharide-binding protein (LBP) as well as apoptotic cells. CD14 plays a role in the immune response towards bacteria.
CD45 30-F11	BD Bio 553076	CD45 protein tyrosine phosphatase activity plays a central role in T-cell activation. CD45 plays an important role in signal transduction inhibition or upregulation of various immunological functions.
CD44 (IM7)	BD Bio 553131	CD44 *antibody* assays have shown that some isoforms play a role in abnormal gene splicing in human cells. In immunobiology, CD44 is a valuable marker for memory cells, since B-cell and T-cell activation in the immune response leads to high expression of CD44. The protein is bound to hyaluronic acid in the extracellular matrix. When an antigen triggers the immune response and activates the T-helper cells, CD44 activity is increased by up-regulation. However, despite its usefulness as a marker protein, its role in the immune response has remained elusive. Recently, scientists at the Sanford-Burnham Medical Research Institute discovered that CD44 can assist a specific subset of T-helper cells, Th1, to actualize immunologic memory. The study showed that in the absence of CD44, Th1 cells tagged to an influenza virus fragment underwent rapid autophagy, thus blocking the development of immunologic memory.
K8	Covance	This gene is a member of the type II keratin family clustered on the long arm of chromosome 12. Type I and type II keratins heteropolymerize to form intermediate-sized filaments in the cytoplasm of epithelial cells. The product of this gene typically dimerizes with keratin 18 to form an intermediate filament in simple single-layered epithelial cells. This protein plays a role in maintaining cellular structural integrity and also functions in signal transduction and cellular differentiation. Mutations in this gene cause cryptogenic cirrhosis [provided by RefSeq].
K13	Covance	Cytokeratin 13 belongs to the intermediate filament family and is a heterotetramer of two type I acidic and two type II basic keratins. It is generally associated with cytokeratin 4. Defects in the KRT13 gene are a cause of white sponge nevus (WSN) of cannon, a rare autosomal dominant disorder which predominantly affects noncornified stratified squamous epithelia and is characterized by the presence of soft, white, and spongy plaques in the oral mucosa.

2. Mass culture dishes can be fixed with ice-cold (−20 °C) acetone:methanol (50:50) for 10–15 min at −20 °C. Dishes may then be processed using standard immunofluorescence (IF) protocols with antibodies of interest.
3. After staining, the sides of the dishes are removed and the bottom of each dish with intact cells can be mounted onto glass slides or cartridges and viewed for microscopic analysis. Using IHC or IF can provide semiquantitative data.

3.3 3T3 Feeder Layer

3.3.1 Initialization of 3T3 Cell Line

1. Quickly thaw one vial containing frozen 3T3 cells from the liquid nitrogen canister by placing vial in 37 °C water bath until slightly thawed. Remove vial when most of the ice has melted. Wipe the tube with a 70 % alcohol swab and in a biosafety cabinet or a laminar flow hood, place the entire contents into a T-150 flask, and rinse the 3T3 vial with 1 ml 3T3 CGM (**Note** 7). Add 30 ml of pre-warmed CGM to the cells slowly. Gently rock flask to evenly spread the cells. Label the flask with cell line, date, and passage number of the cells. Incubate at 37 °C with 5 % CO_2 and 95 % humidified air.
2. Change medium in 24 h to remove dead cells and DMSO cryopreservation agent. After the first medium change, the medium is changed twice weekly. The cells are only allowed to proliferate to 80 % confluence.
3. T-150 flasks are used for culture initialization. T-225 flasks are used for subculture after initialization.

3.3.2 Subculturing the 3T3 Cell Line

1. Remove flask from incubator, aspirate media, and wash twice with cold sterile PBS with gentamicin. Pipet 10 ml of pre-warmed (37 °C water bath) 0.25 % trypsin solution into each flask. Place flask on a 37 °C warming tray. Observe cells every 30 s under an inverted microscope to look for detachment of cells from growth surface. Continue to incubate until many of the cells have detached. Trypsin solution may be cloudy with detached cells. Not all cells need to detach.
2. Pipet the trypsin solution three times, washing the growth surface of the flask. Remove the trypsin solution containing the cells and place in 30 ml of CGM in a 50 ml conical tube. Rewash the growth surface of the flask 3–5 times with 10 ml of the CGM–trypsin–cell mixture from the conical tube. Two flask's contents can be placed in one 50 ml conical tube; if only one flask is used, then place the 10 ml of trypsin/cells into 20 ml CGM in a 50 ml conical tube.
3. Centrifuge at $160 \times g$ for 7 min at 4 °C.
4. Aspirate supernatant fraction and re-suspend cell pellet with 5 ml of CGM triturating gently ten times. Add 10 ml of CGM to bring total volume in the 50 ml conical tube to 15 ml.

Triturate again ten times, and place 5 ml of cell suspension into each of 3T-150 flasks. The subculture ratio is 1:3 in T-150 flasks or 1:4 in T-225 flasks. Add 30 ml of pre-warmed 3T3 CGM to each of the flasks.

5. Label flask with cell line, date, and passage number.

3.3.3 Freezing the 3T3 Cell Line

1. Follow methods of subculturing 3T3 cells up to **step 3**.
2. Remove tube from centrifuge and place on ice. Aspirate supernatant fraction, and re-suspend cell pellet with 1 ml DMSO–DMEM for each flask harvested.
3. Place 1 ml of DMSO–DMEM with cell suspension into each cryovial (one cryovial for each flask harvested). Label vial with passage number, cell line (3T3), and date they were frozen.
4. Place vials into Nalgene cell freezer and place in a –70 °C freezer for 1–2 days. Remove vials and place in liquid nitrogen storage tank for long-term storage. Put cryovial information and location on liquid nitrogen inventory sheet.

3.3.4 Irradiation and Seeding of the 3T3 Feeder Layer

1. One week prior to irradiation of cells, allow cells in flasks to grow to 100 % confluence. The cells used are normally within passages of 120–130.
2. For the clonogenic assay, coating the 60-mm Petri dishes with a Purecol-fibronectin (collagen) coating BEFORE seeding 3T3 cells is necessary. Place just enough of the collagen-coating solution into a dish to coat the bottom (around 2–3 ml), and then remove any excess amounts of the collagen-coating liquid. Place in an incubator at 37 °C and 5 % CO_2 for a minimum of 1 h or a maximum of 6 h (**Note 5**). Dishes do not need to be dry.
3. On the day of irradiation, follow "Subculturing of 3 T3 cells" **steps 1–3**. Re-suspend cell pellet in 50 ml fresh CGM, close conical tube, and seal with parafilm. Use Ziploc plastic bags to double bag the parafilm-sealed tube and place on ice at 2–4 °C. If cells will be on ice for >2 h, then a cold starting temperature of –10 °C works best so that by the end of a 4-h period of time the cells are not likely to warm up above 10 °C.
4. The cells within the 50 ml conical tube are irradiated with 5,000 RADS (50 cGy) using a biological X-ray machine. The entire 50 ml conical tube with medium can be irradiated. Depending on the machine, this procedure can take up to an hour.
5. After irradiation, centrifuge cells at $160 \times g$ for 7 min. Aspirate the supernatant fraction and re-suspend cell pellet with 5 ml of CGM, triturating gently ten times. Add an additional 25 ml of medium to bring the total volume to 30 ml and triturate ten times.

6. Remove approximately 0.5 ml of the cell mixture and place into a small sterile tube. Remove 200 μl of this cell mixture and mix in 200 μl of 0.4 % trypan blue solution. Pipet this mixture three times gently. Place cells within a hemacytometer, and count all nucleated cells. All dark or blue cells are scored as nonviable, whereas small gold cells are scored as viable.
7. Calculate the number of viable cells and the cell concentration.
8. Pipet 1×10^6 cells (a minimum of 7×10^5 cells may be used) in 4 ml of modified high-calcium Williams E medium into 60-mm collagen-coated Petri dishes. Allow cells to attach for 24 h prior to seeding primary keratinocytes for clonogenic assay.

3.3.5 Setup and Maintenance of Clonal Cultures

1. For clonogenic assays, cells are seeded at 1×10^3 cells in 4 ml per 60-mm dish on an irradiated 3T3 feeder layer with collagen coating and modified William's E medium with supplements and serum (**Note 8**).
2. For clonal cultures, the first medium change is 2 days after seeding and three times weekly thereafter. Care needs to be taken during media changes because the 3T3 feeder layer is delicate and can easily be peeled up if media is pipetted too quickly (**Note 9**).
3. Typically, clonal cultures are cultivated for 2- and 4-week intervals. At these time points, the medium is aspirated and the cultures fixed in 10 % buffered formalin overnight.
4. After fixation, cultures are stained for a minimum of 1 h with 0.5 % rhodamine B in distilled water. The stain is then removed, and the dishes are rinsed in cold distilled water until the dishes run clear and no excess stain is present. Colonies are counted when dishes are dry.
5. When the dishes are dry, the total numbers of keratinocyte colonies are recorded. In addition, the diameters of colonies are measured with calipers and recorded as <1 mm, 1–2 mm, and >2 mm.
6. Sterile, sorted clonal cultures may also be performed. Cells are prepared following the FACS procedure below. The sorted keratinocytes can be counted and seeded directly from the BD FACSAria II onto the 60-mm dish.

3.3.6 Analysis of Clonal Cultures (Counting and Measuring Colonies)

1. Fixed and stained keratinocyte colonies 0.5 mm in diameter are counted manually with a Manostat counter. Colonies are verified by light microscopic inspection and by comparison with 3T3-only controls conducted in each experiment. As needed, the diameter of each colony is measured with a caliper, the area is calculated, and a size distribution is determined.
2. In some experiments, clonal cultures may be treated to determine the effects of various biological or xenobiotic agents on

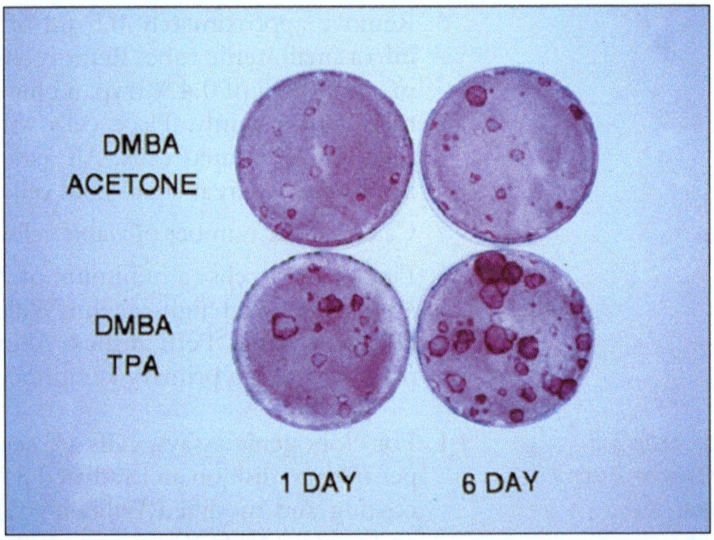

Fig. 3 Assay for ex vivo clonogenic keratinocytes from adult mice. This figure illustrates the results of a typical keratinocyte colony assay where the mice were pretreated with either acetone (control) or DMBA (test group) followed 1 week later by either acetone (control) or the tumor promoter, TPA (test group). Note the effects of the different in vivo treatments on the colony size and number. Such experiments are usually quantified by counting and measuring the colonies

the number and size of the colonies. The colonies are counted and sized as described above. Figure 3 demonstrates one such experiment where the mice were treated with acetone, DMBA, or TPA prior to harvesting and clonal culture.

3.4 Fluorescent-Activated Cell Sorting and Cell Cycle Analysis

3.4.1 Preparation of Keratinocyte Cells

1. Process all harvest and staining steps (for either sterile or non-sterile sorts) in a Class II biological safety cabinet using aseptic technique.
2. At 24 h before sorting: place 4 ml of sterile SMEM + 20 % FBS + 2× gentamicin into 4–8 sterile 5 ml RB tube for sorting collection, put cap on, and place at 4 °C overnight. Remove 3 ml of solution from each tube the next morning, and give the tube to the cytometry technician for cell sorting. Coating the dishes helps to increase viability during the sorting process.
3. Label all control and sample tubes as well as collection tubes prior to staining cells for FACS sorting.
4. Determine the number of sorted cells you will need for your assay. For the typical FACS assay using CD34 and CD49f, calculate and obtain at least a total of 34×10^6 keratinocytes from the harvest (use 2–3 mice). If more cells are required, use the approximate distributions of cells in each population,

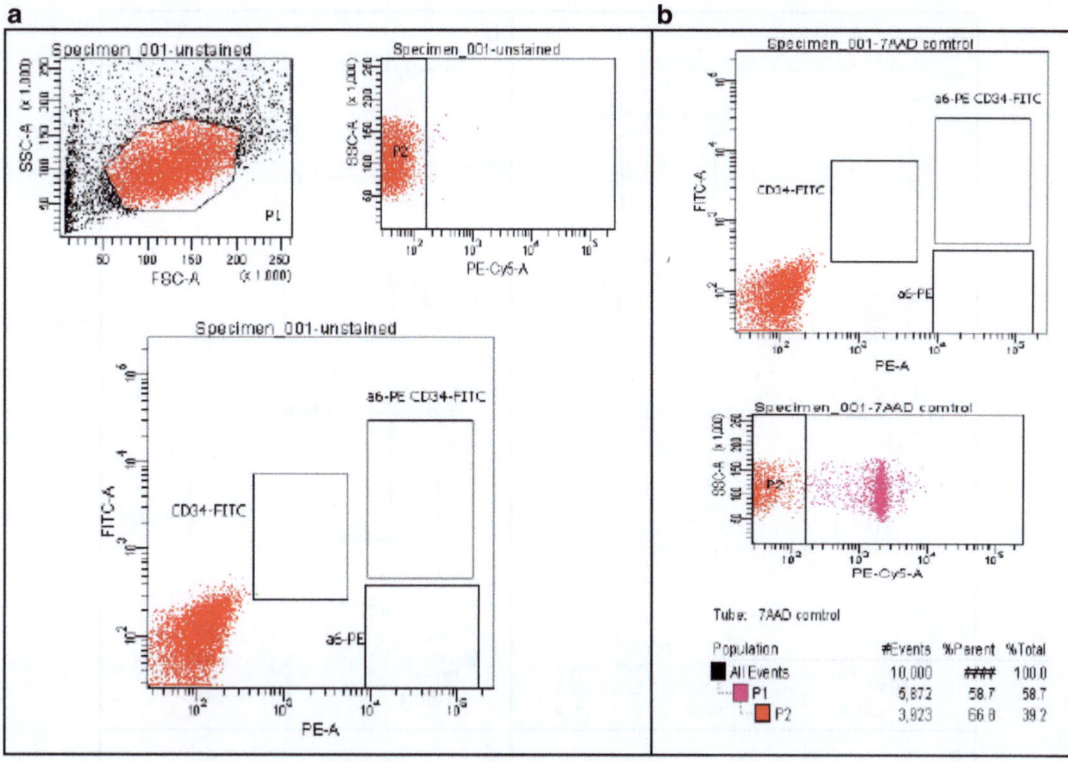

Fig. 4 FACS sorting controls. This figure is a typical scatterplot of unstained epidermal keratinocytes from adult mice (**a**) and keratinocytes stained with 7-AAD to determine viability (**b**). 7-AAD is a fluorescent dye that reacts with compromised or dead cells. Our typical presort viability averages about 73 %, and post-sort viabilities average 77 % for CD49f+/CD34+ hair follicle stem cells, 61 % for CD49f+basal cells alone, and 66 % for CD34+ alone

cell viability, and account for cells used in control tubes to determine the appropriate number of mice needed.

(a) Sort using live cells only. Viability is typically 75–90 % (Fig. 4).

(b) Number of cells required for FACS with CD34 and CD49f (Fig. 5).

- Control tubes: Re-suspend 0.5–1.0 × 10^6 cells/ml in harvesting medium, minimum volume of 500 μl.
- Sample tubes: Re-suspend up to 14.0 × 10^6 cells/ml in harvesting medium, minimum volume of 1 ml.

(c) Approximate distribution of cells for FACS with CD34/CD49f (Fig. 6):

- 1–2 % CD34+/CD49f–
- 3–11 % CD34-/CD49f–

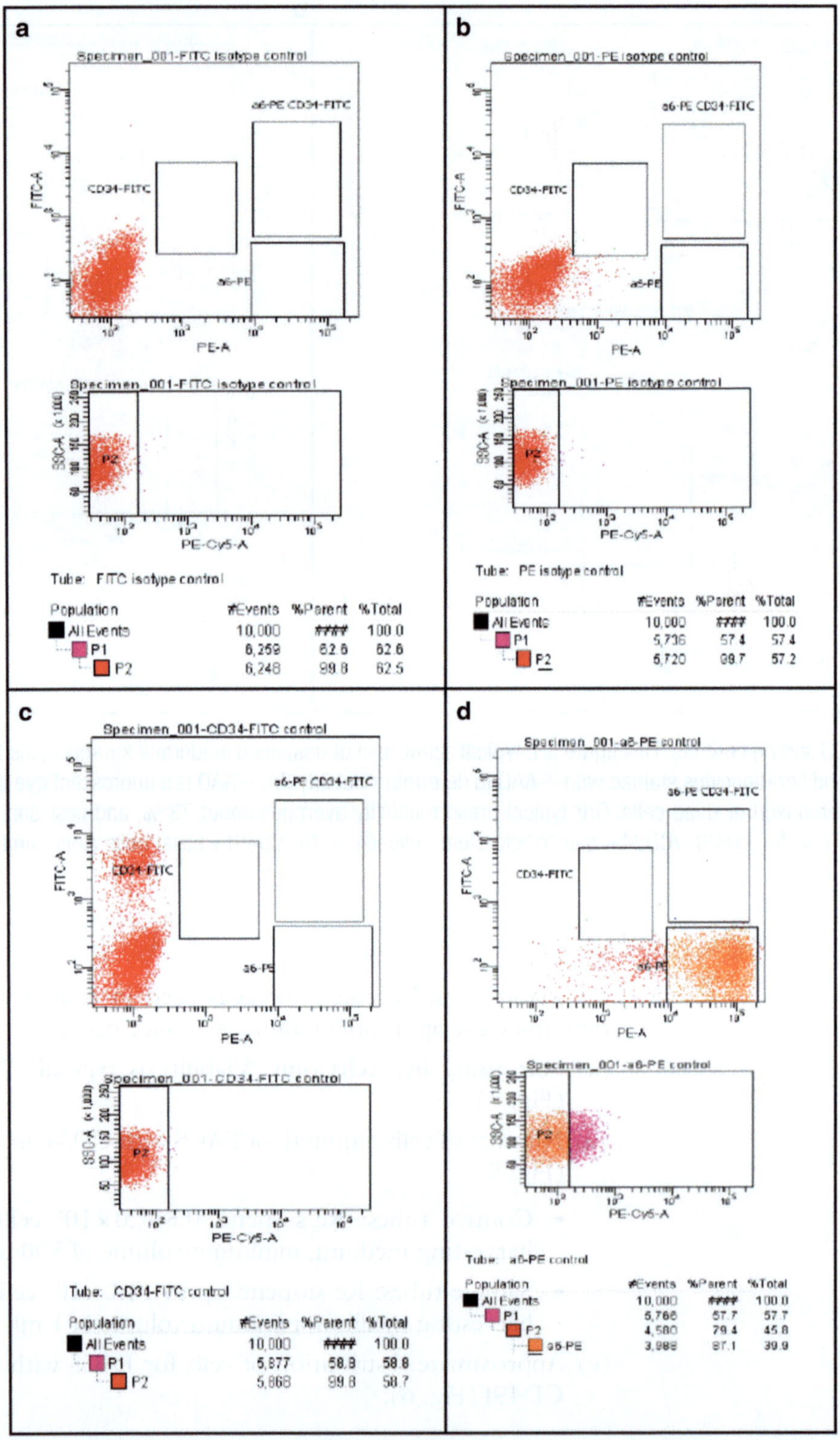

Fig. 5 FACS sorting controls. This figure demonstrates typical FACS sorting isotype controls in preparation for sorting CD49f+/CD34+ epidermal keratinocytes from adult mice. (**a**) FITC; (**b**) PE; (**c**) CD34-FITC alone; (**d**) CD49f-PE alone

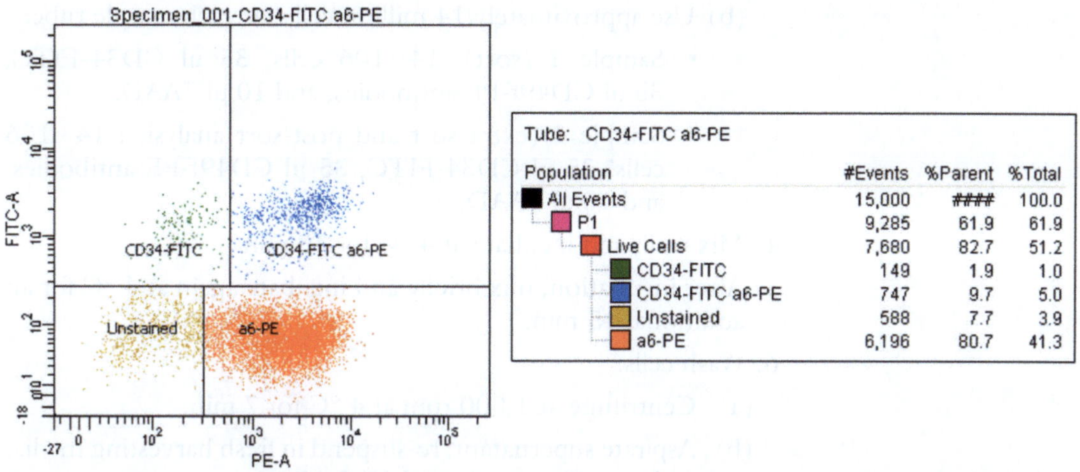

Fig. 6 FACS scatterplot demonstrating the typical distribution of CD34 and CD49f (alpha 6-integrin) immunoreactivities of epidermal keratinocytes. The relative percentages of the four major subpopulations are given in the accompanying chart. Note that the double-stained stem cell population is about 5 % of the total viable cells

- 8–10 % CD34+/CD49f+
- 80–85 % CD34-/CD49f+

5. Harvest epidermal keratinocytes from adult mice as previously mentioned through **step 15**.
6. Centrifuge original tube of epidermal keratinocytes for 7 min at 1,000 rpm at 4 °C.
7. Re-suspend cells in harvesting medium to a concentration of 1×10^6 cells/ml in a 50 ml conical tube.

3.4.2 CD34 and CD49f (Alpha6 Integrin) Staining

1. Items are light sensitive after this step. Protect from light until after sorting process is complete.
2. Add antibodies in the amounts below to corresponding tubes. After aliquoting the antibodies, add the keratinocytes.
3. When staining, numbering the tubes in this order (Fig. 5) is helpful:

   (a) Use 0.5–1×10^6 cells for each control tube:

   - Unstained keratinocyte control: 1 ml cells.
   - 7AAD control (exclusion of dead cells): 1 ml cells and 10 μl 7AAD.
   - PE isotype control: 1 ml cells and 10 μl Rat IgG_{2a}, kappa–PE conjugate.
   - FITC isotype control: 1 ml cells and 10 μl Rat IgG_{2a}, kappa–FITC conjugate.
   - CD49f-PE control: 1 ml cells and 10 μl CD49f-PE.
   - CD34-FITC control: 1 ml + 10 μl CD34-FITC.

(b) Use approximately 14 million cells for each sample tube:
   - Sample 1 (sort): 14×106 cells, 35 µl CD34-FITC, 35 µl CD49f-PE antibodies, and 10 µl 7AAD.
   - Sample 2 (extra sort and post-sort analysis): 14×106 cells, 35 µl CD34-FITC, 35 µl CD49f-PE antibodies, and 10 µl 7AAD.

4. Mix well, and incubate at 4 °C for 45 min.
5. After incubation, mix briefly and incubate again at 4 °C for an additional 45 min.
6. Wash cells:
   (a) Centrifuge at 1,000 rpm at 4 °C for 7 min.
   (b) Aspirate supernatant, re-suspend in fresh harvesting media, and centrifuge again at 4 °C for 7 min.
   (c) Aspirate supernatant fraction, re-suspend control tubes with 1 ml, and sample tubes with 2–4 ml harvesting medium.
7. Filter cells with a flow cytometry cell strainer cap (or 40 µm sterile cell strainer) over a sterile 5 ml RB test tube before sorting.
   (a) Post-sort analysis tube: Remove 0.5 ml of cells from sample 2 (tube 8) and during filtering step place it into a separate sterile 5 ml RB tube, add 1 ml harvesting medium, and label "Post-Sort Analysis."
8. Place all tubes on ICE in a box that protects from light.
9. Take cells to cytometry department for sterile or non-sterile sorting. Non-sterile sorting usually takes about 1–2 h; sterile sorting usually takes 1.5 or more hours.
10. To prevent serious cell aggregation before and during FACS, you may use DNAse or HBSS + 1 % BSA (or 1 % FCS); you may also refilter cells as needed through a new flow cytometry cell strainer cap over a sterile 5 ml round-bottom test tube (**Note 10**).

3.4.3 Setup of Instruments: BD FACS Aria II

1. Sorting is performed on a BD ARIA II Special Order System. Drop delay is set using BD Accudrop beads.
2. 100-µm nozzle is used at a default pressure of 20 psi.
3. Laser delays and area scaling are set using CS&T beats.

3.4.4 Analysis of Cell Cycle

1. Cells are harvested with 0.25 % trypsin + 5 mM EDTA in PBS, with 2.5 % FBS + 5 mM EDTA added when cells are detached.
2. After washing with PBS, the cells are re-suspended in 0.4 ml of PBS and 1 ml of ice-cold absolute ethanol.
3. Cells are fixed and kept at −20 °C for a minimum of 2 h followed by a PBS wash.

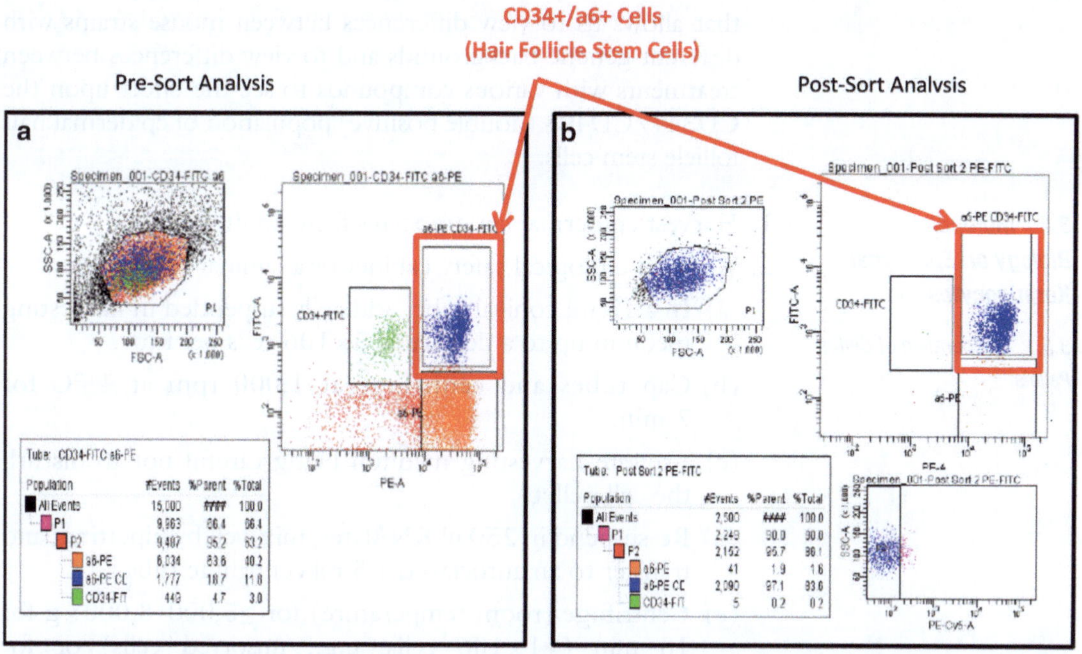

Fig. 7 FACS scatterplots demonstrating the importance of conducting pre- and post-sort analyses. (**a**) Illustrates that about 12 % of the total cells are double positive before the sort but (**b**) are enriched to 84 % after the sort. In some cases, the cells may be sorted again to purify the stem cells further

4. Incubate with 20 μg/ml of propidium iodide and 200 μg/ml of RNase A for 30 min at room temperature in the dark.
5. Cells are analyzed on the BD FACSCalibur flow cytometer. Intact cells are gated in the FSC/SSC plot to exclude small debris. Cell cycle is determined using ModFit software.

3.4.5 Interpreting Scatterplots

1. Cells are analyzed by flow cytometry on a FACSAria II (Becton Dickinson, San Jose, CA). 7-AAD is added to identify cells with permeable membranes (dead cells). Initial gating is set on an FSC-A vs. SSC-A dot plot to exclude debris. Doublets are excluded with SSC-H vs. SSC-W and FSC-H vs. FSC-W dot plots. Membrane-permeable cells are excluded using an SSC-A vs. 7-AAD dot plot (7-AAD ex: 561 nm, detection: 660/20 nm).
2. Post-sort analysis tests the efficiency of the sort and is conducted by sorting the cells and then running each population of sorted cells again to determine the purity of the sample (Fig. 7).
3. Data from FACS sorting with CD34 and CD49f antibodies are useful in many ways. We can see differences between the compositions of cell populations within the CD34/CD49f quadrants with the use of additional antibodies. We can see differences in the percent distribution among the CD34/CD49f quadrants

that allows us to view differences between mouse strains with different genetic backgrounds and to view differences between treatments with various compounds to see the effect upon the CD34+/CD49+ (double positive) population of epidermal hair follicle stem cells.

3.5 Molecular Biology on Epidermal Keratinocytes

3.5.1 Preparation of Cell Pellets

1. Harvest epidermal keratinocytes from adult mice.
2. Within a biological safety cabinet or a laminar flow hood:
   (a) In a 15 ml conical tube, add cells suspended in harvesting medium up to a density of 5 × 106 cells per tube.
   (b) Cap tubes and centrifuge at 1,000 rpm at 4 °C for 7 min.
   (c) Aspirate harvesting medium being careful not to disturb the cell pellet.
   (d) Re-suspend in 250 μl RNAlater, mix well by pipetting, and transfer to an autoclaved 1.5 ml centrifuge tube.
   (e) Centrifuge (room temperature) for ≥5,000–8,000 × g for 10 min (≥1 × 106 cells, e.g., unsorted cells) or for 20–30 min (<1 × 106 cells, e.g., sorted cells).
   (f) Aspirate RNAlater being extremely careful not to disturb the cell pellet.
   (g) Close the cap on the centrifuge tube, and either proceed immediately to RNA isolation or store at –80 °C.
   (h) If needed, the pellet can further be washed using 70 % ETOH and solubilized in nuclease-free water.

3.5.2 Preparation of RNA

1. Make sure that cells are pelleted at concentrations less than 5×10^6 cells.
2. Follow the instructions from Qiagen Sciences (Germantown, MD, USA).
   (a) Use the RNeasy Mini kit (1 × 106 to 5 × 106 cells) for unsorted cells and tissues.
   (b) Use the RNeasy Micro Kit (<1 × 106 cells) for FACS-sorted cells.
   (c) To isolate total RNA, RNAlater is completely removed leaving only the cell pellet in the tube. Trizol reagent is added directly to the cell pellet, and RNA is isolated as per the manufacturer's instructions. The RNA is washed using 70 % ETOH and solubilized in nuclease-free water (Ambion).
3. Once RNA is isolated, ultraviolet spectroscopy is used to calculate the concentration of material. Do this before freezing the sample for the first time to avoid unnecessary freeze–thaw cycles (**Note 11**).

4. UV spectroscopy:
   (a) Add 2 μl RNA sample to 98 μl of RNase-free water and in a separate tube, add only 100 μl of RNase-free water as a "blank."
   (b) Set up spectrometer for single-cell holder, and select single-cell holder on screen.
   (c) Pre-warm the UV lamp for 5 min, and set up computer software to read for RNA.
   (d) Take readings at 260 and 280 nm absorption values.
   (e) Add the contents of the "blank" tube to a clean cuvette.
   (f) Use the software to blank the machine. Once the machine is zeroed, record three readings.
   (g) Load each 100 μl diluted RNA sample into a clean cuvette, and record three readings for each sample.
   (h) Save and print all data when complete; clean up, turn off the UV lamp, and return the machine to default settings.
   (i) To clean cuvettes, aspirate any liquid, add enough 100 % ethanol to fill, let soak for a couple of minutes, and then aspirate again. Next, add enough methanol to fill, let soak for a couple of minutes, then aspirate methanol, and air-dry completely.
5. Determine the concentration of RNA:
   (a) Using the 260 nm absorption values, take the average of the three readings per sample.
   (b) Multiply the average absorbance value at 260 nm by 40 (RNA factor).
   (c) Multiply again by 50 (dilution factor).
   (d) Resulting number will be the concentration of RNA in ng/μl.
   (e) Divide the concentration of RNA in ng/μl by 1,000 for concentration of RNA in μg/ml.
   (f) To determine the entire amount of RNA isolated, multiply the concentration of RNA in ng/ μl by the volume used to elute the RNA from the spin column during the final step of the Qiagen RNeasy protocol.
       - Subtract 2 μl before multiplication to account for loss from determining the concentration of RNA.
       - RNeasy Mini kit elutes with 30 μl of water.
       - RNeasy Micro kit elutes with 14 μl of water, but 2 μl remain on the filter. Realistically, 12 μl are eluted.
   (g) To determine the quality of the RNA, compare the ratio of the 260 nm Abs and 280 nm Abs readings.

*3.5.3 Preparation of DNA (**Note 12**)*

1. For RT-PCR with keratinocytes, use 100 ng (or 0.1 μg) of RNA for cDNA synthesis (**Note 13**).
   (a) Multiply 0.1 μg by the concentration of RNA in μg/ml (measured and calculated from UV spectroscopy).
   (b) This gives you the amount of RNA (in microliters) that needs to be used in the PCR reaction to synthesize cDNA.
2. Synthesize cDNA
   (a) Step 1: Total reaction volume 25 μl.
      - In MicroAmp tube strip, add appropriate mRNA and water as calculated to reach 24 μl volume.
      - Add 1 μl Oligo DT.
      - Put in thermocycler, and set to run at 80 °C for 10 min.

   (b) Step 2: Total reaction volume 40 μl.
      - Place tube strip on ice for 10 min.
      - During incubation, prepare master mix, multiplying the amounts below as necessary for the correct number of reactions:
        - 1 μl RNase Out
        - 4 μl 10× RT buffer
        - 2 μl 10 mM dNTPs
        - 4 μl 0.1 M dTT
        - 1 μl Superscript II enzyme
        - 3 μl MQ H_2O
      - After incubation, add 15 μl of master mix to each reaction tube.
      - Place tube strip in thermocycler at 42 °C for 2 h and then at 85 °C for 5 min.

   (c) Step 3: Total reaction volume 41 μl.
      - Add 1 μl of RNase H to each reaction tube.
      - Place tube strip in thermocycler at 37 °C for 20 min.

   (d) Dilute to working concentration by adding 109 μl RNase-free water to cDNA in a new 2 ml centrifuge tube.
      - The diluted cDNA can be stored at 4 °C for up to a week, –20 ° C for up to 3 months, and at –80 ° C for long-term storage.

3.5.4 Preparation of RT-PCR

1. Plan experiment with intended primer pairs for genes of interest and include a housekeeping gene (GapdH or Actb works well for keratinocytes).

2. Prepare RT-PCR reactions:
   (a) Dilute primers to 15 pmol/μl.
   (b) For each set of primers, prepare a master mix, multiplying the amounts below as necessary for the correct number of reactions. We typically allow for triplicate sampling:
      - 12.5 μl SYBR green
      - 2 μl forward primer (at 15 pmol/μl)
      - 2 μl reverse primer (at 15 pmol/μl)
      - 28.5 μl MQ H_2O
   (c) For control against SYBR green: 12.5 μl SYBR green + 32.5 μl water = 45 μl of master mix.
   (d) For control water use 50 μl ddH_2O (MQ H_2O).
   (e) Using MicroAmp RT-PCR optical tube strips, add 45 μl of master mix or controls to respective wells, allowing for three wells per gene for each cDNA sample.
   (f) Add 5 μl of cDNA to respective sample wells and SYBR green control well for a total of 50 μl of sample per tube.
3. Run RT-PCR:
   (a) Add samples to GeneAmp 9700 RT-PCR machine.
   (b) Determine the appropriate annealing temperatures by averaging the melting temperatures of all the primers in use and subtracting an additional 5 °C (**Note 14**).
   (c) Set up the program to detect SYBR Green and to run the following cycle:
      - 1 repetition of 50.0 °C for 2 min.
      - 1 repetition of 95.0 °C for 10 min.
      - 40 repetitions of 95.0 °C for 15 s, determined annealing temperature for 1 min.
      - 1 repetition of 95.0 °C for 15 s, determined annealing temperature for 1 min, 95.0 °C for 15 s, 60.0 °C for 15 s.

3.5.5 Analysis of RT-PCR

1. Determine the fold change for each gene of interest:
   (a) Determine the average Ct of the housekeeping gene where Ct is the threshold cycle, a relative measure of the concentration of the target in the PCR reaction.
   (b) Take each raw Ct for the genes of interest, and subtract the average of the housekeeping gene. This is the DCt, the difference in the threshold cycle compared to the housekeeping gene.
   (c) Determine [–DCt] by taking $0.5D^{C}t$.

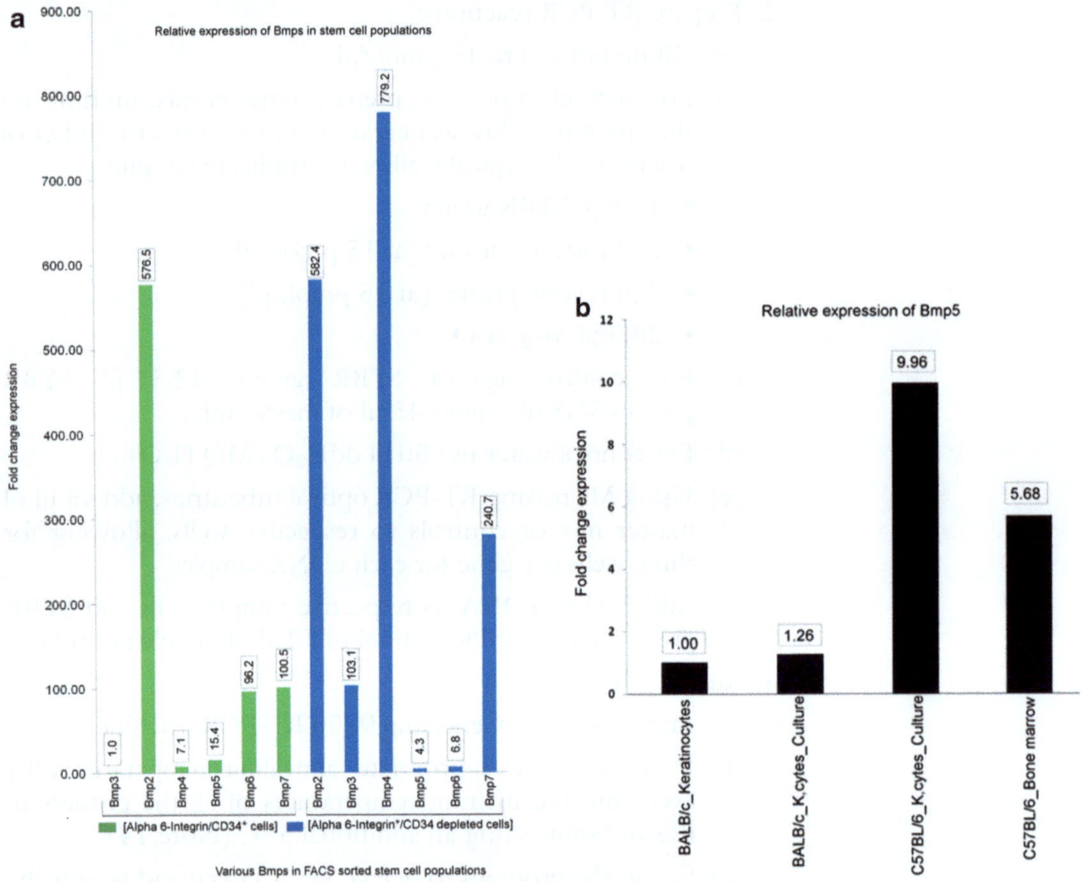

Fig. 8 Quantitative real-time PCR of epidermal keratinocytes. (**a**) Shows the expression of several bone morphogenic proteins (BMPs) in epidermal keratinocytes freshly harvested and FACS sorted from adult mice to enrich for CD49f+/CD34+ double-positive and CD34-depleted subpopulations. (**b**) Illustrates BMP5 expression in epidermal keratinocytes before and after culture

(d) Multiply [−DCt] by 1,000,000 to obtain R.A. R.A. is the relative abundance of the target mRNA expression compared to the housekeeping gene.

(e) Average the R.A. for each gene to give the average fold change.

2. Figure 8 illustrates an example of quantitative real-time PCR applied to FACS-sorted, freshly harvested keratinocytes without culture or following culture.

4 Notes and Troubleshooting

1. If male mice are used, they must be housed singly because otherwise they fight and inflict skin damage that can interfere with culture assays.

2. The outlined procedure can be used for single mice also. The only change to the procedure would be the final dilution of the cell suspension. Instead of 30 ml, use 10 ml for the main suspension and a 1:20 dilution for counting in a hemacytometer.
3. Mice with light fur will retain a yellow color from the iodine that is not noticeable with mice with dark fur. The yellow color does not cause any obvious changes in cell viability or in growth in culture. Do not use iodine scrub because the included detergent will kill the keratinocytes.
4. Trypsinization time and temperature are critical for obtaining good yields of highly culturable cells. Although other methods may provide good yields of viable cells, the culturability of the keratinocytes has been less satisfactory in our hands when trypsinized at 37 °C or at 4 °C overnight.
5. Coating of culture dishes is very important for attachment, spreading, and ultimate growth of epidermal cells from adult mice.
6. During the epidermal scraping step, keeping the blade perpendicular to the skin is imperative. If the blade is angled toward the motion of the blade, a tendency to tear the tissue will occur. If the blade is angled away from the motion of the blade, an insufficient amount of the epidermis will be removed.
7. DMEM purchased from ATCC is formulated with reduced levels of sodium bicarbonate and is intended for use in 5 % CO_2.
8. When performing a quantitative clonal assay, we have found that never pipetting less than 1 ml of cells is helpful. Thus, if cells in the first 30 ml dilution (see Sect. 3.2, **step 14**) are concentrated, then serial dilutions should be made to the cloning dilution.
9. Media should be changed on no more than eight dishes at a time; any more than that and the cells tend to dry out and become stressed. Pipetting fresh media should also be conducted with great care. A rate of 1 ml per 7–10 s is optimal when using a 5 ml pipette.
10. All controls and samples should be kept chilled throughout the entire sorting process.
11. RNA is less stable than cDNA, and the likelihood that sample integrity is weakened increases until synthesized into cDNA; multiple freeze–thaw cycles should be avoided, but if stored properly, purified RNA from RNeasy kits can successfully be stored at –70 °C for about a year without degradation.
12. Our laboratory generally makes cDNA on the same day that the RNA is isolated.

13. The amount of cDNA synthesized is directly proportional to the amount of RNA used. Optimized use with keratinocytes suggests that best performance occurs with one reaction per 100 ng of mRNA.
14. The annealing temperature should be lower than the lowest individual primer melting temperature.

5 Summary

In summary, preparations of freshly harvested epidermal cells from treated or untreated adult mice are useful for downstream applications such as clonal culture, FACS, molecular biology, or other readouts involving adult tissue stem cells in the context of carcinogenesis or chemoprevention. The harvesting methods described here were developed to give reproducible yields of highly culturable cells with the goal of faithfully enabling their functions ex vivo.

References

1. Morris RJ, Tacker KC, Fischer SM, Slaga TJ (1988) Quantitation of primary in vitro clonogenic keratinocytes from normal adult murine epidermis, following initiation, and during promotion of epidermal tumors. Cancer Res 48(22):6285–6290
2. Wu WY, Morris RJ (2005) Method for the harvest and assay of in vitro clonogenic keratinocytes stem cells from mice. Methods Mol Biol 289:79–86
3. Popova NV, Teti KA, Wu KQ, Morris RJ (2003) Identification of two keratinocyte stem cell regulatory loci implicated in skin carcinogenesis. Carcinogenesis 24(3):417–425
4. Popova NV, Tryson KA, Wu KQ, Morris RJ (2002) Evidence that the keratinocyte colony number is genetically controlled. Exp Dermatol 11(6):503–508
5. Tani H, Morris RJ, Kaur P (2000) Enrichment for murine keratinocyte stem cells based on cell surface phenotype. Proc Natl Acad Sci U S A 97(20):10960–10965
6. Trempus CS, Morris RJ, Bortner CD, Cotsarelis G, Faircloth RS, Reece JM, Tennant RW (2003) Enrichment for living murine keratinocytes from the hair follicle bulge with the cell surface marker CD34. J Invest Dermatol 120(4):501–511. doi:10.1046/j.1523-1747.2003.12088.x
7. Morris RJ, Liu Y, Marles L, Yang Z, Trempus C, Li S, Lin JS, Sawicki JA, Cotsarelis G (2004) Capturing and profiling adult hair follicle stem cells. Nat Biotechnol 22(4):411–417. doi:10.1038/nbt950
8. Trempus CS, Dang H, Humble MM, Wei SJ, Gerdes MJ, Morris RJ, Bortner CD, Cotsarelis G, Tennant RW (2007) Comprehensive microarray transcriptome profiling of CD34-enriched mouse keratinocyte stem cells. J Invest Dermatol 127(12):2904–2907. doi:10.1038/sj.jid.5700917
9. Baer-Dubowska W, Morris RJ, Gill RD, DiGiovanni J (1990) Distribution of covalent DNA adducts in mouse epidermal subpopulations after topical application of benzo(a)pyrene and 7,12-dimethylbenz(a)anthracene. Cancer Res 50(10):3048–3054

Chapter 11

Quantitation of Acetaldehyde-DNA Adducts: Biomarkers of Alcohol Consumption

Silvia Balbo and Stephen S. Hecht

Abstract

DNA adduct measurements provide valuable information about DNA damage associated with exposure to specific genotoxicants. N^2-Ethylidene-dGuo, the major DNA adduct formed upon reaction of acetaldehyde with DNA, has been used to investigate mechanisms of alcohol carcinogenesis focusing on the effects of acetaldehyde, the primary metabolite of ethanol. N^2-Ethylidene-dGuo is stable in DNA, but it easily degrades when released as a nucleoside. A liquid-chromatography-electrospray ionization-tandem mass spectrometry-selected reaction monitoring (LC-ESI-MS/MS-SRM) method for the analysis of N^2-Ethylidene-dGuo as its reduced form N^2-ethyl-dGuo has been developed. This assay is based on addition of the reducing agent $NaBH_3CN$ to the DNA before hydrolysis and on the use of a ^{15}N-labeled analog of N^2-ethyl-dGuo as an internal standard. The addition of the reducing agent and internal standard are followed by enzymatic hydrolysis and sample purification and enrichment. This chapter provides detailed step-by-step information on the analysis of N^2-ethyl-dGuo in DNA by LC-ESI-MS/MS-SRM. The protocol described easily can be applied to DNA isolated from different tissues and cell types and on DNA amounts as low as 5–10 μg.

Key words Alcohol, Acetaldehyde, DNA adduct, Enzymatic hydrolysis, Solid-phase extraction, LC-ESI-MS/MS-SRM

1 Introduction

Alcohol consumption is a recognized cancer risk factor. A causal link has been established between alcohol drinking and cancers of the oral cavity, pharynx, esophagus, colon, rectum, liver, larynx, and breast [1]. A recent study estimated alcohol consumption to result in 3.2–3.7 % of all cancer deaths in the USA [2]. Another study focusing on Western Europe has raised the incidence of total cancer attributable to alcohol consumption to 10 % in men and 3 % in women. For selected cancers the figures were 44 and 25 % for upper aerodigestive tract, 33 and 18 % for liver, and 17 and 4 % for colorectal cancer for men and women, respectively, and 5.0 % for female breast cancer [3]. Despite this clear association between

Ann M. Bode and Zigang Dong (eds.), *Cancer Prevention: Dietary Factors and Pharmacology*, Methods in Pharmacology and Toxicology, DOI 10.1007/978-1-4614-9227-6_11, © Springer Science+Business Media New York 2014

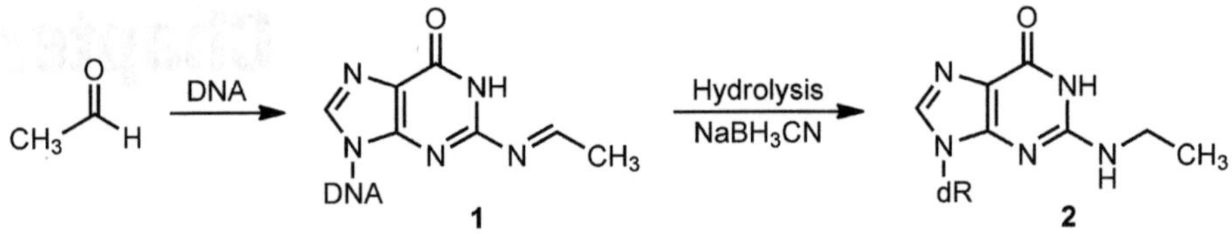

Scheme 1 The major reaction of acetaldehyde with DNA forms compound **1**. This compound is then converted to the reduction product **2**, which is stable when released after DNA hydrolysis

alcohol consumption and cancer, the underlying mechanisms of alcohol-induced carcinogenesis remain unclear. Various mechanisms may come into play depending on the type of cancer. Alcohol may interfere with folate absorption; it may raise estrogen levels; it may act as a solvent helping other harmful chemicals to enter cells; or it may act through its main metabolite acetaldehyde, which is a known genotoxic and carcinogenic compound. The latter hypothesis has prompted studies leading to the classification of acetaldehyde from alcohol consumption as a Group 1 carcinogen by the International Agency for Research on Cancer [4]. Acetaldehyde can react with DNA at various sites forming DNA adducts [4, 5]. The major reaction occurs on the exocyclic amino group of guanine forming the Schiff base N^2-ethylidenedeoxyguanosine (N^2-Ethylidene-dGuo, **1**, Scheme 1). This adduct is stable in DNA, but it easily breaks down when released as a nucleoside. Thus it is detected as its reduced form N^2-ethyldeoxyguanosine (N^2-ethyl-dGuo, **2**). Fang et al. were the first to report the detection of this DNA adduct in the leukocytes of alcoholics. In their work a ^{32}P-postlabelling method was used for the adduct quantitation [6]. Only samples from heavy drinkers showed detectable amounts of N^2-ethyl-dGuo resulting, most likely, from the reduction of N^2-Ethylidene-dGuo by endogenous reducing agents such as ascorbic acid and glutathione [7]. In order to avoid the degradation of N^2-Ethylidene-dGuo during hydrolysis and increase the sensitivity of the method, a new approach was developed by our group [8]. A reducing agent, $NaBH_3CN$, was introduced at the beginning of the assay, when dissolving the DNA in buffer prior to hydrolysis. Additionally, a stable isotope dilution method was used for the quantitation of the DNA adduct by liquid-chromatography-electrospray ionization-tandem mass spectrometry-selected reaction monitoring (LC-ESI-MS/MS-SRM).

The use of this new method allowed detection of N^2-ethyl-dGuo in DNA from all samples analyzed including a range of alcohol exposures as well as endogenous levels. This methodological improvement set the stage for the use of this adduct as a marker for acetaldehyde-induced DNA damage. Since then, N^2-ethyl-dGuo has been measured in DNA from various samples, for the

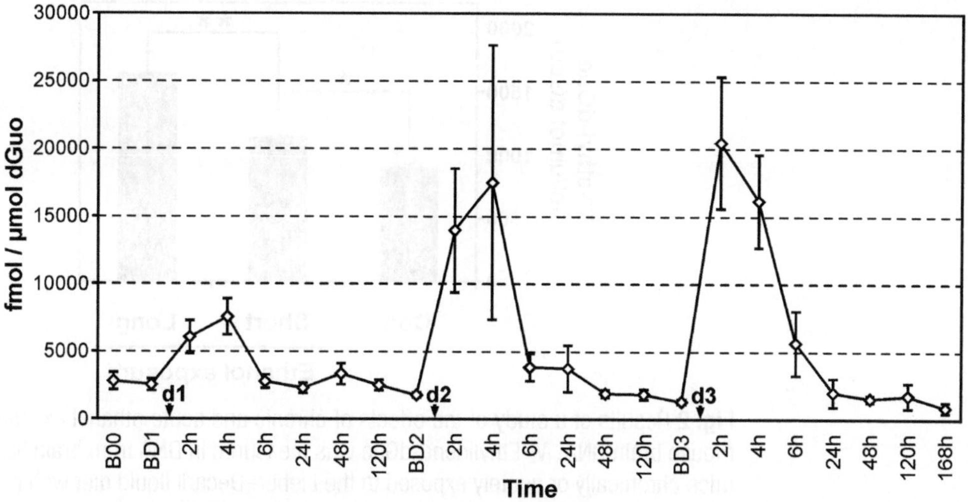

Fig. 1 Summary of the results obtained from a study investigating the effects of consumption of increasing doses of alcohol on oral cell DNA. The study was performed on samples collected from ten subjects who abstained from drinking any alcoholic beverage other than the doses provided over the entire duration of the study. The graph reports the mean levels of N^2-ethyl-dGuo (fmol/µmol dGuo) measured in oral cell DNA at various intervals before and after three increasing alcohol doses. The first time point reported on the *left* (B00) refers to 1 week before consumption of the first alcohol dose. Starting from this time point participants began to abstain from consuming any alcoholic beverage. The next time point (BD1) refers to the baseline level detected 1 week later, 1 h before consumption of the first dose (d1, *lowest*). Subsequently, the graph shows the levels of N^2-ethyl-dGuo measured at the various time points considered after each dose (2–120 h). The DNA adduct levels were measured at the same time points before and after exposure to the next two doses (d2, *intermediate*, and d3, *highest*). Levels of the adduct increased 2 h after exposure even after consumption of the lowest dose and returned to baseline 24 h after exposure. A clear dose–response effect of alcohol on N^2-ethyl-dGuo levels was found. The baseline time points measured 1 h before the dose (BD1, BD2, and BD3) are 7 days apart. Values shown as means ± S.E. Reprinted with permission from Cancer Epidemiol Biomarkers Prev. 2012 Apr; 21(4):601–608. Copyright (2012) American Association for cancer Research

investigation of the effects on DNA of acetaldehyde from different sources. Our group quantified levels of this adduct in human liver [8] and has investigated the effects of cigarette smoking on N^2-ethyl-dGuo in leukocyte DNA. A 28 % decrease in the levels of the DNA adduct was observed in subjects who quit smoking [9]. Singh et al. have applied the method to investigate effects on lung DNA of acetaldehyde deriving from cigarette smoking. N^2-Ethylidene-dGuo was detected in all samples with no evident difference when comparing smokers and nonsmokers; however the quantitation was performed on samples from only four smokers and four nonsmokers [10]. More recently we have used this method to investigate the relationship between alcohol consumption and adduct levels in human granulocyte, monocyte, and oral cell DNA [11, 12]. An increase in the levels of N^2-ethyl-dGuo was observed after alcohol consumption with a particularly evident dose–response effect seen in oral cell DNA as shown in Fig. 1. Abraham et al. used

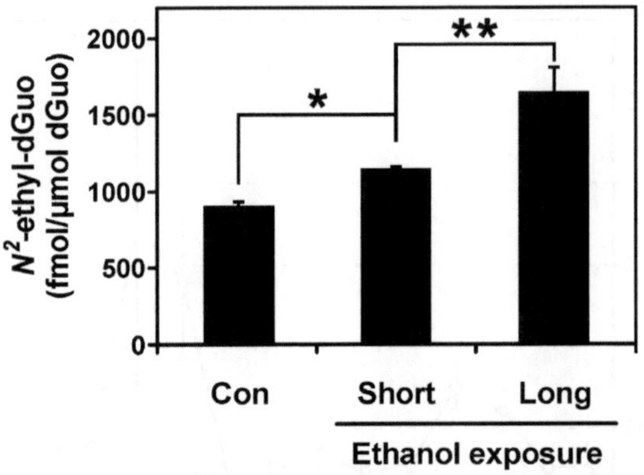

Fig. 2 Results of a study of the effects of chronic and acute ethanol exposure on mouse brain DNA. N^2-Ethylidene-dGuo was measured in DNA from brain tissue of mice chronically or acutely exposed to the Lieber–Decarli liquid diet with or without ethanol (5 %). N^2-Ethylidene-dGuo levels were significantly increased in DNA from mice after long-term ethanol exposure, compared with mice after short-term exposure and control (Con) mice. Values are shown as means ± S.E.; $*p < 0.05$; $**p < 0.001$. Copyright (2012) The AmericanSociety for Biochemistry and Molecular Biology

the quantitation of N^2-ethyl-dGuo to measure ethanol-induced DNA damage in HeLa-ADH1B cells which corresponded to the activation of the Fanconi anemia-breast cancer susceptibility (FA-BRCA) DNA damage response network [13], while Fowler et al. investigated ethanol-induced DNA damage in brain cells of ethanol-treated mice and measured higher levels of N^2-ethyl-dGuo in animals exposed chronically and acutely to ethanol compared to animals not exposed as shown in Fig. 2 [14].

These examples clearly demonstrate how quantitation of N^2-ethyl-dGuo provides information relevant for the investigation of DNA damage associated with acetaldehyde exposure from alcohol consumption. This assay is an extremely valuable tool in the investigation of alcohol-related mechanisms of carcinogenesis.

2 Materials

2.1 Equipment

Descriptions of specific equipment used are given; however, any model of comparable capability can easily be substituted.

Vacuum concentrator. Samples are dried using a Thermo Scientific Savant SpeedVac Plus concentrator, connected to a refrigerated vapor trap and a vacuum pump from Thermo Scientific, Waltham, MA.

DNA quality control spectrophotometer. DNA purity is tested using a Thermo Scientific NanoDrop™ 1000 Spectrophotometer from Thermo Scientific, Waltham, MA.

HPLC-UV. DNA quantitation is performed on an Agilent 1100 capillary flow HPLC with a diode array UV detector set at 254 nm (Agilent Technologies, Palo Alto, CA). A 4.6 mm × 25 cm 5 μm particle size C18 Luna column (Phenomenex, Torrance, CA) is used for the chromatographic separation.

LC-ESI-MS/MS. The N^2-ethyl-dGuo quantitation is performed with an Agilent 1100 capillary flow HPLC (Agilent Technologies) with a 250 mm × 0.5 mm 5 μm particle size Polar RP column (Phenomenex) coupled to a Vantage (Thermoelectron, San Jose, CA) triple-quadrupole mass spectrometer.

2.2 Reagents and Solutions

N^2-Ethylidene-dGuo and $[^{15}N_5]N^2$-ethyl-dGuo are prepared as described [8]. Ethanol is purchased from AAPER Alcohol and Chemical Co. (Shelbyville, KY). Isopropanol is purchased from Acros Organics (Morris Plains, NJ). Puregene DNA purification solutions are obtained from Qiagen (Valencia, CA). Calf thymus DNA is purchased from Worthington Biochemical Corporation (Lakewood, NJ). Alkaline phosphatase (from calf intestine) is obtained from Roche Diagnostics Corporation (Indianapolis, IN). All other chemicals and enzymes are purchased from Sigma-Aldrich (St. Louis, MO).

Aqueous buffer. Prepare a solution of Tris 10 mM (using Trizma preset crystals) and $MgCl_2$ 5 mM. This buffer is used to dissolve DNA and to prepare the solutions of enzymes for DNA hydrolysis.

Solid-phase extraction solutions. Prepare a 0.2 N NaOH solution in H_2O, a 0.01 N NaOH solution in H_2O, a 0.01 N KOH solution in MeOH, a 1 M ammonium acetate solution in H_2O, a solution of 10 % MeOH in H_2O, and a solution of 70 % MeOH in H_2O (**Note 1**).

3 Methods

A summary of the assay is presented in Scheme 2.

3.1 Samples

This assay has been developed and used for the quantitation of N^2-ethyl-dGuo in DNA from numerous sample types. DNA extracted from tissue, blood, oral cells, and cell cultures can be used. Samples should be stored frozen (−20 or −80 °C) until DNA extraction. No heat should be used in the DNA extraction procedure, and, once isolated, DNA should be dried and stored at −20 °C.

3.2 DNA Isolation

DNA is isolated using a kit from Qiagen following the manufacturer's protocol and avoiding any heating step. In particular, cell lysis is performed by incubating the sample at room temperature overnight; and RNA degradation is performed by adding RNase and incubating the sample at room temperature for 2 h (**Note 2**).

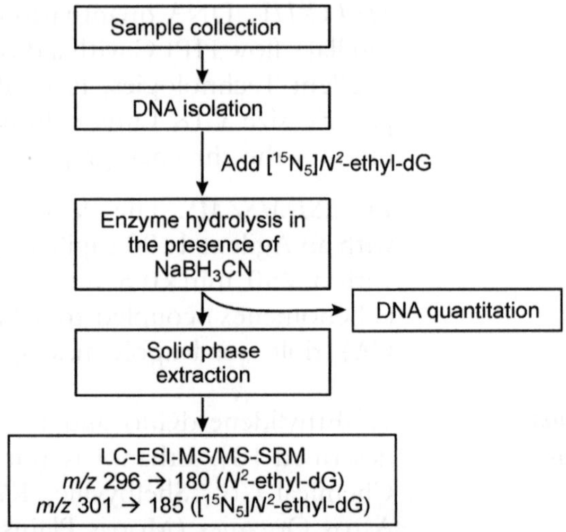

Scheme 2 Outline of the analytical method for determination of N^2-Ethylidene-dGuo in human leukocyte DNA, as N^2-ethyl-dGuo

3.3 DNA Purity

The quality of the DNA isolated can be tested using a Thermo Scientific NanoDrop™ 1000 Spectrophotometer. The purity of the sample can be assessed by measuring UV absorption of the DNA at 230, 260, and 280 nm. The ratio of the absorbance at 260/230 and 260/280 in pure DNA should be 2.4 and 1.8, respectively. If contamination with protein is present, the ratio will be significantly less than the values given above, and accurate quantitation by UV will not be possible.

3.4 DNA Hydrolysis

DNA hydrolysis and sample enrichment and purification are carried out as reported [15]. For enzyme hydrolysis:

1. DNA (0.05–1 mg) is dissolved in 400 μL of 10 mM Tris/5 mM $MgCl_2$ buffer containing [$^{15}N_5$]N^2-ethyl dGuo (50 fmol) and $NaBH_3CN$ (30 mg) (**Note 3**).
2. The pH is adjusted to 7 with 0.1 N HCl.
3. The DNA is initially digested overnight at room temperature with 1,300 U of DNase I (type II, from bovine pancreas) dissolved in 60 μL of 10 mM Tris/5 mM $MgCl_2$ buffer.
4. To the resulting mixture are added 1,300 additional units of DNase I dissolved in 60 μL of 10 mM Tris/5 mM $MgCl_2$ buffer, 0.07 U of phosphodiesterase I (type II, from *Crotalus adamanteus* venom) dissolved in 10 mM Tris/5 mM $MgCl_2$ buffer to obtain a 1 U/mL solution, and 750 U of alkaline phosphatase.
5. The mixture is incubated at 37 °C for 70 min and then allowed to stand overnight at room temperature (**Note 4**).

6. Enzymes are removed by centrifugation at 4,000 rpm for 40 min, using a centrifree MPS device (MW cutoff of 30,000; Amicon, Beverly, MA) (**Note 5**).
7. A 10 μL aliquot is removed and set aside for dGuo analysis and DNA quantitation (**Note 6**).

3.5 Sample Enrichment and Purification by Solid-Phase Extraction

The hydrolysate is desalted and purified using a solid-phase extraction cartridge [Strata-X 33 μm, 30 mg/1 mL (Phenomenex)].

3.5.1 Strata X

1. The cartridge is conditioned with 1 mL MeOH and washed with 1 mL of H_2O.
2. The sample is loaded.
3. The cartridge is washed with 1 mL of H_2O and 1 mL of 10 % MeOH in H_2O.
4. The analyte is eluted with 1 mL of 70 % MeOH in H_2O. This final fraction is collected.
5. The collected fraction is evaporated to dryness (**Note 7**).
6. The sample is dissolved in 1 mL of H_2O.
7. The sample is vortexed and sonicated for 5 min before being ready for the next purification step.

3.5.2 Oasis MAX

The 1 mL solution obtained above is further purified using a mixed mode, anion exchange reversed-phase extraction cartridge (Oasis MAX, 30 mg/cartridge, Waters). This purification step allows for reduction of the background noise and the ion suppression effect that otherwise affect dramatically the final quantitation of N^2-ethyl-dGuo on the LC-ESI-MS/MS-SRM.

1. The cartridge is conditioned with 1 mL of MeOH and then washed with 1 mL of a 0.2 N NaOH solution in H_2O.
2. Before loading the sample onto the cartridge, 300 μL of the same solution (0.2 N NaOH) are added to the 1 mL sample solution (**Note 8**).
3. The sample is loaded onto the cartridge.
4. The cartridge is washed with 1 mL of a 0.01 N NaOH solution in H_2O and 1 mL of a 0.01 N KOH solution in MeOH. These two washing steps eliminate most of the dC and dA from the sample.
5. The cartridge is then neutralized with 1 mL H_2O, 1 mL ammonium acetate buffer (pH 6.8), and 1 mL H_2O.
6. One milliliter of 10 % MeOH in H_2O is used to eliminate most of the dT from the sample.
7. Finally the DNA adduct is eluted with 1 mL of 70 % MeOH in H_2O, and this fraction is collected and evaporated to dryness (**Note 9**).

8. The residue is dissolved in 20 μL of H_2O, and 8 μL aliquots are analyzed by LC-ESI-MS/MS.

3.6 Positive and Negative Controls

Buffer blanks containing internal standard but no DNA are processed as above and analyzed to check the MS instrument baseline and possible contamination. Each set of samples should always be run together with at least one buffer blank. Calf thymus DNA (0.1 mg) with internal standard added as above is used as a positive control to determine inter-day precision and accuracy. Each set of samples is run together with three positive controls (**Note 10**).

3.7 HPLC-UV Analysis

Quantitation of dGuo is conducted using a gradient from 5 to 40 % MeOH in H_2O over the course of 35 min at a flow rate of 10 μL/min. Levels measured in the samples are compared to the levels measured in a calibration curve obtained analyzing solutions of known concentrations of dGuo. The range of concentrations chosen for the calibration curve should include that found in the samples.

3.8 LC-ESI-MS/MS-SRM Analysis

The N^2-ethyl-dGuo quantitation is performed using a solvent elution program with a 10 μL/min gradient from 5 to 40 % MeOH in 35 min at 30 °C. The ESI source is set in the positive ion mode as follows: voltage, 3.7 kV; current, 3 μA; and heated ion transfer tube, 275 °C. The collision energy is 12 eV, and the Ar collision gas pressure is 1.0 mTorr. Adducts are quantified by MS/MS with selected reaction monitoring (SRM) at m/z 296 → m/z 180 ($[M+H]^+ \rightarrow [BH]^+$) for N^2-ethyl-dGuo and at the corresponding transition m/z 301 → m/z 185 for $[^{15}N_5]N^2$-ethyl-dGuo. Typical traces observed for N^2-ethyl-dGuo and its corresponding labeled internal standard are shown in Fig. 3.

A calibration curve is constructed before each analysis using a standard solution of N^2-ethyl-dGuo and $[^{15}N_5]N^2$-ethyl-dGuo. A constant amount of $[^{15}N_5]N^2$-ethyl-dGuo is mixed with differing amounts of N^2-ethyl-dGuo choosing N^2-ethyl-dGuo/$[^{15}N_5]N^2$-ethyl-dGuo ratios in a range that will include the ratios of analyte/internal standard expected to be measured in the samples. Figure 4 represents an example in which 40 fmol of the internal standard were mixed with 4, 8, 16, 32, 128, and 512 fmol of the analyte and analyzed by LC-ESI-MS/MS-SRM.

The accuracy of the method was tested and the results have been reported [9]. This was performed by adding various amounts of N^2-ethyl-dGuo to 0.3 mg calf thymus DNA. The N^2-ethyl-dGuo naturally present in $NaBH_3CN$-treated calf thymus DNA was measured and subtracted from each value. The results are summarized in Table 1. An excellent correlation ($R^2 = 1.0$) was observed between the added and measured amounts of N^2-ethyl-dGuo. The reproducibility of the measurements was excellent,

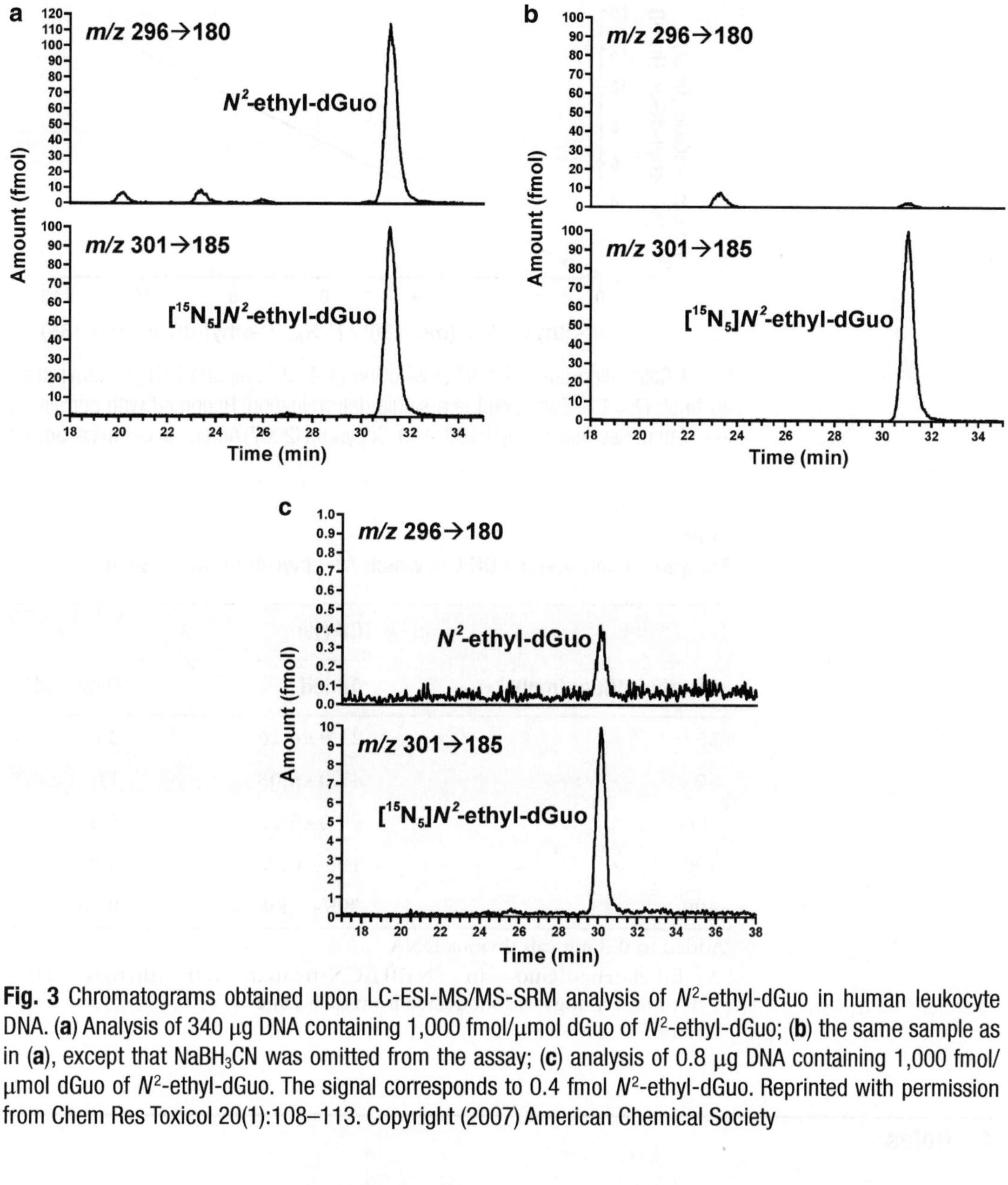

Fig. 3 Chromatograms obtained upon LC-ESI-MS/MS-SRM analysis of N^2-ethyl-dGuo in human leukocyte DNA. (**a**) Analysis of 340 μg DNA containing 1,000 fmol/μmol dGuo of N^2-ethyl-dGuo; (**b**) the same sample as in (**a**), except that $NaBH_3CN$ was omitted from the assay; (**c**) analysis of 0.8 μg DNA containing 1,000 fmol/μmol dGuo of N^2-ethyl-dGuo. The signal corresponds to 0.4 fmol N^2-ethyl-dGuo. Reprinted with permission from Chem Res Toxicol 20(1):108–113. Copyright (2007) American Chemical Society

with RSD ranging from 20 % at the lowest levels added to 0.73 % at the highest.

Analyte recovery for this assay averages 48 %. The limit of detection of N^2-ethyl-dGuo injected on column is 0.05 fmol (S/N = 6). The estimated limit of quantitation of N^2-ethyl-dGuo in DNA is 10 fmol/mg DNA, about three adducts per 10^9 nucleotides, or about 15 fmol/μmol dGuo, starting with 500 μg DNA, and S/N = 4. When the assay is run with amounts of DNA as low as 1 μg, the estimated limit of quantitation is 0.4 fmol.

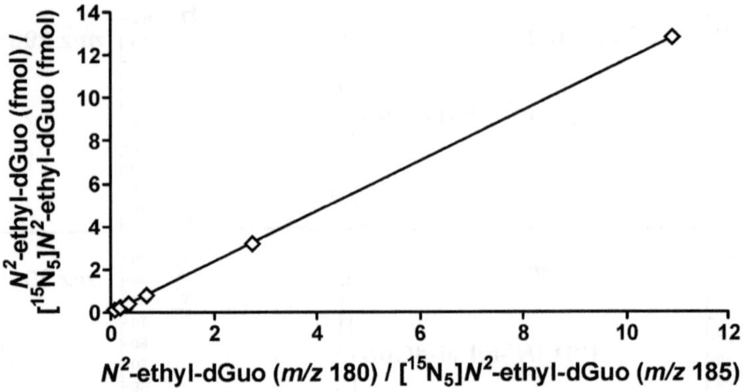

Fig. 4 Calibration curve for N^2-ethyl-dGuo (4–512 fmol) and [$^{15}N_5$]N^2-ethyl-dGuo, 40 fmol; $R^2 = 1.0$. Each point is a single determination. Reprinted with permission from Chem Res Toxicol 20(1):108–113. Copyright (2007) American Chemical Society

Table 1
Analysis of calf thymus DNA to which N^2-ethyl-dGuo was added

N^2-ethyl-dGuo (fmol)[a,b]	Added	CV (%) Detected[c]
25	21.0 ± 4.16	20
50	47.0 ± 5.03	11
100	99.0 ± 5.13	5.2
200	193 ± 4.36	2.3
400	395 ± 2.89	0.73

[a]Added to 0.3 mg calf thymus DNA
[b]N^2-Ethylidene-dGuo in $NaBH_3CN$-treated calf thymus DNA (130 fmol/0.3 mg) was subtracted from each value
[c]Mean ± S.D. ($N = 3$)

4 Notes

1. Solutions for DNA hydrolysis and solid-phase extraction are freshly prepared before each experiment; however, for experiments repeated frequently the solutions for solid-phase extraction can be stored for a couple of weeks (aqueous solutions should be stored at 4 °C).
2. DNA isolation protocols usually include a final ethanol wash step. Particular care should be addressed towards selecting pure ethanol with low traces of acetaldehyde. If information about the acetaldehyde content of the solvent is not available, isopropanol can be used instead.

3. $NaBH_3CN$ treatment converts N^2-Ethylidene-dGuo to N^2-ethyl-dGuo [8]. This is a crucial step to assure the complete conversion of N^2-Ethylidene-dGuo into its stable reduced form.
4. To optimize N^2-ethyl-dGuo recovery any step during DNA hydrolysis that requires heating to temperatures over 37 °C is avoided and substituted with longer incubation time.
5. Samples should be applied to the centrifree filter without forming bubbles over the filter surface in order to avoid incomplete filtration.
6. Aliquots can be stored at −20 °C until HPLC quantitation.
7. Dried fractions can be stored at −20 °C overnight if necessary. Samples should be redissolved in 1 mL H_2O right before proceeding with the next purification step.
8. This step is key to ensure that the DNA adduct is negatively charged, due to removal of the H at the N1 position of dGuo, and able to bind to the cartridge substrate.
9. Dried fractions can be stored at −20 °C for several weeks. Samples should be redissolved in H_2O right before proceeding with the LC-ESI-MS/MS-SRM analysis.
10. The presence of co-eluting peaks in the final analysis is a potential issue that can greatly affect the final adduct quantitation. A high variability of the N^2-ethyl-dGuo levels measured in the positive controls can help in detecting the presence of interfering peaks in the LC-ESI-MS/MS-SRM analysis.

References

1. Baan R, Straif K, Grosse Y, Secretan B, El Ghissassi F, Bouvard V, Altieri A, Cogliano V (2007) Carcinogenicity of alcoholic beverages. Lancet Oncol 8(4):292–293
2. Nelson DE, Jarman DW, Rehm J, Greenfield TK, Rey G, Kerr WC, Miller P, Shield KD, Ye Y, Naimi TS (2013) Alcohol-attributable cancer deaths and years of potential life lost in the United States. Am J Public Health 103(4):641–648. doi:10.2105/AJPH.2012.301199
3. Schutze M, Boeing H, Pischon T, Rehm J, Kehoe T, Gmel G, Olsen A, Tjonneland AM, Dahm CC, Overvad K, Clavel-Chapelon F, Boutron-Ruault MC, Trichopoulou A, Benetou V, Zylis D, Kaaks R, Rohrmann S, Palli D, Berrino F, Tumino R, Vineis P, Rodriguez L, Agudo A, Sanchez MJ, Dorronsoro M, Chirlaque MD, Barricarte A, Peeters PH, van Gils CH, Khaw KT, Wareham N, Allen NE, Key TJ, Boffetta P, Slimani N, Jenab M, Romaguera D, Wark PA, Riboli E, Bergmann MM (2011) Alcohol attributable burden of incidence of cancer in eight European countries based on results from prospective cohort study. BMJ 342:d1584. doi:10.1136/bmj.d1584
4. Secretan B, Straif K, Baan R, Grosse Y, El Ghissassi F, Bouvard V, Benbrahim-Tallaa L, Guha N, Freeman C, Galichet L, Cogliano V (2009) A review of human carcinogens—Part E: tobacco, areca nut, alcohol, coal smoke, and salted fish. Lancet Oncol 10(11): 1033–1034
5. Wang M, McIntee EJ, Cheng G, Shi Y, Villalta PW, Hecht SS (2000) Identification of DNA adducts of acetaldehyde. Chem Res Toxicol 13(11):1149–1157
6. Fang JL, Vaca CE (1995) Development of a 32P-postlabelling method for the analysis of adducts arising through the reaction of acetaldehyde with 2′-deoxyguanosine-3′-monophosphate and DNA. Carcinogenesis 16(9):2177–2185

7. Fang JL, Vaca CE (1997) Detection of DNA adducts of acetaldehyde in peripheral white blood cells of alcohol abusers. Carcinogenesis 18(4):627–632
8. Wang M, Yu N, Chen L, Villalta PW, Hochalter JB, Hecht SS (2006) Identification of an acetaldehyde adduct in human liver DNA and quantitation as N2-ethyldeoxyguanosine. Chem Res Toxicol 19(2):319–324. doi:10.1021/tx0502948
9. Chen L, Wang M, Villalta PW, Luo X, Feuer R, Jensen J, Hatsukami DK, Hecht SS (2007) Quantitation of an acetaldehyde adduct in human leukocyte DNA and the effect of smoking cessation. Chem Res Toxicol 20(1):108–113. doi:10.1021/tx060232x
10. Singh R, Sandhu J, Kaur B, Juren T, Steward WP, Segerback D, Farmer PB (2009) Evaluation of the DNA damaging potential of cannabis cigarette smoke by the determination of acetaldehyde derived N2-Ethylidene-2′-deoxyguanosine adducts. Chem Res Toxicol 22(6):1181–1188. doi:10.1021/tx900106y
11. Balbo S, Meng L, Bliss RL, Jensen JA, Hatsukami DK, Hecht SS (2012) Time course of DNA adduct formation in peripheral blood granulocytes and lymphocytes after drinking alcohol. Mutagenesis 27(4):485–490. doi:10.1093/mutage/ges008
12. Balbo S, Meng L, Bliss RL, Jensen JA, Hatsukami DK, Hecht SS (2012) Kinetics of DNA adduct formation in the oral cavity after drinking alcohol. Cancer Epidemiol Biomarkers Prev 21(4):601–608. doi:10.1158/1055-9965.EPI-11-1175
13. Abraham J, Balbo S, Crabb D, Brooks PJ (2011) Alcohol metabolism in human cells causes DNA damage and activates the Fanconi anemia-breast cancer susceptibility (FA-BRCA) DNA damage response network. Alcohol Clin ExpRes35(12):2113–2120.doi:10.1111/j.1530-0277.2011.01563.x
14. Fowler AK, Hewetson A, Agrawal RG, Dagda M, Dagda R, Moaddel R, Balbo S, Sanghvi M, Chen Y, Hogue RJ, Bergeson SE, Henderson GI, Kruman II (2012) Alcohol-induced one-carbon metabolism impairment promotes dysfunction of DNA base excision repair in adult brain. J Biol Chem 287(52):43533–43542. doi:10.1074/jbc.M112.401497
15. Balbo S, Hashibe M, Gundy S, Brennan P, Canova C, Simonato L, Merletti F, Richiardi L, Agudo A, Castellsague X, Znaor A, Talamini R, Bencko V, Holcatova I, Wang M, Hecht SS, Boffetta P (2008) N2-ethyldeoxyguanosine as a potential biomarker for assessing effects of alcohol consumption on DNA. Cancer Epidemiol Biomarkers Prev 17(11):3026–3032. doi:10.1158/1055-9965.EPI-08-0117

Chapter 12

Imaging Tools in Discovery and Development of Phytochemical Chemopreventive Agents

Marna Ericson

Abstract

This is an exciting era in the development and cross-disciplinary use of new imaging technologies, including single-photon and multiphoton laser scanning microscopy; second- and third-harmonic generation imaging; coherent anti-Raman stokes imaging (CARS); and live-cell, whole-mouse, hyperspectral, and super-resolution microscopy. These imaging technologies provide invaluable tools for developing and validating phytochemical-derived drug discovery and parsing out the molecular mechanisms by which these natural compounds can modulate distinct target proteins involved in oncogenic signaling. This chapter provides detailed steps in preparing relatively thick (e.g., up to 200 μm) tissue samples for microscopy using multiple biomarkers providing unprecedented imaging information on pathophysiology, localization, and co-localization of target structures and signaling components. Examples are presented of these new, next-generation imaging modalities used in discovery and development of phytochemical agents.

Key words Confocal microscopy, Quantitation, Single photon, Co-localization

1 Introduction

A critical step in the development of phytochemical cancer-preventive agents is validating the effects of the agents with a biological assay beginning from the initial stages with the non-purified naturally occurring product. Advances in imaging technologies now enable us to perform target-specific visualization, in vivo, with genetically modified fluorescent reporters in animal models, site-specific recombinase technology, cells, and molecules. With single- and/or multiphoton microscopy optical sectioning of multi-stained tissues, we can visualize 3-dimensional (3-D) organization and morphology with respect to the target tissue and identification and quantification of physiologically important structures.

Historically, formalin-fixed, paraffin-embedded thin (4–6 μm) tissue sections have been and still are the most common technique for studying tissue pathology. Differences in binding affinity of dyes provide contrast to tissues, cells, and subcellular components

Ann M. Bode and Zigang Dong (eds.), *Cancer Prevention: Dietary Factors and Pharmacology*, Methods in Pharmacology and Toxicology, DOI 10.1007/978-1-4614-9227-6_12, © Springer Science+Business Media New York 2014

in bright field microscopy. The most commonly used dye combination is hematoxylin and eosin (H&E stain) [1]. H&E-stained tissues are observed using bright field microscopy wherein white light is transmitted through the tissue. Structures that have accumulated more dye are denser and appear darker.

Whereas in bright field illumination, sample contrast comes from absorbance of light in the sample, in dark field illumination, the sample contrast comes from light scattered by the sample. Phase contrast microcopy takes advantage of the fact that light will pass through different parts of the sample and the surrounding medium at different speeds. The phase microscope converts the phase shifts in light waves passing through a transparent specimen to brightness changes in the image using a transparent phase plate to visualize an otherwise transparent object. When the incident light is polarized, the interference of that unidirectional light can be interrupted by tissue structures, providing contrast. In super-resolution light microscopy, the diffraction-limited resolution of light, 250 nm, is surpassed by taking advantage of the nonlinear response to excitation of many fluorophores, thereby enhancing resolution.

Another variation in dark field microscopy is hyperspectral analysis and may also include epifluorescence. In the hyperspectral imaging (HSI) configuration, the optical spectrum of each pixel within a $1{,}024 \times 1{,}024$ field of view is acquired every 1.5 nm from 400 to 1000 nm, thus creating a spectral fingerprint for the object of interest. This microspectrophotometry is based on NASA satellite imaging technology, and the associated Environment for Visualizing Images (ENVI) software is the same used for remote sensing and target detection. Using HSI, Siddiqi et al. [2] could distinguish normal, precancerous, and cancerous cervical cells on Pap-test slides, which is a valuable prescreening test for chemopreventive therapies in the fight against cervical cancer [3].

In conventional epifluorescence microscopy, out-of-focus fluorescence from the sample obscures resolution, and reduction of epifluorescent light intensity and photobleaching of the fluorophores are common. In laser scanning confocal microscopy (LSCM), the out-of-focus light appears black because illumination and detection are limited to the same *z*-plane of focus in a well-defined optical section. Because only in-focus light is collected, contrast, clarity, and detection sensitivity are greatly enhanced and 3-D image stacks can be acquired [4]. Whereas in single-photon confocal microscopy the excitation and emission light are confined to a single plane, in multiphoton microscopy the excitation and emission light are confined to a single point. The duration of illumination at that single spot is much shorter with higher energy, thereby reducing internal heating and damage. In particular, multiphoton microscopy has opened a new vista of imaging techniques with wide-ranging possibilities to image up to 1 mm into tissue with very little interference and to image living tissue in real time because of reduced localized heating generated by the laser excitation beam. Additionally, because multiphoton microscopy uses pulsed laser light at high frequencies, the nonlinear optical properties of some non-stained native structures such as collagen fibrils and myosin have a strong signal and can be detected without staining. This chapter provides detailed instructions for processing and multi-staining tissues for single- and multiphoton imaging.

2 Materials

2.1 Equipment

1. Cryostat: Adjustable to cut up to 200 μm thick samples.
2. Welled Glass Dishes (Fisher Scientific #72208S, 6 pk #171.77).
3. Ceramic coverslip boat racks (Thomas Scientific, 1-800-345-2100, Phil USA).
4. Conventional Epifluorescence Microscope fitted with high-resolution camera and also with multiple filter sets for viewing in UV, green, red, and far-red channels (**Note 1**).
5. Single-photon laser scanning confocal microscope (LSCM) (**Note 2**).
6. Multiphoton laser scanning microscope (MLSM).
7. Software: Photoshop or Image J and Excel or Prism.

2.2 Reagents and Solutions

1. Zamboni's Biopsy Fixative [5]: 0.03 % (w/v) picric acid and 2 % (w/v) paraformaldehyde in Millonig's buffer (Sigma-Aldrich, St. Louis, MO) (**Notes 3, 4**).
2. Sodium Phosphate Buffered Saline (PBS) (Sigma-Aldrich, St. Louis, MO) (**Note 5**).
3. Biopsy storage buffer/cryo-preservative (**Note 6**).
4. Optimal cutting temperature (OCT) (Electron Microscopy Science, Hatfield, PA).
5. PBS with 0.3 % Triton-X100 (TPBS) (Sigma-Aldrich, St. Louis, MO) (**Note 7**).
6. PBS with 5 % normal serum (NTPBS) in 0.5× PBS, aliquot (500 μl) (**Note 8**).
7. Nuclear stains: For example, DAPI, Hoechst, YOYO (1:10,000–1:50,000) (Life Technologies, Grand Island, NY).
8. Antibody solutions: Store antibodies at −20 °C in 50 % glycerol/PBS at 1:10 dilution and aliquot (**Note 9**).
9. Lectins conjugated to fluorescent reporters, e.g., *Ulex europaeus*—FITC (Vector Labs, Burlingame, CA).

10. Agar: 1.35–1.5 % Noble Agar in dH_2O (Sigma-Aldrich, St. Louis, MO) (**Note 10**).
11. Methyl salicylate (Sigma-Aldrich, St. Louis, MO) (**Note 11**).
12. Mountant: DEPEX (Electron Microscopy Science, Hatfield, PA).

3 Methods

3.1 Tissue Acquisition

For large pieces of human skin, a local hospital surgical suite may be able to provide breast reduction or abdominoplasty skin with prior patient consent and Institutional Review Board (IRB) approval. Human or animal skin biopsies can be acquired under local anesthesia or whole-animal anesthesia, respectively. Patient consent and IRB approval or IACUC approval is a prerequisite. Use extreme care when handling tissue to avoid damaging the tissue. All samples are immediately drop-fixed in cold (4 °C) Zamboni's fixative (**Notes 12, 13**).

3.2 Fixation and Storage

Fix tissue in Zamboni's fixative for 24–48 h in vials at 4 °C. The time depends on tissue size, e.g., 4-mm human skin tissues require 24 h and a whole mouse foot requires 48 h. Decant Zamboni's from tissue into small beaker and then transfer Zamboni's to a hazardous waste bottle in a fume hood. Cover tissue in cryopreservative and store at 4 °C (**Note 14**).

3.3 Immunostaining with Multiple Primary and Secondary Antibodies

The protocol described below has been maximized to achieve an optimal epifluorescent signal from biomarkers. To facilitate using this protocol, the steps are presented in chronological order. Likewise, precautions are taken to minimize endogenous tissue fluorescence and reduce nonspecific binding. The protocol is similar for triple or single antibody, pre-conjugated antibody, or direct labeling/staining, e.g., fluorescent-conjugated lectin, DAPI, YOYO, and Polymyxin-Oregon Green (**Note 15**).

1. Day 1

   Cryo-section—Rinse a Pyrex 9-well glass dish. Mount tissue in OCT on a precooled specimen mounting stand (i.e., chuck) and cut on cryostat into sections of desired thickness (60–200 μm) (**Notes 16, 17**). To envisage the entire length of, e.g., the hair follicle of cut vertical sections, which are perpendicular to the epidermal surface, gently lift and place cut sections in a sequential manner (1 section/well if possible) into wells of the Pyrex 9-well glass dish pre-filled with PBS.

   Normal serum—After all sections are cut, decant PBS, fill wells with TPBS, and then decant TPBS. Incubate in 100 μl of 5 % normal serum in TPBS (5 % NTPBS) overnight at room temperature (RT) with gentle gyro-rotatory shaking (**Notes 18, 19**).

2. Day 2

Primary antibody—Most often, primary antibodies can be added together, although sequential addition is fine as well. All new lots of antibodies and each combination of antibodies must be titrated to determine the strongest fluorophore signal with the least amount of background (**Notes 20, 21**). Remove 5 % NTPBS, and apply 50–200 μl primary antibody(ies) in 1 % NTPBS to predetermined working dilutions (**Note 22**). Incubate for 8 h to overnight at RT with gentle gyro-rotatory shaking. Be certain that your solutions do not escape the wells while shaking. Use a new pipette tip for each well. For negative controls, leave two wells with no primary(ies), and use buffer only. One well will receive no secondary antibody(ies), and the other well will have neither primary or secondary antibody(ies) (**Note 23**). To possibly determine the binding specificity of the primary antibody, run a pre-absorption staining experiment wherein the antigen peptide is preincubated with the antibody before applying to sample.

3. Day 3—a.m.

Wash—Remove primary antibody solution and do a rapid 5-min rinse and then three 1-h washes of 500 μl of 1 % NTPBS per well. Washing overnight is fine as well.

Day 3—p.m.

Secondary antibody—Draw off 1 % NTPBS, and incubate all sections in 100 μl of the appropriate secondary antibody(ies) at a predetermined dilution for 8 h to overnight at RT with gentle gyro-rotatory shaking. Protect sample from light from this point on.

4. Day 4

Wash—Wash sections with minimum of two changes in 1 % TPBS and incubate overnight at RT in PBS buffer with gentle gyro-rotatory shaking.

5. Day 5

Wash—Wash sections with PBS a minimum of 2×—30 min each.

Incubate tissue in nuclear stain (if desired)—After first PBS wash, apply nuclear stain (e.g., DAPI-1:50,000; Hoechst; YOYO) and incubate samples for 30 min. Wash sections 2× in PBS for 30 min. Use a generous amount of PBS to wash sections.

Mount—Prepare agar, which is the support medium for sections, place agar in a beaker of water on a slide warmer, and remove any debris. Position dissecting microscope over the slide warmer surface to facilitate screening wells and to aid in mounting tissue pieces onto cover slips. Use "canned air" to blow dust off of cover slip immediately prior to mounting. Place cover slip onto the slide warmer under the microscope. The goal is to have the sample lying directly on the cover slip with no agar between sample and cover slip. Place a bubble of agar on the cover slip, and carefully submerge tissue in agar. Pipette off any excess agar leaving enough agar to cover the entire sample while reducing the agar bubble height as much as possible (**Note 24**). Additional agar might need to be added to avoid agar dehydration. Cool on bench top, tissue side up, for about 1 min. Be very careful to maintain tissue orientation and well number.

Dehydrate and clear—Load cover slips into ceramic boats with tissue sections facing forward, and be mindful of orientation as the sections become almost invisible to the human eye after incubation in methyl salicylate (**Notes 25**, **26**). In a fume hood, immerse cover slip boat in 75 % EtOH for 30+ min, then 95 % EtOH for 30+ min, and then move to 100 % EtOH for 30+ min, and finally immerse cover slip boat in methyl salicylate.

Mount cover slips onto slides—Pre-label slides with date, experiment number, and slide number. Do not use permanent marker because it will be washed off by the mounting media. In a fume hood gently apply a liberal amount of DEPEX mounting medium to the microscope slide. Invert cover slip, sample side down, onto DEPEX puddle one edge at a time to avoid crushing the specimen and to avoid air bubble formation. Dry slides, undisturbed in the hood, protected from light, for 48 h. Store slides flat in cardboard slide file folder at room temperature—indefinitely (**Note 27**). Samples do not lose their fluorescence and are very durable against laser quenching.

3.4 Image Acquisition

The staining of the target tissue in the test organism is crucial to understand the changes in expression of specific proteins, signaling molecules, and receptors. Through methodical preparation of thick samples and systematic acquisition of image data using laser scanning microscopy, not only can the 3-D architecture and time-course of changes in tissue structures and physical interactions be observed, but also biomarkers can be quantified and the effects of chemopreventive agents determined. Several image capture and quantitation scenarios are presented to illustrate the application of these techniques in a variety of tissues including human and mouse skin, mouse dorsal root ganglion, the whole foot of the mouse, and rat mammary tumors.

3.4.1 Antibody Specificity

To monitor and detect nonspecific binding by fluorescent-labeled secondary reporter antibodies, representative tissue sections are stained as described in the Methods section (Sect. 3.3, Day 2), but the primary antibodies are omitted. Tissue sections that received both primary and secondary antibodies show robust staining of the, e.g., axons, while no signal is observed in tissue sections that received only the secondary antibody. Using the baseline image capture settings from these primary-only sections when capturing image data from all samples is critical (**Note 28**). Far-red irradiation, although not visible to the naked eye, is preferable because

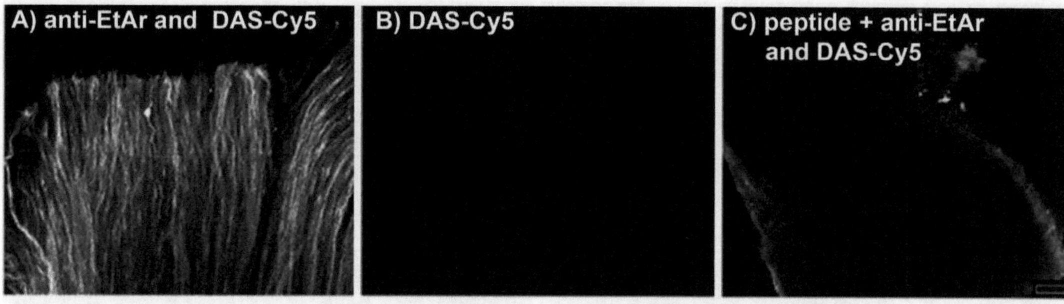

Fig. 1 LSCM image montage showing primary and secondary antibody specificity. No epifluorescence is observed in the LSCM image of a murine sciatic nerve tissue stained only with the Cy5 secondary antibody compared to a section that received primary and secondary antibodies. Fixed, whole sections of excised sciatic nerve were labeled (**a**) with or (**b**) without 1:100 anti-endothelin A receptor (EtAr) made in sheep (Research Diagnostics Inc.) and 1:2,000 donkey-anti-sheep (DAS) IgG conjugated to Cyanine 5.18 (Cy5, far-red channel) (Jackson ImmunoResearch, Inc.). (**c**) The polyclonal EtAr antibody is first incubated (60 °C, 2 h) with a 1,000-fold excess of the peptide antigen used to generate the polyclonal EtAr antibody. Nerve tissue is then incubated overnight with the antigen–EtAr complex followed by DAS–Cy5 secondary antibodies, and no epifluorescence is observed in the far-red channel. Objective: Olympus 20× PlanApo/0.08 oil. Scale bar = 50 μm

fewer endogenous compounds, such as NADPH and hemoglobin, that fluoresce in the far red are present (**Note 29**). To verify the specificity of the primary antibody for the target epitope, the primary antibody is preincubated with a 100-fold excess of the peptide antigen and tissue sections are then incubated with this complex. Little or no signal should be detected in this example (Fig. 1).

3.4.2 Target Specificity: Knockouts

Knockout models can be crucial for ascertaining biological mechanisms of target proteins. In studies with topically applied phytochemicals, studying full-thickness vertical skin sections provides us with valuable information on transdermal penetration, activity, and biomarker localization within the layers of the skin as well as changes in morphology and architecture. In studies to ascertain the mechanism of the capsaicin receptor (TRPV1) in skin cancer, the TRPV1 knockout mouse proved invaluable in demonstrating that the TRPV1 suppresses skin carcinogenesis (Fig. 2; [6]).

3.4.3 Fluorescent Reporters

Treatment effects on morphology and metastasis can be observed by transfecting cancer cell lines with plasmids resulting in the expression of fluorescent reporter proteins. These stable fluorescent biomarkers can be imaged in live animals. The tissue can also be multi-stained to observe tissue interactions with proteins and structures of interest (Fig. 3).

3.4.4 Co-localization and Visualization of Multiple Fluorescent Biomarkers in a Single Section

Capsaicin, a natural-occurring substance, is often used to block pain signals in epidermal nerve fibers, and it does so by binding to the TRPV1 receptor. However capsaicin can act as a cocarcinogen not through TRPV1 binding but by activating the epidermal

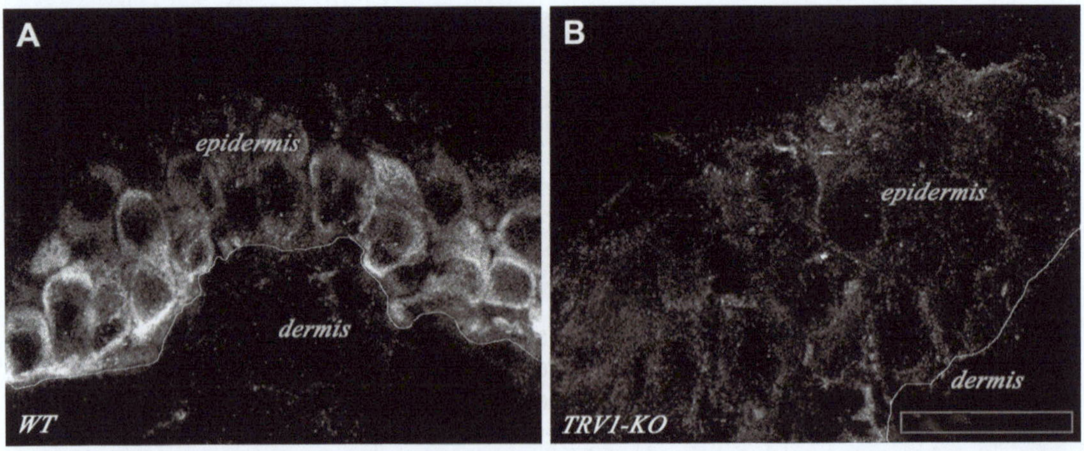

Fig. 2 LSCM image projections of TRPV1 immmunoreacity in the wild-type and the TRPV1 knockout mouse. Expression of the capsaicin receptor is high in the epidermis of dorsal skin from (**a**) TRPV1 WT mice compared with no expression in skin from (**b**) TRPV1 KO mice. The image was captured with LSCM. Sections were immunostained with anti-TRPV1 (1:100, made in guinea pig, Santa Cruz Biotech) and the secondary reporter anti-guinea pig IgG Cy2 (1:200, made in donkey, Jackson ImmunoResearch). Scale bar = 50 μm

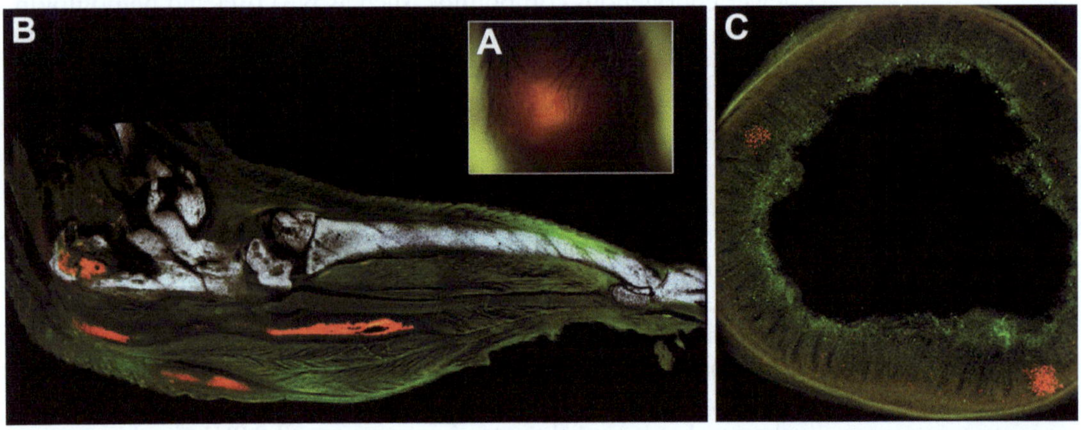

Fig. 3 Fluorescent reporters DsRed2 transfected into cancer cell lines readily visible in the live mouse and in tissue sections. Stable fluorescent cancer cells are readily identified in murine tissues. (**a**) DsRed2-transfected fibrosarcoma cells implanted into and around the calcaneus bone of the C3H/He mice post-implantation day 10 in vivo and (**b**) in fixed heel section. Transfections of the DsRed2 cancer cells were generated using the sleeping beauty transposase methodology [11,12]. (**c**) The metastatic patterns of the murine DsRed2 leukemia cell line were examined and found in numerous organs including the intestinal tract. Note that with this DsRed2 cell line, small clumps or individual cells are visible. **a** has been reproduced with permission of the International Association for the Study of Pain® (IASP). The figures may NOT be reproduced for any other purpose without permission)

growth factor receptor (EGFR) signaling pathway [7]. Using a chemical carcinogenesis model, mice were treated with DMBA/TPA to induce tumor growth. Triple staining a tumor-bearing region of the dorsal skin revealed, as expected, that TRPV1 co-localizes with a subset of nerves in the skin and that the EGFR is highly expressed in and around hair follicles. The EGFR is also abundant in the papilloma itself although very little co-localization of TRPV1 with EGFR was observed (Fig. 4).

3.4.5 Quantifying Density/Expression of Select Biomarker/Structures in Tissue

A morphometric approach to quantifying immunolabeled structures, which do not rely on fluorescence intensity, can yield quantitative comparisons of structural biomarkers, e.g., relative nerve or blood vessel density within the target tissue. Stereology is the study of 3-D geometric relationships between structures projected in 2-D images [8]. This is an unbiased method for collecting information about the number, length, surface area, and volume of structures and whole organs by examining a minor part of it [9]. LSCM images must be acquired in a uniform, unbiased, and systematic manner.

This step-by-step protocol can quantify nerves and blood vessels in a rodent tumor model using stereology principles with image data from LSCM. Two-hundred micron thick sections of the entire mouse foot were cryo-sectioned and immunostained for vasculature and nerves, using the staining protocol described earlier (Sect. 3.3). Images were captured in the green channel (CD31-ir blood vessels), red channel (DsRed2 tumor cells), and far-red channel (calcitonin gene-related peptide (CGRP)-ir nerves; Fig. 5). Two-photon laser scanning microscopy (LSM) was used to capture bone images in the ultraviolet channel (**Note 30**).

1. At the tumor site, LSCM serial optical section data sets were collected. All image projections were 50 μm thick composed of six 10-μm optical sections captured in the *z*-plane stack of focus at 100× magnification. All acquisition parameters were the same, and all images for a specific treatment were imaged during the same session to avoid any differences in the microscope lasers or detectors that might occur from day to day.
2. Merged green–red–blue projections were generated using the confocal software.
3. The color images were opened in Photoshop and by viewing only the red channel, the red tumor was selected with the lasso tool, its area measured, and the nerves and blood vessels outside the tumor excluded from counting. Having established and measured the region of interest, e.g., the DsRed2 tumor, either the green channel vessels or the blue nerves were singularly displayed and only image data within the previously established tumor boundaries were included in the measurements.
4. A geometric probe, a cycloid grid, was applied and merged onto each projection. Observers counted the points of intersections (i.e., hits) between the grid and discrete nerve fiber/bundles (Cy5 in the far-red channel) or blood vessels (Cy2 in the green channel).

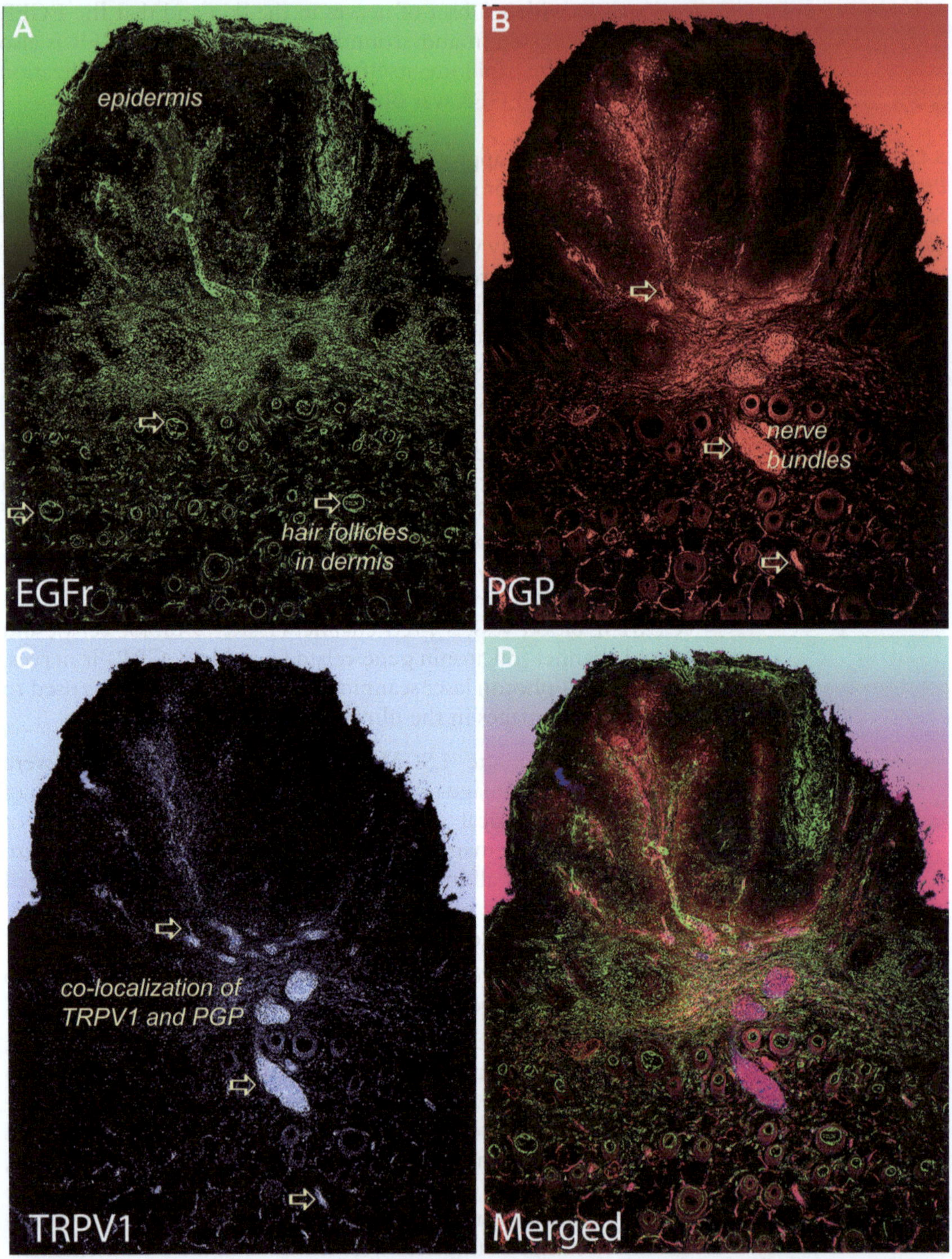

Fig. 4 Co-localization and visualization of multiple fluorescent biomarkers in a mouse skin cancer model. Immunoreactivity of (**a**) EGFR, (**b**) PGP, (**c**) TRPV1, and (**d**) merged in a rodent chemical carcinogenesis model. The almost "volcanic" nature/abundant expression captured using LSCM of a critical signaling factor; EGFR (*green*) is evident in a rodent skin lesion. EGFR is also abundant in the outer root sheath of the hair follicles (*arrows*, (**b**, **c**, **d**)). TRPV1 immunoreactive nerves are a subset of PGP immunoreactive nerves and nerve bundles.

5. Because the size of the tumor varied between samples, the numbers of hits were normalized for percent area of projection occupied by the tumor.
6. Nerve and blood vessel density within the tumor is reported as number of hits per normalized 1,024c × 1,024 pixel field.
7. To achieve statistical significance, three mice per time point per treatment were analyzed. From each mouse, we studied four sagittal sections (200 mm thick), two immunostained with antibodies against CD31 and PGP9.5, and two against CD31 and CGRP. Image data of two 200 μm thick tissue sections per mouse were collected.
8. Mean withdrawal response frequency to mechanical stimuli and tumor size measurements were analyzed by repeated measures ANOVA. This was followed by Bonferroni protected least significant difference (PSLD) post hoc comparison for significance to control for multiple group comparisons over several time points. All data were presented as means ± standard error of the mean (S.E.M.) for treatment groups and analyzed using StatView 5.0 (SAS Institute).

4 Notes

1. Even though far-red light is invisible to the human eye, sensitive CCD cameras can pick up the epifluorescent signal.
2. Acquisition of signals, with LSCM from tissues stained with multiple fluorophores, must be acquired in sequential mode and with appropriate cutoff filters to avoid bleed-through of fluorescent signals.
3. Zamboni's: Add 3 g (hydrated) picric acid to 150 ml distilled H_2O (dH_2O) to make a saturated aqueous solution. Stir for 1 h, and filter with a 0.2 μm filter. Add 20 g paraformaldehyde to 100 ml dH_2O and heat to 60 °C. Add several drops of 2.5 % NaOH while stirring continuously. Filter, cool, and mix with picric acid solution. Make up paraformaldehyde/picric acid solution to a final volume of 1 l with Millonig's sodium phos-

Fig. 4 (continued) Samples were immunostained with (1) anti-TRPV1 (1:20, made in goat, Santa Cruz Biotechnology) plus anti-goat IgG Cy2 (1:200, Jackson ImmunoResearch); (2) anti-pan-neuronal biomarker PGP9.5 (1:500, made in mouse, AbD Serotec, Raleigh, NC) plus anti-rabbit IgG Cy3 (1:1,000, Jackson ImmunoResearch); and (3) anti-EGFR (1:200, made in rabbit, Santa Cruz Biotechnology) plus anti-rabbit IgG Cy5 (1:500, Jackson ImmunoResearch). The image is a montage of two fields of view from Z-stack projections of twenty-four 2-μm optical sections using laser scanning confocal microscopy

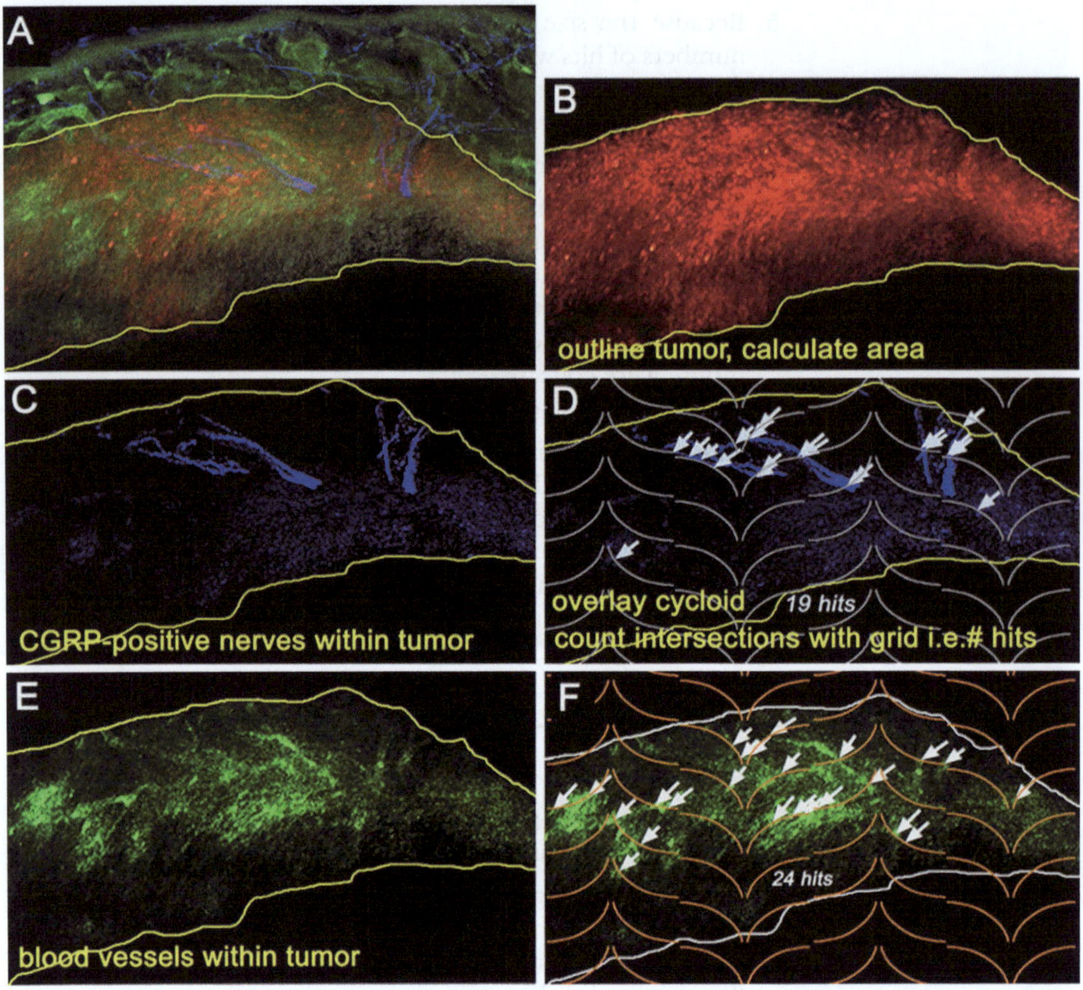

Fig. 5 Quantitation of nerves and vessel density within soft tissue DsRed2 fibrosarcomas. Relative nerve and blood vessel density within a DsRed2 fibrosarcoma soft tissue mass at a hyperalgesic testing site was determined. Stereology cycloid was applied to 3-D LSCM image data set projections. All images are taken similarly in that the *Z* series is 60 μm at 10-μm steps. Sections are stained with either a PGP9.5 or CGRP antibody (*blue*) or a CD31 antibody (*green*). (**a**) Merged LSCM projection (green vessels, red tumor, and blue nerves) of murine plantar surface immunostained with a CGRP antibody (*blue*) and a CD31 antibody (*green*). The red tumor boundary is outlined in *yellow*. (**b**) Isolation of the red channel image allows for exclusion of all but tumor area (*yellow boundary line*) under study. (**c**) The far-red channel is isolated, and the blue nerves within the tumor mass boundary line are visible. (**d**) A cycloid grid is applied, and points of intersection (*hits*) between grid and nerves are counted (*arrows*). (**e**) The green channel is isolated, and the green CD31-ir vessels within the tumor mass boundary line are visible. (**f**) A cycloid grid is applied, and points of intersection (*hits*) between grid and vessels within tumor boundary are counted (*arrows*). UplanFL10×/0.30. These data revealed that tumors from hyperalgesic mice are more densely innervated although vascularization is reduced when compared with tumors from non-hyperalgesic mice. (**a**, **b**, **d**, and **f** have been reproduced with permission of the International Association for the Study of Pain® (IASP). The figures may NOT be reproduced for any other purpose without permission)

phate buffer (PBS). Millonig's buffer for Zamboni's fixative (1 l): 1.80 g NaH_2PO_4–H_2O, 23.25 g $NaHPO_4$ $7H_2O$, and 5.00 g NaCl and store at 4 °C.

4. Picric acid is highly explosive when dry. Clean up all spills.
5. PBS: Purchase 10× pre-made stock. Make fresh weekly.
6. Biopsy/tissue storage buffer (cryo-preservative): Add 20 g sucrose to 100 ml of 0.5× PBS (no triton) for a 20 % sucrose solution. Add 0.5 g sodium azide for a final concentration of 0.05 % azide. Store at 4 °C.
7. TPBS: Add 3 ml Triton-X100 to 1 l PBS and store at 4 °C.
8. Normal serum: Reconstitute normal serum and store at 4 °C. Normal serum is from the animal in which secondary antibodies were raised, and pretreatment of tissue will reduce nonspecific binding of secondary antibodies to endogenous binding sites in tissue. Purchase from same vendor that supplied the secondary antibodies.
9. Use caution with antibodies because they can be very fragile and should be aliquoted into glycerol to avoid damaging freeze/thaw cycles. Use a positive-displacement pipette when drawing up the glycerol, and use only high-grade glycerol.
10. Agar: Add 0.38 g noble agar into 25 ml dH_2O into a 50 ml Erlenmeyer flask. Place mixing flask in a beaker of boiling water until dissolved.
11. Methyl salycilate: It is a clearing agent that improves confocal images by reducing refractive index differences between objective, immersion oil, and mounting media.
12. When harvesting mouse dorsal skin from euthanized animal for analysis of hair follicles, carefully excise skin and avoid touching the center of the piece of skin following the procedure of Peters et al. [10]. Briefly, excise a rectangle of skin down the vertebral column. Staple the edges of cephalad and caudal ends of the dorsal skin to a poster board before *gently* submersing in Zamboni's fixative or immediately freeze outer pieces in liquid nitrogen for protein or RNA extraction.
13. Acquisition and fixation of biopsy tissue require gentle handling. Organs and tissues from a perfused animal should be fixed for only 24 h more in Zamboni's. The volume of fixative should be 15× the tissue volume for adequate fixation. Be gentle! Do not jam tissue into too small of a fixation vial. If fixative solution becomes very cloudy within the first hour, decant and add new solution. This can be the case with heart, kidney, or spleen. The picric acid in Zamboni's fixative causes blood to precipitate. Some protocols fix tissues at room temperature or even a 37 °C fixative as opposed to 4 °C. The reduced temperature of 4 °C may reduce endogenous protease action.

Conversely, the reduced temperature may induce microtubule depolymerization, thereby destroying native cytoskeleton architecture. Do not fix longer than 48 h because the antigenic sites within the tissue can become cross-linked with prolonged fixation and the epitope will not be accessible to the antibody. This is especially critical for the monoclonal antibody against the protobacteria *Bartonella henselae.*

14. Theoretically, a sample can be stored indefinitely, but staining as soon as possible is probably better. However, batch-processing samples to reduce intra-experiment differences is more important.
15. Pretreating tissue with heat and/or citrate buffer to unmask antigens might be necessary.
16. Orient skin biopsy tissue with epidermis in the northeast corner of the chuck for more uniform cuts. Skin punch biopsies often have a cone shape, and therefore a great deal of patience is required to assure that the sections are not cut transversely by adjusting the angle of the cutting blade. However, in our hands better results were obtained by adding small amounts of OCT and a short burst of spray freeze and adjusting the angle of punch relative to the mounting chuck. For mouse skin tissue, the head-to-tail orientation must be maintained or hairs will be cut transversely.
17. Some cryostats indicate a maximum cutting thickness of up to 100 μm. Therefore you must "trick" the cryostat into cutting thicker sections. Section thickness is selected by setting the index scale. Thick sections may be obtained by rocking the hand wheel. Start with the handle at 12 o'clock, and move to 3 o'clock and then back to 12 o'clock. Each forward movement advances the specimen (an audible click will be heard) without a pass by the knife. To section at 180 μm, for example, set the index at 60 μm, rock the hand wheel two times, and then section on the third movement.
18. To keep tissues from drying out, put dishes into a lidded plastic container with a couple of layers of *fresh* wet paper towels on the bottom. Cover with foil when secondary antibodies have been added. Wash after each experiment.
19. You may also want to add a nonspecific blocking agent like BSA or fish gelatin.
20. As with all new antibodies, you will need to titrate each new batch and each combination of antibodies to determine the strongest fluorophore signal with the least amount of background. Just prior to adding the antibody, remove an aliquot from the freezer and "flick" the tube several times with fingers to mix. The antibody stock is quite viscous because antibodies are reconstituted and diluted 1:10 in 50 % glycerol aliquots and stored at −20 °C. Be careful to mix VERY thoroughly—

use a positive-displacement pipette when drawing up the glycerol, and use only high-grade glycerol.

21. Just prior to adding the primary antibodies, spin the diluted antibodies in a microcentrifuge for 3 min, and then be very careful not to disturb any pellet that may have formed when decanting the solution.
22. For a single 80-μm mouse skin tissue piece, 50 μl is adequate, but use greater volume for larger tissue or with multiple sections per well.
23. Negative controls are critical to determine acquisition settings when imaging stained samples.
24. Orientation can be critical when analyzing structures that run throughout the sample, e.g., hairs or ducts.
25. Cover slip should be smaller than the slide. You can do multiple tissue slices on each cover slip if desired.
26. For very thick sections (160 μm and up), use gasketed cover slips (Sigma).
27. As opposed to DPX, DEPEX contains phthalate resulting in a more flexible end product, which can be beneficial for deep optical sectioning. DEPEX, like all mounting media, will have about a 3–5 % shrink rate, and therefore adding more DEPEX at 24 and 48 h may be necessary. You may also want to add more DEPEX to the edges to be certain no bubbles form. The DEPEX is easy to remove with a sharp razorblade when the slide is dry. When DEPEX is almost empty, it may be too tacky to work with or have too many bubbles, and therefore opening a new one is recommended. Set the slide on top of a rack with open spaces, and be certain that the rack is level or the cover slips may slip off of the slide. Samples can be stored in slide boxes after 6 months, but store boxes on their sides so that cover slips are on top of the microscope slides.
28. Single- and multiphoton image capture settings, which must be used for each set and each scanning session, include scan rate, laser power, dwell time, laser intensity, gain, offset, simultaneous or sequential acquisition of multiple fluorophores, and filter sets.
29. A fluorescent reporter that emits in the green, red, or far-red channels should result in the same signal, although endogenous tissue fluorescence may contribute to the epifluorescent signal.
30. Using Adobe PhotoShop software the epidermis was selected. Total area pixel count of the entire selected epidermis was obtained. The area pixel count of the CGRP-ir (green channel) and PGP-ir (red channel) nerve fibers in the selected epidermal area was calculated by first thresholding the respective grayscale images.

References

1. Coleman R (2006) The long-term contribution of dyes and stains to histology and histopathology. Acta Histochem 108(2):81–83. doi: http://dx.doi.org/10.1016/j.acthis.2006.04.001
2. Siddiqi AM, Li H, Faruque F, Williams W, Lai K, Hughson M, Bigler S, Beach J, Johnson W (2008) Use of hyperspectral imaging to distinguish normal, precancerous, and cancerous cells. Cancer Cytopathol 114(1):13–21. doi:10.1002/cncr.23286
3. Beach JM (2009) A richer view of bio structures. BioOptics 2/3:2
4. Lee MH, Buterbaugh K, Richards-Kortum R, Anandasabapathy S (2012) Advanced endoscopic imaging for Barrett's Esophagus: current options and future directions. Curr Gastroenterol Rep 14(3):216–225. doi:10.1007/s11894-012-0259-3
5. Stefanini M, De Martino C, Zamboni L (1967) Fixation of ejaculated spermatozoa for electron microscopy. Nature 216(5111):173–174
6. Bode AM, Cho YY, Zheng D, Zhu F, Ericson ME, Ma WY, Yao K, Dong Z (2009) Transient receptor potential type vanilloid 1 suppresses skin carcinogenesis. Cancer Res 69(3):905–913. doi:0008-5472.CAN-08-3263 [pii] 10.1158/0008-5472.CAN-08-3263 [doi]
7. Hwang MK, Bode AM, Byun S, Song NR, Lee HJ, Lee KW, Dong Z (2010) Cocarcinogenic effect of capsaicin involves activation of EGFR signaling but not TRPV1. Cancer Res 70(17):6859–6869. doi:0008-5472.CAN-09-4393 [pii]10.1158/0008-5472.CAN-09-4393
8. Mayhew TM (1996) Adaptive remodelling of intestinal epithelium assessed using stereology: correlation of single cell and whole organ data with nutrient transport. Histol Histopathol 11(3):729–741
9. Hartoft-Nielsen ML, Rasmussen AK, Feldt-Rasmussen U, Buschard K, Bock T (2005) Estimation of number of follicles, volume of colloid and inner follicular surface area in the thyroid gland of rats. J Anat 207(2):117–124. doi:JOA442 [pii] 10.1111/j.1469-7580.2005.00442.x
10. Peters EM, Ericson ME, Hosoi J, Seiffert K, Hordinsky MK, Ansel JC, Paus R, Scholzen TE (2006) Neuropeptide control mechanisms in cutaneous biology: physiological and clinical significance. J Invest Dermatol 126(9):1937–1947. doi:5700429 [pii]10.1038/sj.jid.5700429
11. Hackett PB, Ekker SC, Largaespada DA, McIvor RS (2005) Sleeping beauty transposon-mediated gene therapy for prolonged expression. Adv Genet 54:189–232. doi:S0065-2660(05)54009-4 [pii]10.1016/S0065-2660(05)54009-4
12. Ivics Z, Hackett PB, Plasterk RH, Izsvak Z (1997) Molecular reconstruction of Sleeping Beauty, a Tc1-like transposon from fish, and its transposition in human cells. Cell 91(4):501–510. doi:S0092-8674(00)80436-5 [pii]

Chapter 13

Designing the Chemoprevention Trials of Tomorrow: Applying Lessons Learned from Past Definitive Trials

Karen Colbert Maresso and Ernest Hawk

Abstract

Chemoprevention represents an important part of cancer medicine's future. The identification of chemopreventive agents holds tremendous promise for reducing the burden of cancer. Currently, 13 agents are FDA approved for the treatment of precancerous lesions or to reduce the risk of invasive cancer. The identification and availability of safe and effective chemopreventive agents rely upon their rigorous evaluation in phase I–IV clinical trials. Five critical elements must be considered in the design and conduct of any clinical trial: (a) agent or intervention to be tested for its ability to suppress the incidence of precancerous or cancerous lesions, inhibit their progression, or induce their regression; (b) biomarkers evaluated at the level of a tissue, cell, or biochemical product as secondary endpoints to evaluate the underlying biology of the preinvasive neoplastic lesion and/or the mechanisms underlying an agent's efficacy and/or toxicities; (c) the cohort of individuals at risk for cancer who are enrolled to participate in the trial; (d) design specifying how the various components are combined, implemented, and monitored; (e) endpoint—the primary goal of the trial that drives the sample size and power estimates. These elements can be remembered by the pneumonic "ABCDE." In this chapter, we discuss each of the five cardinal elements of trial design and evaluate previous trials in the context of these cardinal elements to glean lessons that can inform and enhance the design and conduct of future trials.

Key words Chemoprevention, Clinical trials, Cancer, Prevention

1 Introduction

Chemoprevention represents an important opportunity for cancer medicine's future. The identification and application of chemopreventive agents hold tremendous promise for reducing the burden of cancer, which has been amply demonstrated by preventive agents applied to reduce cardiovascular risks. While the focus in cancer medicine has been and is still largely treatment oriented, an increasing cancer burden and escalating treatment costs necessitate a shift towards prevention. The power of prevention in cancer medicine is illustrated in the setting of cervical cancer, where use of the pap test led to a greater than 60 % reduction in cervical cancer death rates in the USA between 1955 and 1992 [1] and where the HPV

Ann M. Bode and Zigang Dong (eds.), *Cancer Prevention: Dietary Factors and Pharmacology*, Methods in Pharmacology and Toxicology, DOI 10.1007/978-1-4614-9227-6_13, © Springer Science+Business Media New York 2014

Agent	Biomarkers	Cohort	Design	Endpoint
▪ More target-driven approach	▪ Need for early biomarkers	▪ High-risk *vs.* Average risk	▪ Rigorous preclinical toxicity testing	▪ Difficult to access in prevention trials
▪ Need to balance efficacy vs. safety	▪ Risk marker *vs.* Response marker	▪ Need for more careful patient selection	▪ Phase I - Phase IV Clinical Trials in Humans	▪ Need intermediate measures of benefit

Fig. 1 The "ABCDEs" of clinical prevention trials

vaccine may reduce cervical cancer death rates worldwide by a similar amount, in addition to potentially reducing deaths due to anal, vulvovaginal, penile, and oral cancers [2].

Only relatively recently have compelling rationales and opportunities emerged for a true chemopreventive approach towards cancer. We now have refined insights into cancer etiology and early pathogenesis, successful risk assessment models, and enhanced screening strategies that are increasingly applied due to successful public education campaigns and reduced financial barriers through the enactment of the Affordable Care Act. Furthermore, we have an established track record of 13 FDA-approved preventive agents and additional agents with apparent broad efficacy (e.g., aspirin) in common diseases of aging Western populations that have not required FDA's consideration or endorsement.

The identification of additional novel preventive agents that are both safe and efficacious relies upon rigorous testing in well-designed clinical trials. The goals in clinical preventive trial design include exploring dosing and toxicity in phase I, establishing preliminary evidence of efficacy and associated mechanisms in phase II, establishing definitive evidence of efficacy and relative safety in phase III leading to agent approval, and exploring less common or severe toxicities and establishing definitive evidence of effectiveness in phase IV trials. Five critical elements must be considered in the design and conduct of any clinical trial: (a) agents or the intervention to be tested for its ability to suppress incident precancerous or cancerous lesions, inhibit their progression, or induce their regression; (b) biomarkers evaluated at the level of a tissue, cell, or biochemical product as secondary endpoints to evaluate the underlying biology of the preinvasive neoplastic lesion and/or the mechanisms underlying an agent's efficacy and/or toxicities; (c) the cohort of individuals at risk for cancer who are enrolled to participate in the trial; (d) design specifying how the various components are combined, implemented, and monitored; and (e) endpoint—the primary goal of the trial, which drives the sample size and power estimates. These elements can be remembered by the pneumonic "ABCDE" (Fig. 1).

In Sect. 2 that follows, we outline important points and recommendations for improving upon each of these five cardinal elements so as to enhance the design and conduct of future chemopreventive trials. These points and recommendations are based upon lessons learned from past definitive trials, which are elaborated upon in Sect. 3. Applying these and other lessons to the design of future chemoprevention trials should facilitate the translation of novel agents exhibiting preventive potential into the clinic.

2 Methods

2.1 Improving Agents

In the past, chemopreventive agents were generally classified by their proposed mechanism of action, which was primarily described at the cellular or the tissue level. This classification yielded categories such as anti-mutagens/antioxidants (e.g., tocopherols, isothiocyanates, sulforaphane); antiproliferatives (e.g., eflornithine, retinoids); pro-apoptotics (e.g., corticosteroids); anti-hormonals (e.g., tamoxifen, raloxifen, aromatase inhibitors); anti-inflammatories (e.g., aspirin, nonsteroidal anti-inflammatories); or nutritional supplements (e.g., calcium, carotenoids, selenium, fiber). However, more recently, greater molecular insights into the early stages of carcinogenesis have enabled agent identification to assume a more target-driven approach focused on key molecular aberrancies or pathway alterations that are common in neoplastic initiation and progression. For example, more molecularly targeted agents, such as erlotinib or dutasteride, are now making their way into chemopreventive applications. Several key criteria are met by compelling targets or pathways for cancer prevention (Fig. 2). Perhaps most important to chemopreventive agent development thus far has been the need to balance the risks and benefits of an applied intervention. Thirteen agents (Table 1) have been approved to treat precancerous lesions or reduce cancer risks, but most of these are only rarely used because of concerns over side effects, which can be severe and unpredictable for some of the agents (e.g., tamoxifen, which reduces noninvasive and invasive breast cancer incidence by as much as 50 % but also increases patients' risks of uterine cancer and serious thromboembolic events). Because concerns over toxicities have reduced interest in taking preventive agents, considering how one might improve the therapeutic index of an effective agent is crucial to the field of chemoprevention.

At least five strategies can be employed to make an effective agent safer and more acceptable (Fig. 3).

1. Adjust the method by which the agent is administered to maximize concentrations of the drug in a targeted location, and minimize systemic exposure. Adjust the dose, route, frequency, or duration as needed to provide the greatest chance of efficacy

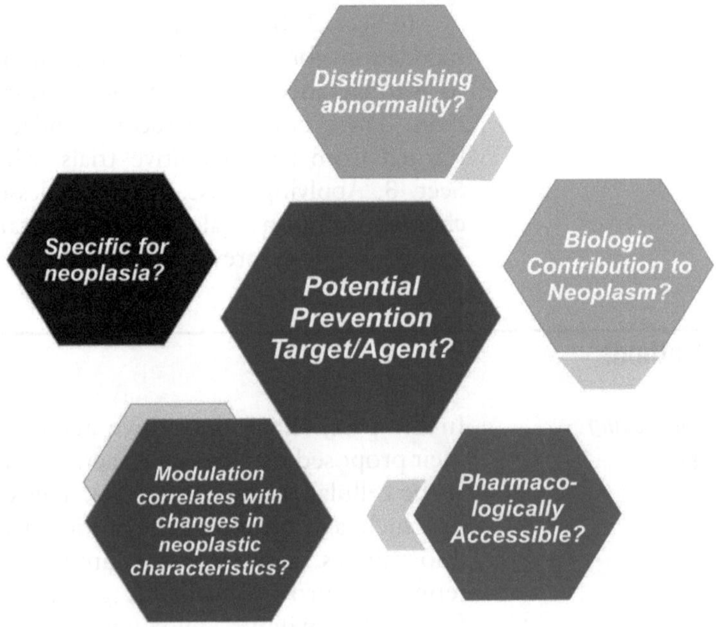

Fig. 2 The five key criteria for a potential preventive target/agent to fulfill. First, a potential target should exhibit an aberrant level of expression or be an abnormal protein in early human neoplasia relative to the normal epithelium. Second, the target should demonstrate an unequivocal biologic contribution to the initiation, maintenance, or progression of a neoplasm in a model system. Third, it must be pharmacologically accessible. Fourth, modulation of the potential target should correspond with reductions in neoplastic (i.e., pre-cancer or cancer) incidence, histopathologic grade, and/or other pathologic evidence. Finally, it should be relatively specific for neoplasia rather than the normal tissues from which cancers arise

while minimizing risks. In the skin, this has been achieved through topical administration of 5-fluorouracil or diclofenac, both of which have a range of toxicities when applied systemically but which are quite tolerable when applied directly to a precancerous lesion, such as an actinic keratosis.

2. If an agent's anticipated dose-limiting or common toxicities are known, administer the chemopreventive agent with a prophylactic agent that can minimize the occurrence and/or frequency of side effects. This approach is best exemplified by the use of H2-blockers or proton pump inhibitors along with aspirin or other nonsteroidal anti-inflammatories to reduce risks of upper gastrointestinal ulceration. This strategy has met with reasonable success, at least in settings other than cancer prevention, per se.
3. If the mechanisms of efficacy and toxicity are known and they differ in one or more regards, identify agents that can more

Table 1
FDA-approved agents for the treatment of precancerous lesions or cancer risk reduction in associated cohorts

Agent	Targeted cohort in indication	Endpoint in indication
Tamoxifen	Women with DCIS following breast surgery and radiation	Reduces the risk of invasive breast cancer
Tamoxifen	Women at high risk for breast cancer ("high risk" defined as women at least 35 years of age with a 5-year predicted risk of breast cancer ≥1.67 %, as calculated by the Gail Model)	Reduces the incidence of breast cancer
Raloxifene	Postmenopausal women at high risk for invasive breast cancer ("high risk" defined as at least one breast biopsy showing lobular carcinoma in situ or atypical hyperplasia, one or more first-degree relatives with breast cancer, or a 5-year predicted risk of breast cancer ≥1.66 % (based on the modified Gail model))	Reduction in the risk of invasive breast cancer (Note: EVISTA does not eliminate the risk of breast cancer. Patients should have breast exams and mammograms before starting EVISTA and should continue regular breast exams and mammograms in keeping with good medical practice after beginning treatment with EVISTA)
HPV vaccine (Cervarix)	Females 9 through 25 years of age	The prevention of the following diseases caused by oncogenic human papillomavirus (HPV) types 16 and 18: Cervical cancer Cervical intraepithelial neoplasia (CIN) grade 2 or worse and adenocarcinoma in situ CIN grade 1
HPV vaccine (Gardasil)	Girls and women 9 through 26 years of age	The prevention of the following diseases caused by human papillomavirus (HPV) types included in the vaccine: Cervical, vulvar, vaginal, and anal cancer caused by HPV types 16 and 18 And the following precancerous or dysplastic lesions caused by HPV types 6,11, 16, and 18: CIN grade 2/3 and cervical adenocarcinoma in situ (AIS) CIN grade 1 Vulvar intraepithelial neoplasia (VIN) grade 2 and grade 3 Vaginal intraepithelial neoplasia (VaIN) grade 2 and grade 3 Anal intraepithelial neoplasia (AIN) grades 1, 2, and 3

(continued)

Table 1 (continued)

Agent	Targeted cohort in indication	Endpoint in indication
HPV vaccine (Gardasil)	Boys and men 9 through 26 years of age	The prevention of the following diseases caused by HPV types included in the vaccine: Anal cancer caused by HPV types 16 and 18 And the following precancerous or dysplastic lesions caused by HPV types 6, 11, 16, and 18: AIN grades 1, 2, and 3
Photodynamic therapy (PDT) with Photofrin	Males and females with high-grade dysplasia (HGD) in Barrett's esophagus	Ablation of HGD in Barrett's esophagus (BE) patients who do not undergo esophagectomy
Celecoxib[a]	Males and females ≥18 years old with familial adenomatous polyposis (FAP)	Reduction in the number of adenomatous colorectal polyps in FAP, as an adjunct to usual care (e.g., endoscopic surveillance, surgery)
Bacillus–Calmette–Guerin (BCG)	Males and females with carcinoma in situ (CIS) of the urinary bladder	Intravesical use in the treatment and prophylaxis of CIS of the urinary bladder and for the prophylaxis of primary- or recurrent-stage Ta and/or T1 papillary tumors following transurethral resection (TUR)
Valrubicin	Males and females with BCG-refractory CIS	Intravesical therapy of BCG-refractory CIS of the urinary bladder in patients for whom immediate cystectomy would be associated with unacceptable morbidity or mortality
Fluorouracil	Males and females with multiple actinic or solar keratoses	Topical treatment of multiple actinic or solar keratoses
Diclofenac sodium	Males and females with actinic keratoses	Topical treatment of actinic keratoses
PDT with 5-aminolevulinic acid	Males and females with actinic keratoses of the face or the scalp	Topical treatment of minimally to moderately thick actinic keratoses of the face or the scalp
Masoprocol[b]	Males and females with actinic (solar) keratoses	Topical treatment of actinic keratoses
Ingenol mebutate	Males and females with actinic keratoses on the face, scalp, trunk, and extremities	Topical treatment of actinic keratoses

[a]FDA labeling voluntarily withdrawn by Pfizer, February 2011
[b]Withdrawn from the US market, June 1996

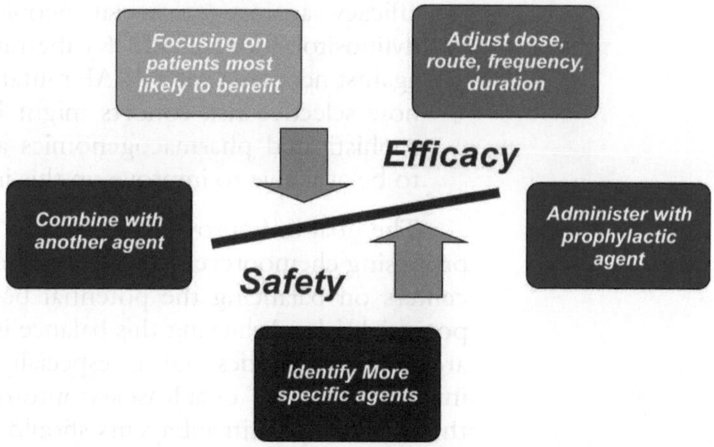

Fig. 3 Improving an agent's therapeutic index. Five strategies are proposed to improve the safety and acceptability of an effective agent. First, adjust how the agent is administered to maximize concentrations of the drug in targeted location and to minimize systemic exposure. Thus the dose, route, frequency, or duration of an agent can be adjusted as needed to provide the greatest chance of efficacy while minimizing risks. Second, if we have a good idea of an agent's anticipated dose-limiting or common toxicities, we can administer the chemopreventive agent with a prophylactic agent that can minimize the occurrence and/or frequency of side effects. Third, if we know the mechanisms of efficacy and of toxicity, and they differ in one or more regards, we may be able to identify agents that can more specifically target the pathologic mechanism without perturbing normal physiology. Fourth, an effective agent may be made more tolerable by administering it in combination with another agent, hopefully with synergistic efficacy, but no greater toxicity. And finally, an effective agent may be demonstrated to be more tolerable with careful patient selection focused on identifying those most likely to benefit and/or least likely to be harmed by a preventive compound

specifically target the pathologic mechanism without perturbing normal physiology (more details in Sect. 3).

4. Combine the agent with another efficacious agent, with the goal of achieving synergistic efficacy, but with no greater toxicity (an example of this concept is provided in Sect. 3). Whether targeting two levels of the same pathway is better than targeting two different pathways remains to be determined.
5. Careful selection of those patients most likely to benefit from, and/or least likely to be harmed by, a preventive compound, which may make an agent more tolerable: This has not yet been tested prospectively in the clinic, although most prevention trials involve cohorts at increased risk of cancer. This strategy is largely due to the notion of applying these agents first in patients most likely to benefit or more likely to tolerate minor toxicities. The recent post hoc analysis of aspirin's selective

efficacy against colorectal neoplasia harboring phosphatidylinositol 3-kinase (PI3-K) aberrations and its lack of efficacy against neoplasia with BRAF mutations are recent examples of how selective risk cohorts might be identified [3, 4]. More sophisticated pharmacogenomics assessments are anticipated to be available to improve on this in the near future.

The goal of improving upon both the quality and quantity of promising chemopreventive agents entering phase III clinical trials centers on balancing the potential benefits of an agent with its potential risks. Achieving this balance is critically important in any area of therapeutics but is especially so in prevention, which involves "healthy," or at least asymptomatic, individuals. To achieve this balance, prioritized agents should demonstrate powerful efficacy in preclinical studies, with cross-model and cross-investigator replication. Dose, duration, and toxicities should be optimally defined by preclinical and phase II studies; and synergy between agents can lead to lower doses, improved efficacy, and fewer and/or less severe toxicities. For these reasons, agent combinations are likely to be very important in the future in cancer prevention, as they are in other areas of medicine (e.g., management of hypertension, osteoporosis, or diabetes).

2.2 Identifying Better Biomarkers

Within the last 30 years, very few chemopreventive agents have been approved by the FDA. This is due, in part, to a lack of validated and practical biomarkers for use in chemopreventive trials. Biomarkers are intended to provide early insights into agent responses that will later translate into clinically meaningful preventive endpoints (e.g., delays or reductions in cancer incidence or mortality). Biomarkers may be considered by their intended application, as risk markers, which estimate the probability of a later event (e.g., exposure, susceptibility, diagnostic, or prognostic biomarkers), or response markers, which measure changes following an intervention. In prevention, an ideal response biomarker is accurate, reliable, and amenable to quantitation; differentially expressed in high-risk (versus normal) tissues; causally related to cancer development; modulated by an intervention, associated with a relatively short latency to invasive cancer; correlated with cancer incidence; and obtainable through noninvasive means.

Biomarkers may also be classified by their biologic level (e.g., DNA, RNA, protein). Generally, although molecular markers provide essential mechanistic information, tissue-level markers are more decisive indicators of cancer risk because they integrate individual molecular markers and more faithfully predict for invasive cancer and are closer to the ultimate goal of intervention, which is, of course, a clinical benefit. The *Bcr-Abl* oncogene in chronic myelogenous leukemia provides a rare example of a molecular defect that is both pathognomonic of the disease and determines clinical management. More often, multiple molecular defects are required to initiate, maintain, and promote carcinogenesis, and no single defect reliably predicts cancer development. Therefore, prevention trials typically assess multiple response biomarkers within any given trial in order to query and confirm neoplastic determinants and agent mechanisms of action across several biologic levels, hopefully providing insights from several different vantage points such as those outlined below.

1. Measuring circulating blood-based biomarkers allows for determination of the plasma drug concentration and blood pharmacodynamics.
2. Assessing germline genomics can allow for the identification of DNA markers that may influence the metabolism of the agent (e.g., single-nucleotide polymorphisms in *CYP* drug-metabolizing genes) and can therefore inform a more personalized or pharmacogenomically driven approach to the development or the application of the agent in question.
3. Examining biomarkers in the target tissue is rarely performed but is needed to confirm adequate dosing as well as to permit greater insight into the agent's mechanism(s) of action.
4. Assessing biomarkers in a tissue anticipated to experience toxic side effects of the intervention can provide information regarding the optimal dosing and pharmacodynamics of the agent.
5. Determining biomarkers in a surrogate tissue, that is, one that is neither the target tissue nor the anticipated toxic tissue, can further provide important correlations with an agent's efficacy or toxicity.
6. Standardizing and improving all aspects of specimen acquisition, handling, transportation, storage, assay, interpretation, and analysis to reduce potential causes of error and noise.
7. Studying the natural history of a marker and how it relates with cancer risk cross-sectionally and over time to validate the use of a particular biomarker: In a prevention trial that involves a placebo arm, many times that arm can be used to confirm a marker's natural history and association with cancer risk (i.e., as a prognostic marker), while the treatment arm provides preliminary evidence of the agent's efficacy (i.e., as a predictive marker).

2.3 Building and Enhancing Cohorts

The type of cohort in which to evaluate an agent is another important element of trial design. A group's underlying risk of preinvasive neoplasia and its progression to cancer permits stratified classifications into average- and increased-risk categories. Historically, the cohorts involved in chemoprevention trials were generally of average risk and therefore large in number and costly to follow over the extended time required for endpoint determinations. However, the more recent trend is to move away from this type of design towards smaller, less expensive cohorts of individuals at increased risk of cancer due to inherited or cumulative environmental risks (e.g., unhealthy lifestyle choices such as smoking, physical inactivity, unhealthy diets, or occupational exposures). Using germline and somatic markers of risk is a promising approach to enrich a cohort for those at increased risk of a cancer or a premalignancy. Individuals with germline susceptibilities tend to develop neoplasia earlier and have an accelerated rate of progression. A family history of cancer in a first-degree relative, especially if it was diagnosed at an early age or occurred in more than one relative, may increase cancer risks twofold, even in the absence of an identified or a specific genetic cause. An alternative approach to enriching a cohort for those at increased risk is based on a history of exposure to any number of environmental hazards (e.g., tobacco, radiation, exogenous hormones, infections with hepatitis B, hepatitis C, *H. pylori*, Epstein–Barr, or human papilloma viruses) that adversely affect the genome or its expression. Selecting individuals at increased risk requires careful characterization and quantification of cancer risks based on questions about one's lifestyle habits, personal history of exposures, prior neoplasia (invasive or noninvasive), family history of neoplasia or associated risk factors, and, increasingly, biospecimen collection reflecting an individual's germline genetics and cumulative systemic exposures (e.g., blood) or evaluations of specific target organs. More recently, a variety of more specific and quantitative models have been produced for risk assessment of various cancers [5–7].

Employing germline, familial, or increased-risk cohorts compared to individuals at average risk (i.e., general population) can provide substantial benefits.

1. Increased-risk cohorts offer more patients that are informative regarding agent efficacy, thereby increasing trial efficiency and reducing the required sample size.
2. Higher risk cohorts offer more power than do cohorts of average-risk individuals over a shorter time frame, reducing the need for long, expensive trials and facilitating the trend towards faster, cheaper trials.
3. In addition, individuals at higher risk for a cancer or a premalignancy will typically receive greater personal benefit from an efficacious agent and will likely be more tolerant of side effects, increasing motivation to adhere to an intervention and its associated evaluations.

An example of the ability of a single, small trial to inform is provided in Sect. 3.

2.4 Improving Elements of Overall Trial Design

Improving the overall design of clinical trials depends upon a host of factors, not the least of which is an appreciation of the importance of the randomized, placebo-controlled design and the relatively recent increased reliance upon preclinical testing before moving into human testing. Optimal trial designs isolate the agent as the primary study variable, holding all other variables constant. Factors that can significantly influence trial design and outcome include the following listed below.

1. The use of a placebo arm within a trial because this allows for determination of the natural history of the disease and of biomarkers and facilitates toxicity assessments, which are critical to an agent's ultimate appeal and acceptance as a preventive agent (an example of the importance of the placebo arm in a trial is provided in Sect. 3).
2. Basing trial prioritization on a converging premise of strong preclinical data, agent and mechanistic screening, and observational efficacy. Preclinical data and agent/mechanistic studies are typically in vitro or in vivo in nature, whereas observational data are obtained from large population-based epidemiological studies. Combined, these data can be used to support clinical testing in humans, where preliminary efficacy, safety, further mechanistic insights, and dose, route, frequency, and duration are determined in phase II studies, with definitive efficacy tested in phase III trials (Fig. 4).
3. Long-term follow-up and monitoring of both efficacy and safety with sufficient rigor to meet FDA requirements and promote acceptance in the marketplace.
4. Sponsorship, because private investment can yield more discretionary resources but with frequent and important concerns regarding potential bias.
5. Adherence measures, because evaluating dropouts, drop-ins, and their impact on the study's power related to various primary and secondary endpoints over time is essential.
6. Target organ accessibility, with trials involving relatively inaccessible organs (e.g., breast, ovary, prostate, kidney, pancreas, liver, and brain) typically requiring larger sample sizes, longer follow-up durations, and an increased reliance on clinical, rather than biological, efficacy measures. Greater heterogeneity in tissue-based biomarkers is also seen with relatively inaccessible organs. Of the 13 FDA-approved chemopreventive agents, just 2 are approved for use in a relatively inaccessible organ (i.e., tamoxifen and raloxifene for use in breast cancer).

2.5 Establishing Endpoints

Selecting endpoints for use in chemopreventive agent development and trial design is challenging and highly controversial. Reduction in the development of newly identified cancers versus usual care (most often, placebo) in the context of an acceptable risk–benefit balance has been the "gold standard" for regulatory consideration of cancer-preventive agents [8, 9]. However, the time course over which most cancers typically develop precludes the use of incidence and mortality as feasible endpoints given the limited time and

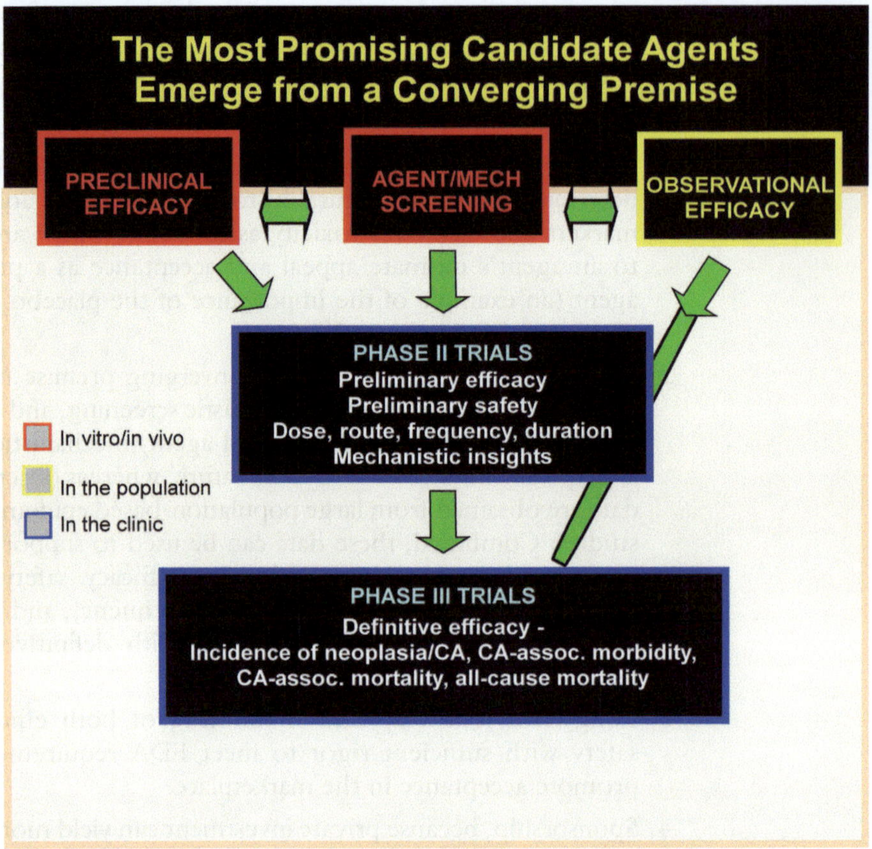

Fig. 4 Schematic demonstrating the types of data and studies comprising a strong premise upon which to build clinical trials. In vitro and in vivo studies are shown in *red*, population-based studies are shown in *yellow*, and clinical studies are shown in *blue*

resources of the typical clinical trial. Improvements in the duration of life, quality of life, or both are also unambiguous efficacy endpoints that are agreed upon by regulatory authorities, scientists, and patients. However, while these outcomes are important, they are also longer term goals, much like reductions in incidence and mortality, and so do not truly address the issue of having more immediate and practical endpoints that can be consistently evaluated within the framework of a typical trial.

Despite the ambiguities and challenges, most phase II and phase III trials of chemopreventive agents involve reductions in the number, size, or grade of intraepithelial neoplastic lesions or patients with these lesions, if not incident invasive cancers, as their primary endpoints. In addition, most trials include a variety of additional biomarkers as secondary or tertiary endpoints, with the intention of bolstering biologic and mechanistic insights into the agent's efficacy and/or incidentally identified toxicities. These endpoints provide pharmacodynamic and pharmacokinetic insights and may indicate the molecular status of residual lesions to try to assure that the progression of the disease has been sufficiently interrupted and to provide insights into the potential long-term implications of the agent.

Because endpoints drive interest and investment in agent development, particularly of the private sector, progress in chemoprevention is expected to be slow until the field of cancer prevention has reasonably validated efficacy endpoints.

3 Discussion

Following are descriptions of landmark proof-of-principle prevention trials that have demonstrated the feasibility and challenges of chemopreventive drug development. We highlight lessons learned from these trials in the context of the ABCDEs.

3.1 The ATBC and CARET Trials in Lung Cancer and the SELECT Trial in Prostate Cancer

In the 1970s and 1980s, beta-carotene was suggested to reduce lung cancer risks based on several different observational studies suggesting strong and consistent associations between dietary intake of carotene-containing fruits and vegetables and reduced lung cancer incidence and mortality. Before suggesting widespread adoption, two randomized, controlled trials were conducted—the CARET trial and the ATBC trial [10, 11]. These trials focused on evaluations of the hypothesis that carotene supplementation would reduce the risk of lung, and possibly other cancers, in high-risk individuals. However, both trials identified increased, and not reduced, risks of lung cancer following treatment with beta-carotene [10, 11].

This same experience was more recently repeated in the Selenium and Vitamin E Cancer Prevention Trial (SELECT) for prostate cancer, which randomized over 35,000 relatively healthy men to receive either oral selenium (200 μg/day from L-selenomethionine) and a matched vitamin E placebo, vitamin E (400 IU/day of all rac-α-tocopheryl acetate), and matched selenium placebo, selenium–vitamin E, or placebo + placebo for a planned follow-up of a minimum of 7 years and a maximum of 12 years. Results showed that selenium and vitamin E, neither in combination nor alone, prevented prostate cancer; and in fact, a non-statistically significant 17 % increased risk for prostate cancer was observed among those in the vitamin E group [12]. The premise for the SELECT trial was largely based on associations between alpha-tocopherol and prostate cancer in the ATBC trial, as well as selenium's potential effect on prostate cancer incidence, as described as a promising secondary efficacy measure from a large RCT involving patients at risk for skin cancer [11, 13].

These counterintuitive findings of the ATBC, CARET, and SELECT were both surprising and sobering, suggesting that rigorous and careful clinical studies of all preventive agents should be undertaken prior to assuming efficacy or safety or suggesting widespread adoption of even the most presumably benign of agents. These three trials moved directly from epidemiological observations to phase III trials without compelling mechanistic data or phase I and II data. They demonstrated the need for thorough preclinical and early-phase work in order to better understand mechanisms and minimize the risk of toxicities before undertaking large and expensive phase III trials. They emphasized the need for selecting agents for further evaluation based on a converging premise of evidence that includes not only observational data but also preclinical data and phase I and II clinical trial data.

3.2 The PCPT and REDUCE Trial in Prostate Cancer

The Prostate Cancer Prevention Trial (PCPT) randomized over 18,000 relatively healthy men to receive either 5 mg of finasteride daily or placebo for 7 years. Results demonstrated a significant 28 % reduction (RR = 0.75; 95 % CI: 18.6–30.6) in the prevalence of prostate cancer over the 7 years in those taking finasteride [14]. However, high-grade tumors (Gleason scores 7, 8, 9, or 10) were significantly more common in this group ($p = 0.005$), as were sexual side effects ($p < 0.001$) [14].

The Reduction by Dutasteride of Prostate Cancer Events (REDUCE) trial randomized over 8,000 men aged 50–75 at high risk for prostate cancer (i.e., elevated PSA level and previous suspicion of prostate cancer leading to a prostate biopsy) to receive either 0.5 mg of dutasteride daily or placebo for 4 years [15]. Results revealed a 23 % reduction in risk (RR = 0.77; 95 % CI: 15.2–29.8) of incident prostate cancer over the 4-year period [15].

PCPT and REDUCE together show an overall relative reduction of 23–25 % in prostate cancer diagnoses. However, subsequent analyses determined that this observed reduction was largely due to a decrease in incidence of only low-grade tumors (Gleason score ≤6)—tumors that were unlikely to ever become clinically significant [16]. Additionally, these analyses identified a slight increase in the incidence of high-grade tumors in the chemoprevention group of both trials [16]. Ultimately, the Federal Drug Administration did not approve the use of either finasteride or dutasteride for prostate cancer risk reduction because of concerns over the drugs' risk–benefit profiles [16]. Although the PCPT and REDUCE trial did not lead to approval of chemopreventive agents for the most common cancer in men, they emphasized the FDA's imperative of appropriately balancing risks and benefits in a chemopreventive setting.

3.3 The BCPT and STAR Trial in Breast Cancer

The Breast Cancer Prevention Trial (BCPT) randomized over 13,000 women aged 35–70 who were at risk for breast cancer (as determined by the Gail model) to 20 mg/day tamoxifen or placebo for 5 years, with the primary endpoint being occurrence of breast cancer [8]. The study was closed early after an interim analysis revealed a 49 % reduction in invasive breast cancer incidence and a 50 % reduction in noninvasive breast cancer incidence for those on tamoxifen. Subsequently, the Study of Tamoxifen Against Raloxifene (STAR) trial randomized nearly 20,000 postmenopausal women at increased risk of breast cancer to either 20 mg/day tamoxifen or 60 mg/day raloxifene for 5 years, with the occurrence of breast cancer as the primary endpoint [9, 17]. STAR demonstrated that while these two agents had similar efficacy (~50 % reduction in breast cancers), raloxifene had far fewer side effects (fewer uterine cancers, thrombosis, and hot flashes) than did tamoxifen. Raloxifene demonstrated a nearly 50 % reduction in the rate of uterine cancers at 8 years compared to tamoxifen [9, 17]. The BCPT and STAR demonstrate that safety of a chemopreventive agent can be improved in iterative generations of agents and trials.

3.4 Trials of Nonsteroidal Anti-inflammatory Drugs in Colorectal Cancer

A number of clinical trials have tested the nonsteroidal anti-inflammatory drugs (NSAIDs), aspirin and celecoxib, for risk reduction and prevention in the setting of colorectal cancer (CRC) and adenomas. Over 6 years, beginning in 2000 with the publication of results from the landmark Celecoxib in FAP randomized controlled trial (RCT), these studies led to a number of important discoveries and lessons regarding the ABCDEs.

The Celecoxib in FAP trial randomized 83 patients with familial adenomatous polyposis (FAP) and prevalent adenomas to receive either 100 or 400 mg twice daily or placebo twice daily for 6 months. The study revealed a significant 28 % ($p = 0.003$) reduction in polyp number and a nearly 31 % ($p = 0.001$) reduction in polyp burden in those receiving the 400 mg/BID dose when compared to those receiving the placebo [18]. Despite the small size and short time frame of this trial, its impact was substantial. Not only did it demonstrate a new adjunctive pharmacologic approach for the management of FAP patients, it provided a much-needed stimulus for additional research in this area and, perhaps more importantly, for private investment in chemoprevention in general. It also served as the scientific premise for additional research with cyclooxygenase (COX)-2 inhibitors in other at-risk cohorts and validated the mechanism-driven approach to cancer prevention. The Celecoxib in FAP trial serves as an excellent example of the ability of a single small trial to inform broadly and supports the current trend of designing smaller, shorter, and more high-powered trials of those at increased risk.

In 2003, results of two large, randomized trials demonstrated significant protective effects of aspirin on the development of adenomas in those with a history of CRC [19] and in those with a history of previous adenomas [20]. Sandler et al. randomized 625 patients with a prior history of CRC to receive either 325 mg/day or placebo for 1 year and found a significantly lower mean number of adenomas in the aspirin group than in the placebo group ($p = 0.003$) as well as a significantly reduced risk of adenoma recurrence (RR = 0.65; 95 % CI: 0.46–0.91) [19]. Baron et al. randomized 1,121 patients with a recent history of adenomas to receive either 81 or 325 mg of aspirin daily, or placebo, for 3 years and also identified significantly reduced risks for adenoma recurrence (RR = 0.81; 95 % CI: 0.69–0.96) and advanced lesions (RR = 0.59; 95 % CI: 0.38–0.92) among those taking the lower dose of aspirin [20].

In 2006, results of the National Cancer Institute- and Pfizer-supported Adenoma Prevention with Celecoxib (APC) trial were published [21]. This RCT randomized over 2,000 patients with prior sporadic adenomas to receive either 200 or 400 mg of celecoxib or placebo, twice daily, for 3 years. Ninety-one clinical sites from across the USA, Canada, Australia, and the UK were included. Results identified a significant 33 % reduction ($p < 0.001$) in the risk of recurrent adenomas among those taking 200 mg of celecoxib twice daily and a significant 45 % reduction ($p < 0.001$) among those taking 400 mg twice daily [21]. However, findings also revealed that the use of celecoxib was associated with a significantly increased risk (RR in low-dose group, 2.6; 95 % CI: 1.1–6.1; RR in high-dose group, 3.4; 95 % CI: 1.5–7.9) of serious cardiovascular events, precluding its use as an effective agent for the prevention of colorectal adenomas [21]. Importantly, the APC trial revealed the imperative for broad, sensitive toxicological and human safety assessments. Subsequent pooled analyses of upper gastrointestinal and cardiovascular risks of celecoxib confirmed its potential risks but placed it in a broader context of similar effects across a broad range of nonsteroidal anti-inflammatories and COX-2 inhibitors [22, 23].

Interestingly, additional recent placebo-controlled trials of celecoxib and other COX-2 inhibitors in other settings have also revealed the increased cardiovascular risks associated with these agents. These cardiovascular risks of COX-2 inhibitors originally went undetected in early trials because they had only initially been tested against traditional NSAIDs and not placebos. Comparing coxibs to NSAIDS masked the cardiovascular toxicity of coxibs because of the high background rate of cardiovascular events in the tested populations and because both agents may cause them. Further experimentation has demonstrated that coxibs, although intended to be highly specific for COX-2, may actually inhibit a variety of other targets at pharmacologic doses, casting some question on the entire notion of the specificity of targeted agents and underscoring the opportunity for proper placebo-controlled trials of most agents along with broad toxicological and human safety assessments.

In an additional study focusing on a high-risk cohort with previous adenomas, another NSAID, sulindac, was tested in combination with difluoromethylornithine (DFMO), a polyamine synthesis inhibitor [24]. These two agents had been previously shown to interact additively to inhibit the growth and viability of human colon cancer cells [25]. This RCT randomized 374 patients with a history of resected adenomas to receive a low-dose combination of 500 mg DFMO and 150 mg sulindac once daily or placebo for 3 years. This trial serves as the first example of a study examining two potential chemopreventive agents in combination. Results were dramatic. Compared to the placebo group, those given the DFMO and sulindac combination demonstrated a significant 70 % reduction in the risk of recurrent adenomas, a significant 92 % reduction in the risk of one or more advanced adenomas, and a significant 95 % reduction in the risk of multiple adenomas [24]. This trial clearly highlights the potential synergy that can be achieved through agent combinations, resulting in the use of lower doses, improved efficacy, and fewer or less severe toxicities. The results suggest the use of agent combinations as a promising strategy in the future of chemoprevention. In support of this concept, recent preclinical studies suggest that combinations of a tumor necrosis factor (TNF)-related apoptosis-inducing ligand (TRAIL) agonist with a retinoid may demonstrate similar synergies [26].

NSAIDs are one of the most powerful and broadly applicable classes of drugs available; however, at least some members of this class confer an increased risk of adverse cardiovascular events. To enable their use as chemopreventive agents, additional research needs to be directed at improving their risk/benefit balance. Moreover, integrative assessments of the risks and benefits of NSAIDs across multiple diseases (e.g., risks and benefits assessed across cardiovascular disease and cancer) may be needed to tip the risk/benefit ratio in favor of their chemopreventive use.

4 Conclusion

Translational science has largely driven the transformation of medicine from the twentieth century, where disease was treated based on the appearance of symptoms and loss of normal function, to the twenty-first century, where cellular and molecular insights have afforded significant opportunities for disease prevention. Chemoprevention represents an important part of cancer medicine's future. The identification of chemopreventive agents holds tremendous promise in reducing the burden of cancer. A number of potential preventive agents have entered clinical trials and 13 have received FDA approval for treatment of precancerous lesions or to reduce the risk of invasive cancer. When evaluated in the context of the cardinal elements of clinical trial design—agent, biomarkers, cohort, design, and endpoint—many of these previous trials offer important lessons that can inform and enhance the design and conduct of future trials. Important lessons learned regarding agents come from ATBC and CARET, which demonstrated the need for more preclinical and early-phase work in order to better understand mechanisms and minimize the risk of toxicities before undertaking large and expensive phase III trials; from BCPT and STAR, which showed that safety can be improved in iterative generations of agents and trials; from the APC, FAP, and aspirin in adenoma prevention trials, which highlighted the benefit of preclinical and phase II testing as well as the imperative for broad, sensitive toxicological and human safety assessments; and finally the DFMO and sulindac combination trial, which demonstrated that synergy between agents can lead to lower doses, improved efficacy, and fewer or less severe toxicities. Regarding cohorts, we have learned that substantial benefits can be gained by employing germline, familial, or increased-risk cohorts compared to individuals at average risk. Higher risk cohorts offer more power over a shorter time frame, as illustrated in the Celecoxib in FAP trial; and high-risk patients are typically more tolerant of side effects and have increased motivation to adhere to an intervention. An assessment of the endpoints in trials that have resulted in the approval of a preventive agent reveals that nearly all have been approved on the basis of the treatment of intraepithelial neoplasia rather than cancer prevention, per se, particularly in accessible organs. Lessons gleaned regarding the overall design of clinical trials underscore the importance of the randomized and placebo-controlled designs, because they allow for determination of the natural history of disease and facilitate toxicity assessments, as well as the need for long-term follow-up and rigorous monitoring to meet FDA requirements and promote acceptance in the marketplace. Applying these and other lessons to the design of future chemoprevention trials should facilitate the translation of novel agents exhibiting preventive potential into the clinic.

References

1. NIH NIoH (2010) Cervical cancer fact sheet. http://report.nih.gov/NIHfactsheets/ViewFactSheet.aspx?csid=76. Accessed 14 June 2013
2. CDC CfDCaP (2011) Human papillomavirus vaccines fact sheet. Accessed 14 June 2013 http://www.cdc.gov/vaccinesafety/vaccines/HPV/Index.html
3. Liao X, Lochhead P, Nishihara R, Morikawa T, Kuchiba A, Yamauchi M, Imamura Y, Qian ZR, Baba Y, Shima K, Sun R, Nosho K, Meyerhardt JA, Giovannucci E, Fuchs CS, Chan AT, Ogino S (2012) Aspirin use, tumor PIK3CA mutation, and colorectal-cancer survival. N Engl J Med 367(17):1596–1606. doi:10.1056/NEJMoa1207756
4. Nishihara R, Lochhead P, Kuchiba A, Jung S, Yamauchi M, Liao X, Imamura Y, Qian ZR, Morikawa T, Wang M, Spiegelman D, Cho E, Giovannucci E, Fuchs CS, Chan AT, Ogino S (2013) Aspirin use and risk of colorectal cancer according to BRAF mutation status. JAMA 309(24):2563–2571. doi:10.1001/jama.2013.65991700495 [pii]
5. Gail MH, Brinton LA, Byar DP, Corle DK, Green SB, Schairer C, Mulvihill JJ (1989) Projecting individualized probabilities of developing breast cancer for white females who are being examined annually. J Natl Cancer Inst 81(24):1879–1886
6. Wen CP, Lin J, Yang YC, Tsai MK, Tsao CK, Etzel C, Huang M, Hsu CY, Ye Y, Mishra L,

Hawk E, Wu X (2012) Hepatocellular carcinoma risk prediction model for the general population: the predictive power of transaminases. J Natl Cancer Inst 104(20):1599–1611. doi:10.1093/jnci/djs372djs372 [pii]

7. Thompson IM, Ankerst DP, Chi C, Goodman PJ, Tangen CM, Lucia MS, Feng Z, Parnes HL, Coltman CA Jr (2006) Assessing prostate cancer risk: results from the prostate cancer prevention trial. J Natl Cancer Inst 98(8):529–534. doi:98/8/529 [pii]10.1093/jnci/djj131
8. Fisher B, Costantino JP, Wickerham DL, Redmond CK, Kavanah M, Cronin WM, Vogel V, Robidoux A, Dimitrov N, Atkins J, Daly M, Wieand S, Tan-Chiu E, Ford L, Wolmark N (1998) Tamoxifen for prevention of breast cancer: report of the national surgical adjuvant breast and bowel project P-1 study. J Natl Cancer Inst 90(18):1371–1388
9. Vogel VG, Costantino JP, Wickerham DL, Cronin WM, Cecchini RS, Atkins JN, Bevers TB, Fehrenbacher L, Pajon ER Jr, Wade JL III, Robidoux A, Margolese RG, James J, Lippman SM, Runowicz CD, Ganz PA, Reis SE, McCaskill-Stevens W, Ford LG, Jordan VC, Wolmark N (2006) Effects of Tamoxifen vs. Raloxifene on the risk of developing invasive breast cancer and other disease outcomes: the NSABP study of Tamoxifen and raloxifene (STAR) P-2 trial. JAMA 295(23):2727–2741. doi:295.23.joc60074 [pii] 10.1001/jama.295.23.joc60074
10. Omenn GS, Goodman GE, Thornquist MD, Balmes J, Cullen MR, Glass A, Keogh JP, Meyskens FL Jr, Valanis B, Williams JH Jr, Barnhart S, Cherniack MG, Brodkin CA, Hammar S (1996) Risk factors for lung cancer and for intervention effects in CARET, the beta-carotene and retinol efficacy trial. J Natl Cancer Inst 88(21):1550–1559
11. The effect of vitamin E and beta carotene on the incidence of lung cancer and other cancers in male smokers. The Alpha-Tocopherol, Beta Carotene Cancer Prevention Study Group (1994) N Engl J Med 330:1029–1035
12. Lippman SM, Klein EA, Goodman PJ, Lucia MS, Thompson IM, Ford LG, Parnes HL, Minasian LM, Gaziano JM, Hartline JA, Parsons JK, Bearden JD III, Crawford ED, Goodman GE, Claudio J, Winquist E, Cook ED, Karp DD, Walther P, Lieber MM, Kristal AR, Darke AK, Arnold KB, Ganz PA, Santella RM, Albanes D, Taylor PR, Probstfield JL, Jagpal TJ, Crowley JJ, Meyskens FL Jr, Baker LH, Coltman CA Jr (2009) Effect of selenium and vitamin E on risk of prostate cancer and other cancers: the selenium and vitamin E cancer prevention trial (SELECT). JAMA 301(1):39–51. doi:10.1001/jama.2008.864
13. Clark LC, Combs GF Jr, Turnbull BW, Slate EH, Chalker DK, Chow J, Davis LS, Glover RA, Graham GF, Gross EG, Krongrad A, Lesher JL Jr, Park HK, Sanders BB Jr, Smith CL, Taylor JR (1996) Effects of selenium supplementation for cancer prevention in patients with carcinoma of the skin. A randomized controlled trial. Nutritional Prevention of Cancer Study Group. JAMA 276(24):1957–1963
14. Thompson IM, Goodman PJ, Tangen CM, Lucia MS, Miller GJ, Ford LG, Lieber MM, Cespedes RD, Atkins JN, Lippman SM, Carlin SM, Ryan A, Szczepanek CM, Crowley JJ, Coltman CA Jr (2003) The influence of finasteride on the development of prostate cancer. N Engl J Med 349(3):215–224. doi:10.1056/NEJMoa030660/NEJMoa030660 [pii]
15. Andriole GL (2010) Effect of dutasteride on the risk of prostate cancer. N Engl J Med 362:1192–1202
16. Theoret MR, Ning YM, Zhang JJ, Justice R, Keegan P, Pazdur R (2011) The risks and benefits of 5alpha-reductase inhibitors for prostate-cancer prevention. N Engl J Med 365(2):97–99. doi:10.1056/NEJMp1106783
17. Vogel VG, Costantino JP, Wickerham DL, Cronin WM, Cecchini RS, Atkins JN, Bevers TB, Fehrenbacher L, Pajon ER, Wade JL III, Robidoux A, Margolese RG, James J, Runowicz CD, Ganz PA, Reis SE, McCaskill-Stevens W, Ford LG, Jordan VC, Wolmark N (2010) Update of the national surgical adjuvant breast and bowel project study of tamoxifen and raloxifene (STAR) P-2 trial: preventing breast cancer. Cancer Prev Res (Phila) 3(6):696–706. doi:1940-6207.CAPR-10-0076 [pii] 10.1158/1940-6207.CAPR-10-0076
18. Steinbach G, Lynch PM, Phillips RK, Wallace MH, Hawk E, Gordon GB, Wakabayashi N, Saunders B, Shen Y, Fujimura T, Su LK, Levin B (2000) The effect of celecoxib, a cyclooxygenase-2 inhibitor, in familial adenomatous polyposis. N Engl J Med 342(26):1946–1952. doi:10.1056/NEJM200006293422603
19. Sandler RS, Halabi S, Baron JA, Budinger S, Paskett E, Keresztes R, Petrelli N, Pipas JM, Karp DD, Loprinzi CL, Steinbach G, Schilsky R (2003) A randomized trial of aspirin to prevent colorectal adenomas in patients with previous colorectal cancer. N Engl J Med 348(10):883–890. doi:10.1056/NEJMoa021633348/10/883 [pii]
20. Baron JA, Cole BF, Sandler RS, Haile RW, Ahnen D, Bresalier R, McKeown-Eyssen G, Summers RW, Rothstein R, Burke CA, Snover DC, Church TR, Allen JI, Beach M, Beck GJ,

Bond JH, Byers T, Greenberg ER, Mandel JS, Marcon N, Mott LA, Pearson L, Saibil F, van Stolk RU (2003) A randomized trial of aspirin to prevent colorectal adenomas. N Engl J Med 348(10):891–899. doi:10.1056/NEJMoa 021735348/10/891 [pii]

21. Bertagnolli MM, Eagle CJ, Zauber AG, Redston M, Solomon SD, Kim K, Tang J, Rosenstein RB, Wittes J, Corle D, Hess TM, Woloj GM, Boisserie F, Anderson WF, Viner JL, Bagheri D, Burn J, Chung DC, Dewar T, Foley TR, Hoffman N, Macrae F, Pruitt RE, Saltzman JR, Salzberg B, Sylwestrowicz T, Gordon GB, Hawk ET (2006) Celecoxib for the prevention of sporadic colorectal adenomas. N Engl J Med 355(9):873–884. doi:355/9/873 [pii]10.1056/NEJMoa061355
22. Solomon SD, Wittes J, Finn PV, Fowler R, Viner J, Bertagnolli MM, Arber N, Levin B, Meinert CL, Martin B, Pater JL, Goss PE, Lance P, Obara S, Chew EY, Kim J, Arndt G, Hawk E (2008) Cardiovascular risk of celecoxib in 6 randomized placebo-controlled trials: the cross trial safety analysis. Circulation 117(16):2104–2113. doi:10.1161/CIRCULATIONAHA.108.764530CIRCULATION AHA.108.764530 [pii]
23. Patricio JP, Barbosa JP, Ramos RM, Antunes NF, de Melo PC (2013) Relative cardiovascular and gastrointestinal safety of non-selective non-steroidal anti-inflammatory drugs versus cyclo-oxygenase-2 inhibitors: implications for clinical practice. Clin Drug Investig 33(3):167–183. doi:10.1007/s40261-013-0052-6
24. Meyskens FL Jr, McLaren CE, Pelot D, Fujikawa-Brooks S, Carpenter PM, Hawk E, Kelloff G, Lawson MJ, Kidao J, McCracken J, Albers CG, Ahnen DJ, Turgeon DK, Goldschmid S, Lance P, Hagedorn CH, Gillen DL, Gerner EW (2008) Difluoromethylornithine plus sulindac for the prevention of sporadic colorectal adenomas: a randomized placebo-controlled, double-blind trial. Cancer Prev Res (Phila) 1(1):32–38. doi:10.1158/1940-6207.CAPR-08-0042
25. Lawson KR, Ignatenko NA, Piazza GA, Cui H, Gerner EW (2000) Influence of K-ras activation on the survival responses of Caco-2 cells to the chemopreventive agents sulindac and difluoromethylornithine. Cancer Epidemiol Biomarkers Prev 9(11):1155–1162
26. Zhang L, Ren X, Alt E, Bai X, Huang S, Xu Z, Lynch PM, Moyer MP, Wen XF, Wu X (2010) Chemoprevention of colorectal cancer by targeting APC-deficient cells for apoptosis. Nature 464(7291):1058–1061. doi:nature08871 [pii]10.1038/nature08871

Index

Ann M. Bode and Zigang Dong (eds.), *Cancer Prevention: Dietary Factors and Pharmacology*, Methods in Pharmacology and Toxicology, DOI 10.1007/978-1-4614-9227-6, © Springer Science+Business Media New York 2014

D

E

F

G

H

I

K

L

M

N

P

MIX
Papier aus verantwortungsvollen Quellen
Paper from responsible sources
FSC® C105338

If you have any concerns about our products,
you can contact us on
ProductSafety@springernature.com

In case Publisher is established outside the EU,
the EU authorized representative is:
Springer Nature Customer Service Center GmbH
Europaplatz 3, 69115 Heidelberg, Germany

Printed by Libri Plureos GmbH
in Hamburg, Germany